Critical Care Medicine MCQs Practice Book

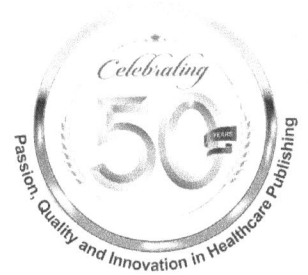

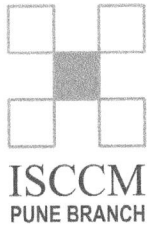

ISCCM
PUNE BRANCH

Critical Care Medicine MCQs Practice Book

Second Edition

Editors

Kapil Zirpe MD FCCM FICCM
Director and Head, Neurotrauma Unit
Grant Medical Foundation, Ruby Hall Clinic
Pune, Maharashtra, India
Immediate Past President ISCCM
President SAARC Critical Care Societies

Subhal Dixit MD FCCM IDCCM FICCM FICP
Consultant, Department of Critical Care
Director, Intensive Care Unit
Sanjeevan and MJM Hospital
Pune, Maharashtra, India

Sushma K Gurav
MBBS DA DNB (Anes) IDCCM Postgraduation in Medicolegal Concepts
Consultant, Neurotrauma Unit, Ruby Hall Clinic
Pune, Maharashtra, India

Balasaheb Pawar MD IDCCM
Consultant, Pulmonologist and Intensivist
Department of Critical Care Medicine (ICU)
Deenanath Mangeshkar Hospital
Pune, Maharashtra, India

Forewords
Yatin Mehta
Shirish Prayag

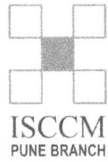

ISCCM
PUNE BRANCH

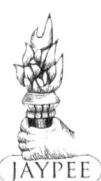

JAYPEE BROTHERS MEDICAL PUBLISHERS
The Health Sciences Publisher
New Delhi | London | Panama

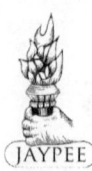

Jaypee Brothers Medical Publishers (P) Ltd

Headquarters
Jaypee Brothers Medical Publishers (P) Ltd
4838/24, Ansari Road, Daryaganj
New Delhi 110 002, India
Phone: +91-11-43574357
Fax: +91-11-43574314
Email: jaypee@jaypeebrothers.com

Overseas Offices

J.P. Medical Ltd
83, Victoria Street, London
SW1H 0HW (UK)
Phone: +44 20 3170 8910
Fax: +44 (0)20 3008 6180
E-mail: info@jpmedpub.com

Jaypee-Highlights Medical Publishers Inc
City of Knowledge, Bld. 235, 2nd Floor, Clayton
Panama City, Panama
Phone: +1 507-301-0496
Fax: +1 507-301-0499
E-mail: cservice@jphmedical.com

Jaypee Brothers Medical Publishers (P) Ltd
Bhotahity, Kathmandu, Nepal
Phone: +977-9741283608
E-mail: kathmandu@jaypeebrothers.com

Website: www.jaypeebrothers.com
Website: www.jaypeedigital.com

© 2020, Jaypee Brothers Medical Publishers

The views and opinions expressed in this book are solely those of the original contributor(s)/author(s) and do not necessarily represent those of editor(s) of the book.

All rights reserved. No part of this publication may be reproduced, stored or transmitted in any form or by any means, electronic, mechanical, photocopying, recording or otherwise, without the prior permission in writing of the publishers.

All brand names and product names used in this book are trade names, service marks, trademarks or registered trademarks of their respective owners. The publisher is not associated with any product or vendor mentioned in this book.

Medical knowledge and practice change constantly. This book is designed to provide accurate, authoritative information about the subject matter in question. However, readers are advised to check the most current information available on procedures included and check information from the manufacturer of each product to be administered, to verify the recommended dose, formula, method and duration of administration, adverse effects and contraindications. It is the responsibility of the practitioner to take all appropriate safety precautions. Neither the publisher nor the author(s)/editor(s) assume any liability for any injury and/ or damage to persons or property arising from or related to use of material in this book.

This book is sold on the understanding that the publisher is not engaged in providing professional medical services. If such advice or services are required, the services of a competent medical professional should be sought.

Every effort has been made where necessary to contact holders of copyright to obtain permission to reproduce copyright material. If any have been inadvertently overlooked, the publisher will be pleased to make the necessary arrangements at the first opportunity. The **CD/DVD-ROM** (if any) provided in the sealed envelope with this book is complimentary and free of cost. **Not meant for sale.**

Inquiries for bulk sales may be solicited at: jaypee@jaypeebrothers.com

Critical Care Medicine MCQs: Practice Book
First Edition: 2019
Second Edition: **2020**
ISBN: 978-93-89188-46-2

Contributors

Abdul Samad Ansari MBBS MD FNB IDCCM
Director
Department of Critical Care
Nanavati Super Speciality Hospital
Mumbai, Maharashtra, India

Abhijit Baheti
MD (Medicine) DM (Clinical Hematology)
Consultant
Department of Hematology
Ruby Hall Clinic
Pune, Maharashtra, India

Ajith Kumar AK MD DNB EDIC FICCM
Senior Consultant
Department of Intensive Care
Manipal Hospitals
Bengaluru, Karnataka, India

Anand Tiwari
MBBS DA DNB (Anes) IDCC FNB (Critical Care Medicine)
Chief Intensivist
Department of Critical Care
Inamdar Multispeciality Hospital
Pune, Maharashtra, India

Anish Gupta MD FNB EDIC
Consultant
Department of Critical Care Medicine
Max Super Speciality Hospital
Saket, New Delhi, India

Balasaheb Pawar MD IDCCM
Consultant, Pulmonologist and Intensivist
Department of Critical Care Medicine (ICU)
Deenanath Mangeshkar Hospital
Pune, Maharashtra, India

Balkrishna D Nimavat
MBBS MD (Anes) DNB (Anes) IDCCM
FNB (Critical Care) EDAIC EDIC
Consultant
Ruby Hall Clinic
Pune, Maharashtra, India

Deeksha Singh Tomar DA IDCCM IFCCM EDIC
Consultant
Department of Critical Care
Narayana Superspeciality Hospital
Gurugram, Haryana, India

Deepak Govil MD EDIC FCCM
Director
Institute of Critical Care and Anesthesiology
Gurugram, Haryana, India

Deven Juneja
DNB FNB EDIC FCCP IFCCM FCCM
Associate Director
Department of Critical Care Medicine
Max Super Speciality Hospital
Saket, New Delhi, India

Dhruv Chaudhary
MD DNB (Medicine) DM (Pulmonary and Critical Care Medicine) FICPI SICCM
Senior Professor and Head
Department of Pulmonary Medicine
Post Graduate Institute of Medical Sciences (PGIMS)
Rohtak, Haryana, India

Divyesh Patel MD IDCC EDIC
Chief Intensivist
Tricolour Hospitals
Vadodara, Gujarat, India

Gaurav Kakkar
MBBS (AFMC) FCARCSI CCT (UK) Fellow
(The Walton Centre for Neurosciences, Liverpool, UK)
Associate Director
Department of Neuroanesthesia and Neurocritical Care
Medanta—The Medicity
Gurugram, Haryana, India
Visiting Consultant
The Walton Centre for Neurosciences
Liverpool, UK

Harish MM MBBS MD DM IDCCM DNB EDICM
Consultant–Incharge
Department of Critical Care Medicine
Mazumdar Shaw Medical Center, Bengaluru
Narayana Hrudayalaya
Bengaluru, Karnataka, India

Jacob George Pulinilkunnathil
MD IDCCM FCCP EDIC
Senior Resident, DM Critical Care Medicine
Department of Anesthesiology
Critical Care and Pain
Tata Memorial Hospital
Mumbai, Maharashtra, India

Jignesh Shah
MD DNB (Anes) IDCCM IFCCM EDIC
Associate Professor
Department of Critical Care Medicine
Bharati Vidyapeeth (Deemed to be) University
Medical College
Pune, Maharashtra, India

Khalid Ismail Khatib MD (Medicine) FICCM
Professor
Department of Medicine
Smt Kashibai Navale Medical College
Medical College
Pune, Maharashtra, India

Moturu Dharanindra MD (Anes)
Senior Resident
Department of Critical Care Medicine
Bharati Vidyapeeth (Deemed to be) University
Medical College
Pune, Maharashtra, India

Natesh Prabu R
MD DNB (Anesthesiology) DM
(Critical Care Medicine) EDIC
Assistant Professor
Department of Critical Care Medicine
St John's Medical College Hospital
Bengaluru, Karnataka, India

Neha Gupta MD FNB (ID)
Consultant ID Physician
Medanta—The Medicity
Gurugram, Haryana, India

Nithya CA MD FNB (Critical Care)
Junior Consultant, ICU
Mazumdar Shaw Medical Centre
Narayana Health City
Bengaluru, Karnataka, India

Omender Singh MD FCCM
Director
Department of Critical Care Medicine
Max Super Speciality Hospital
Saket, New Delhi, India

Palepu B Gopal
MD FRCA FCCM IFCCM
Head
Department of Critical Care Medicine
Continental Hospitals
Hyderabad, Telangana, India

Prasanna Pradip Murudwar
MBBS MD (Anesthesiology) FNB
(Critical Care Medicine 2nd year)
Fellow—Critical Care Medicine
Deenanath Mangeshkar Hospital and
Research Centre
Pune, Maharashtra, India

Rajeev Soman MD FIDSA
Consultant ID Physician
Jupiter Hospital, Pune
Dinanath Mangeshkar Hospital, Pune
Bharati Vidyapeeth (Deemed to be) University
Medical College, Pune
Hinduja Hospital
Mumbai, Maharashtra, India

Rajiv J Shah
FNB (Critical Care) IDCCM DNB (Medicine)
Consultant Intensivist
Nanavati Superspeciality Hospital
Mumbai, Maharashtra, India

Ramya BM MBBS MD
Junior Consultant
Department of Anesthesia
Mazumdar Shaw Medical Center
Narayana Hrudayalaya
Bengaluru, Karnataka, India

Ripenmeet Salhotra
MD (Anesthesiology) IDCCM IFCCM EDIC
Consultant
Department of Critical Care Medicine
Fortis-Escorts Hospital
Faridabad, Haryana, India

Sachin Gupta MD IDCCM IFCCM EDIC FCCM FICCM
Head
Department of Critical Care
Narayana Superspeciality Hospital
Gurugram, Haryana, India

Shrikant Srinivasan MD DNB FNB FICCM EDIC
Consultant and Head
Department of Critical Care Medicine
Manipal Hospital
Dwarka, New Delhi, India

Shubhendu Bajpai MD
FNB Fellow
Medanta—The Medicity
Gurugram, Haryana, India

Subhal Dixit MD FCCM IDCCM FICCM FICP
Consultant, Department of Critical Care
Director, Intensive Care Unit
Sanjeevan and MJM Hospital
Pune, Maharashtra, India

Sudhindra P Kanavehalli MBBS MD
Fellow
Department of Critical Care Medicine
Mazumdar Shaw Medical Center
Narayana Hrudayalaya
Bengaluru, Karnataka, India

Suhail Sarwar Siddiqui
MD Fellow (Critical Care)
DM (Critical Care Medicine) EDIC
Assistant Professor
Department of Critical Care Medicine
King George's Medical University
Lucknow, Uttar Pradesh, India

Sunil Karanth MD FNB EDIC FCICM (Aus/NZ)
Chairman of Critical Care Services
Manipal Health Enterprises (P) Ltd, Bengaluru
Chair of HICC
Member of Medical Advisory Board
Treasurer Bangalore Chapter ISCCM
Adjunct Professor of Critical Care Medicine
Manipal University
Karnataka, India

Sunitha Binu Varghese
DNB (Medicine) IDCCM EDIC
Head
Department of Critical Care
Niramaya Hospital
Pune, Maharashtra, India

Supradip Ghosh
Diplomate National Board (Internal Medicine) EDIC
Director and Head
Department of Critical Care Medicine
Fortis-Escorts Hospital
Faridabad, Haryana, India

Sushil Kumar Yadav MD (Anes) IDCCM FNB
Consultant
Neuro Trauma Unit
Ruby Hall Clinic
Grant Medical Foundation
Pune, Maharashtra, India

Sushma K Gurav
MBBS DA DNB (Anes) IDCCMC Postgraduation in
Medicolegal Concepts
Consultant, Neurotrauma Unit
Ruby Hall Clinic
Pune, Maharashtra, India

Ujwala Mhatre
DNB DA (Anesthesiology) IDCCM
Junior Consultant
Nanavati Superspeciality Hospital
Mumbai, Maharashtra, India

Foreword

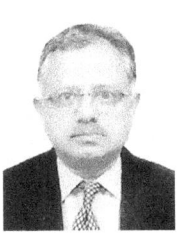

It is with great pleasure that I am writing this foreword for the *Critical Care Medicine MCQs: Practice Book* by Drs Kapil Zirpe, Subhal Dixit, Sushma K Gurav and Balasaheb Pawar. Critical care is recognized now as a superspecialty by Medical Council of India (MCI) (long awaited) and we have multiple training and certification courses by ISCCM, NBE and a few universities (DM) and ESICM (EDIC). All these have both regular assessment and exit examinations which have MCQs. This book has been a stupendous effort by the Pune team who despite their busy clinical, ISCCM and BOB schedules have come out with a great book!

I congratulate them and urge the PG's to go through this book to help them get through the examinations!

Yatin Mehta
MD MNAMS FRCA FAMS FIACTA FICCM FTEE
Past President ISCCM
Chairman
Medanta Institute of Critical Care and Anesthesiology
Medanta—The Medicity
Gurugram, Haryana, India

Foreword

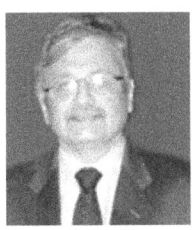

It is with a great degree of pleasure and pride that I am writing this foreword.

Critical care in India has spread far and wide and has reached great heights over the last 25 years. Although isolated foci of excellence in critical care existed in India in individual centers 25 years ago, there was no organized professional activity. Training in this evolving field was non-existent. It is then in 1992, that organized platform for discussions in small group was started in Pune, Maharashtra, India under the banner of Critical Care Society. In 1993, the National Indian Society of Critical Care Medicine (ISCCM) was born and this local activity in Pune merged with ISCCM as its first city branch.

Over the last almost 25 years of activity, Pune Branch of ISCCM has remained in the forefront of academic activities of ISCCM and the critical care world in India. There have been innumerable activities, and all this has led to Pune being awarded the Best Branch award for many consecutive years.

We have always believed in giving something different, unique and enriching to the world of critical care in India. The workbooks for various workshops are therefore a part of this continuing process of dynamic output from this branch.

Way back in 1996-1997, ISCCM decided to take on itself the responsibility of training the budding Intensivists. Initial efforts included the process of setting the standards, identifying units for training and defining the curriculum. The "written "or the theory part of the exit examination was appropriate for that era and consisted of short answer kind of questions.

Over the years, the examination pattern has evolved with time and multiple choice questions (MCQs) have become the way to test the theory knowledge. The preparation of students for their theoretical knowledge, thus has now gets a direction in toning them up with MCQs.

This book is a compilation of these sets of MCQs, so essential for the preparation of any candidate, tested out by experienced examiners. This is being issued in conjunction with the annual review course of ISCCM Pune Branch.

I am sure ISCCM Pune will continue to light the path of all future generations of intensive care doctors through knowledge which is appropriate for that generation.

Shirish Prayag MD FCCM
Director
Department of Critical Care
Prayag Hospital
Pune, Maharashtra, India

Preface to the Second Edition

Dear colleagues, it gives us a great pleasure of publication the second edition of *Critical Care Medicine MCQs: Practice Book* at Best of Brussels Symposium 2019, Pune, Maharashtra, India.

Response to our first edition of this book was phenomenal. The purpose of first edition was to share knowledge among critical care trainees and get them ready for competitive examinations in critical care medicine.

From the feedback we received of first edition and as per expectations of critical trainees, we have decided to add few more features in the second edition of the book. Accordingly second edition has 28 chapters and 668 MCQs related to critical care medicine. We have added fresh 300 + MCQs along with few new sections like imaging, pharma therapy, etc. Even theory paper of 50 questions has been added for practice purpose at the end of book. We have selected contributors from respective areas who are experts in those subjects from all over India. Emphasis has been attributed to tropical diseases, respiratory system, hemodynamic, sepsis, infection control, neurocritical care, trauma and mechanical ventilation. *The answers have been given for MCQs along with explanations at the end of every chapter.* The MCQs on subject have been created with a view to explain concept clearly and intended to enable students to plan their studies. MCQs will help the students to make a self-assessment of the knowledge about critical care medicine. *This book will surely* meets the expectations of the students as it answers the queries in their mind. The contents have been so designed as to include the maximum syllabus of critical care medicine training courses.

This book will be user-friendly and will provide information in structured manner.

We hope the students will find it very user-friendly and meets their expectations.
Best wishes!

Kapil Zirpe
Subhal Dixit
Sushma K Gurav
Balasaheb Pawar

Preface to the First Edition

Dear friends, it gives us a great pleasure in announcing the launch of *Critical Care Medicine MCQs: Practice Book* as the annual review course book at Best of Brussels Symposium at Pune, Maharashtra, India.

The main purpose of this book is to spread knowledge among critical care trainees. The book caters to the need of students aspiring for competitive MCQ-based examinations.

This book has 27 sessions and 486 MCQs related to critical care medicine. Contributors are expertise from all over India. Emphasis has been attributed to tropical diseases, infection control, neurocritical care, trauma and mechanical ventilation. *The answers have been given for MCQs along with explanations at the end of every chapter.* The MCQs on subject have been created with a view to explain concept clearly and intended to enable students to plan their studies. Examples have been given in the text to help the students to understand the application of these concepts in real life situations. MCQs will help the students to make a self-assessment of the knowledge about critical care medicine. This book is highly interactive and meets the expectations of the students as it answers the queries in their mind. The contents have been so designed as to include the syllabus of critical care medicine training courses.

This book is user-friendly and provides information in a structured manner.

We hope the delegates enjoy using this book during the review course and beyond.

Kapil Zirpe
Balasaheb Pawar
Sushma K Gurav

Acknowledgments

On behalf of the Indian Society of Critical Care Medicine (ISCCM), Pune Branch, I sincerely appreciate the contribution of each and every author for timely completing their chapters. Everyone's contribution has added more credibility to this second edition of *Critical Care Medicine MCQs: Practice Book*. I really appreciate sincere efforts of editors in bringing this edition within short time. I thank all critical care trainees for their continued trust on Pune Branch and look forward to doing such activity in the future.

I appreciate the contribution of Shri Jitendar P Vij (Group Chairman), Mr Ankit Vij (Managing Director), Ms Chetna Malhotra Vohra (Associate Director—Content Strategy), and the staff of M/S Jaypee Brothers Medical Publishers (P) Ltd, New Delhi, India, for tireless follow-up and finishing the book within the timeline.

Jyoti Shendage
Chairperson ISCCM
Pune Branch

Contents

Chapter 1: Overview of MCQs Based Critical Care in India — 1
Deepak Govil, Shubhendu Bajpai

Chapter 2: Airway Management — 4
Abdul Samad Ansari, Ujwala Mhatre, Rajiv J Shah

Chapter 3: Cardiopulmonary Resuscitation — 13
Balkrishna D Nimavat

Chapter 4: Shock and Resuscitation — 27
Palepu B Gopal

Chapter 5: Mechanical Ventilation — 45
Sachin Gupta, Deeksha Singh Tomar

Chapter 6: Respiratory System — 54
Balasaheb Pawar

Chapter 7: Hemodynamic Monitoring — 60
Harish MM, Suhail S Siddiqui, Jacob George Pulinilkunnathil, Sudhindra P Kanavehalli

Chapter 8: Infection Control — 92
Ripenmeet Salhotra, Supradip Ghosh

Chapter 9: Infectious Diseases — 104
Rajeev Soman, Neha Gupta

Chapter 10: Gastrointestinal System — 114
Ajith Kumar AK, Nithya CA

Chapter 11: Nutrition — 124
Subhal Dixit, Khalid Ismail Khatib

Chapter 12: Endocrine and Metabolic System — 131
Anand Tiwari

Chapter 13: Neurocritical Care — 142
Sunil Karanth, Gaurav Kakkar

Chapter 14: Trauma — 166
Sushil Kumar Yadav

Chapter 15: Cardiovascular System — 179
Divyesh Patel

Chapter 16: Renal — 191
Sunitha Binu Varghese

Chapter 17: Toxicology — 198
Omender Singh, Anish Gupta, Deven Juneja

Chapter 18:	Obstetric Critical Care	215
	Prasanna Pradip Murudwar	
Chapter 19:	End-of-Life/Ethics/Transplant	226
	Jignesh Shah, Moturu Dharanindra	
Chapter 20:	Oncology	242
	Deven Juneja, Anish Gupta, Omender Singh	
Chapter 21:	Hematology	253
	Abhijit Baheti	
Chapter 22:	Postoperative Critical Care	266
	Sushma K Gurav	
Chapter 23:	Tropical Diseases	277
	Dhruv Chaudhary	
Chapter 24:	Critical Care Pharmacology 2019	285
	Natesh Prabhu R	
Chapter 25:	HRCT Thorax	301
	Balasaheb Pawar	
Chapter 26:	Chest X-Ray	311
	Subhal Dixit, Khalid Ismail Khatib	
Chapter 27:	Arterial Blood Gases	320
	Sushma K Gurav	
Chapter 28:	USG and ECHO	325
	Shrikant Srinivasan	

Exam Paper 341
Khalid Ismail Khatib

CHAPTER 1

Overview of MCQs Based Critical Care in India

Deepak Govil, Shubhendu Bajpai

INTRODUCTION

Multiple Choice Questions (MCQs) are generally recognized as the most widely applicable and useful format for evaluating one's knowledge, judgment, understanding, and problem solving. MCQs were introduced in medical examinations in 1950s and have been shown to be more reliable in testing knowledge than the traditional essay questions. The MCQ is an objective question for which there is prior agreement to what is the correct answer. They are good for measuring knowledge, comprehension and could be designed to measure application and analysis. The MCQ tests are quick and simple to mark (electronic marking). This ease of marking permits rapid turn-round and personalized feedback in a very short time. Particularly where there is a language problem, MCQ tests reduce reliance on skills of writing and self-expression. For all these reasons, MCQ tests are increasingly being used in the educational assessment of health professionals.

For any test to be legally defensible, it should meet two standards:
1. *Validity:* The test must measure what students are expected to know. This is accomplished by writing test questions that align with the objectives.
2. *Reliability:* The test must produce consistent results time after time, i.e. the test should produce same score if given to same students repeatedly.

ANATOMY OF A GOOD MCQ

Multiple choice questions consist of two parts:
1. Stem
2. Alternatives

Designing the stem of the multiple choice questions:
- The stem should express the full problem
- All the relevant material must be in the stem (use most words in the stem)
- Use simple sentence structure and precise wordings
- Eliminate excessive wording and irrelevant information from the stem.

Designing the alternatives:
- Usually there are 3–5 alternatives per question
- Make sure there is only one best answer
- Make sure the distractions (the incorrect alternatives) are appealing and plausible
- The alternatives must be grammatically consistent with the stem

- Place the alternatives in a meaningful order
- Randomly distribute the correct alternative (mix up the order of correct alternative in the entire question paper)
- Avoid overlapping the choices
- Try to keep alternatives of same length
- Avoid using words like all of the above, none of the above, all, none, always, never.

PREPARE A QUESTION BANK

It is important that when preparing a question bank the whole breadth of the published curriculum is covered. Different parts of the curriculum will be weighed on the basis of their importance and relevance. The validity of each question should be checked by the subject matter experts (SME).

Item analysis in MCQs: Item analysis provides a way of measuring the quality of questions—seeing how appropriate they are for the candidates, and how well they measure their ability. It also provides a pool of evaluated items that could be reused repeatedly in different tests with prior knowledge of how they are going to perform.

Difficulty factor: This is essentially the proportion or percentage of students who answered the question correctly. It is based on either the total number of students (the percentage who answered correctly) or it could be based on a sample of upper and lower scores as follows:

$$\text{Difficulty factor} = \frac{Ru + Rl}{T}$$

Where Ru = number selecting the correct option in the upper scoring group, Rl = number selecting the correct option in the lower group, T = total of examinees in upper and lower groups. It is rather confusing because the higher the difficulty factor the easier the question.

Discrimination index (DI): Item analysis programs provide the numbers and proportions of examinees scoring in the top, middle, and bottom thirds (or the upper quartile versus lower quartile) who select each option. The DI is calculated by subtracting the proportion of students who scored correctly in the lower group from the proportion who scored correctly in the upper group:

$$\text{Discrimination index} = \frac{Ru + Rl}{\frac{1}{2}T}$$

Where Ru = number selecting the correct option in the upper scoring group, Rl = number selecting the correct option in the lower group, T = total number of examinees in upper and lower groups.

PREPARE A BLUEPRINT OF THE EXAMINATION

Blueprinting is the planning of the test against the learning objectives of a course or competencies essential to a specialty. It is a guide used for creating balanced examination and consists a list of domains (various organ systems—CNS, CVS, renal, etc.), topics (hypertension, MI, AKI, etc.), context (physical examination, diagnosis, investigations, treatment, etc.) and weightage of each that should be tested in the examination. It is an important task for the exam setting group to select an appropriate number of questions reflecting the relative importance of the different topics within the curriculum. The entire test consists of questions divided into 2 sets: (1) Must know questions (20–30%) and (2) Differentiators (60–70%).

POST TEST EVALUATION

Two broad categories of standards are used in interpretation of test results:
1. *Norm referenced standard:* These are designed to provide a measure of performance that is interpretable in terms of an individual selective standing in some known group. An example of these is the selection examination for admission to medical school (designed to pass only the best of the best).
2. *Criterion referenced standard:* These are designed to provide a measure of performance that is interpretable in terms of clearly defined reference or criterion. An end of course test, which assesses whether the students have mastered specific learning objectives or domains of the course, exemplifies this (standard is established before the exam all can pass or all can fail). Cut score is a score at which a student passes or fails.

Two methods of establishing cut-off score:
1. *Angoff method:* Each reviewer (subject matter expert) individually estimates what percentage of minimally acceptable entry level students would answer the question correctly. The average of those numbers then becomes the cut score for that item. The cut score for the exam is an average of the individual cut scores for each item in the exam.
2. *Nedelsky method:* Three subject matter experts individually assign a probability that a minimally qualified candidate would be able to rule out incorrect options. The Nedelsky value is then calculated by taking the reciprocal of the remaining items. Suppose a minimally qualified student could be expected to rule out 2 out of 4 distractors, this leaves the student with 2 answers to choose from, so the Nedelsky value for this case would be:

$$\tfrac{1}{2} = 0.5.$$

The cut score of the exam is calculated by adding up the average Nedelsky values for each item. Another method to derive cut off score is to have at least 6–8 subject matter experts sit together and discuss each question for validity, difficulty and appropriateness of the question for given test, and they give weightage to each question separately and then the final cut off is derived.

CHAPTER 2

Airway Management

Abdul Samad Ansari, Ujwala Mhatre, Rajiv J Shah

QUESTIONS

1. Indications of capnography are all *except*:
   a. Evaluation of end tidal CO_2
   b. It does not predict adequacy of pulmonary, systemic and coronary blood flow
   c. Estimation of effective (nonshunted) pulmonary capillary blood flow by a partial rebreathing method
   d. As an adjunctive tool to screen for pulmonary embolism

2. Positive pressure inspiration causes all *except*:
   a. Increased intrathoracic pressure
   b. Increased right atrial pressure
   c. Reduces LV afterload
   d. Increases pressure gradient for venous return and RV filling

3. All of the following are predictors of noninvasive ventilation success in patients with acute respiratory failure *except*:
   a. Lower acuity of illness (APACHE Score)
   b. Less air leakage
   c. Improvement of gas exchange, heart rate and respiratory rate within first 2 hours
   d. $PaCO_2 > 95$ mm Hg

4. Factors that influence aerosol delivery in mechanically ventilated patients are all *except*:
   a. Position of administration device in the circuit
   b. Humidification can decrease aerosol delivery
   c. Drug delivered during inspiratory phase
   d. Smaller tidal volumes ensure optimal delivery

5. Pulmonary hypertension treatment includes all *except*:
   a. Epoprostenol
   b. Inhaled iloprost
   c. Ambrisentan
   d. Latanoprost

6. A 65-year-old male was intubated with double lumen tube in OT in view of lung abscess. Following flow-volume loop was seen. What does it indicate?

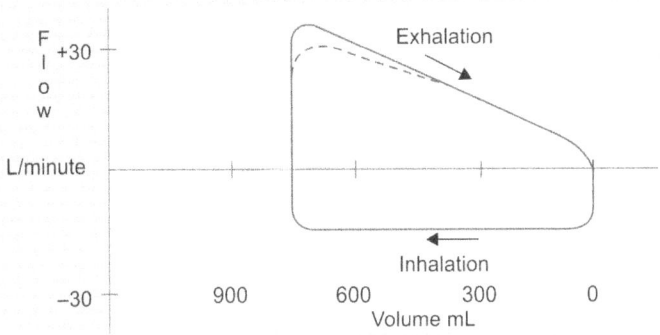

a. Bronchial intubation
b. Secretions in the endotracheal tube
c. Kinking of tube
d. Disconnection of ET tube

7. A 56-year-old man, suffering from Guillain-Barre syndrome, had his ventilator alarms constantly beeping. Following loops were seen by the doctor. What is the cause?
a. Leak
b. Intrinsic PEEP
c. Endotracheal tube is obstructed
d. Overshoot loop

8. The following capnograph indicates:

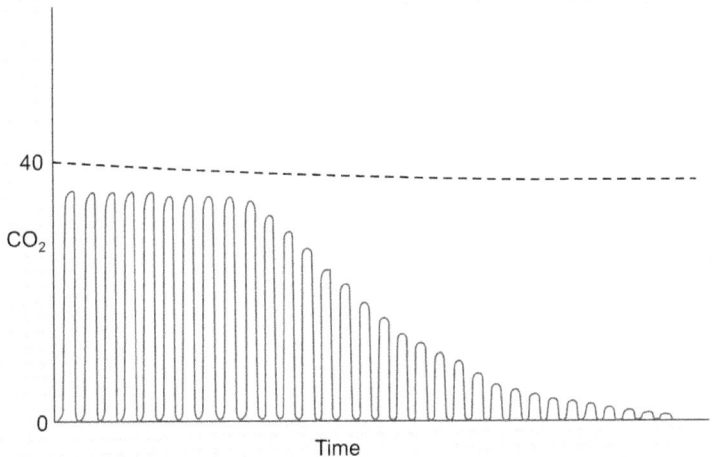

a. Sudden hypotension
b. Circulatory arrest with continued pulmonary ventilation
c. Pulmonary embolism
d. All of the above

9. According to ASTM Standard; a bag mask resuscitator for adults:
   a. Should deliver an inspired oxygen concentration of at least 40% when connected to an oxygen source supplying not more than 15 L/min
   b. Should deliver an inspired oxygen concentration of at least 85% with oxygen enrichment device supplied by manufacturer
   c. Both of the above
   d. None of the above

10. Hazards of suctioning:
    a. Hypoxemia
    b. PEEP loss
    c. Increased ICP
    d. All of the above

11. A 36-year-old male underwent high speed motor vehicle collision. Brought to A and E with SpO_2 = 82%, BP = 100/80 mm Hg, HR = 116/min and GCS = 8. Also suffers from severe facial and head injury. Which of the following maneuver should not be performed?
    a. Chin lift head tilt
    b. Noninvasive ventilator trial should be avoided
    c. Jaw thrust and manual inline stabilization
    d. High flow oxygen by mask

12. Identify the following condition:

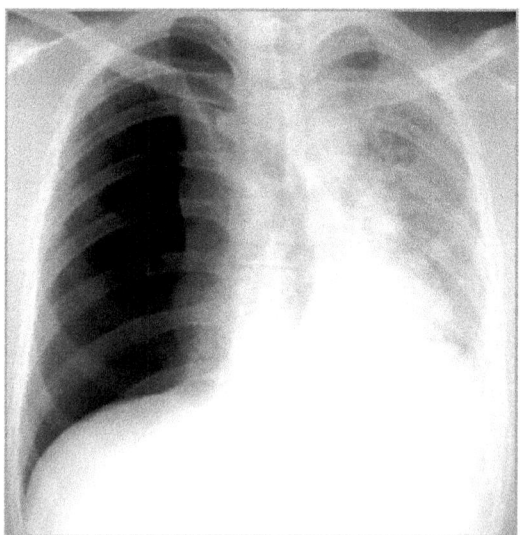

   a. Cardiac tamponade
   b. Left ventricular failure
   c. Pneumothorax
   d. ARDS

13. A 36-year-old male patient had a motor vehicle collision. Presented to A and E with shortness of breath and an open wound over right chest. How will you treat this condition?
    a. Close the defect with sterile occlusive dressing completely
    b. Close the defect with sterile occlusive dressing on 3 sides
    c. Put an ICD through an open wound
    d. Do not close the wound

14. A 24-year-old pregnant patient is admitted with shortness of breath and pedal edema. Which of the following is true?
    a. Minute ventilation decreases
    b. $PaCO_2$ between 35 and 40 indicates impending respiratory failure during pregnancy
    c. Oxygen consumption decreases
    d. Increased residual volume

15. In the mnemonic FAST HUGS BID; second "S" represents:
    a. Suction
    b. Sedation
    c. Spontaneous breathing trial
    d. SIMV

16. All of the following are weaning procedures *except*:
    a. Pressure support ventilation
    b. Spontaneous breathing trial
    c. Automatic tube compensation
    d. High frequency oscillation

17. Maximum inspiratory pressure is:
    a. Amount of negative pressure a patient can generate in 20 sec when inspiring against an occluded measuring device
    b. Measure of ventilatory muscle strength
    c. Measure of weaning
    d. All of the above

18. As per Plan B of DAS 2015 guidelines for difficult intubation:
    a. Cricothyroidotomy should be done
    b. Give muscle relaxant
    c. Supraglottic airway device insertion
    d. 4 attempts of laryngoscopy

19. The endotracheal tube cuff pressure should be:
    a. 30–40 cm H_2O
    b. 20–25 cm H_2O
    c. 40–50 cm H_2O
    d. 26–30 cm H_2O

20. Contraindications for using speaking valve are all *except*:
    a. Laryngeal stenosis
    b. Severe tracheal stenosis
    c. Vocal cord paralysis
    d. Bronchial asthma

21. Sugammadex is all except:
    a. Cyclodextrin molecule
    b. Reverses moderate to deep neuromuscular block
    c. Forms very tight complexes at a 1:1 ratio with aminosteroid muscle relaxants
    d. Binds to plasma proteins

22. A 46-year-old male patient had a high speed motor vehicle collision injuring his both lower extremities. As GCS was low, patient was intubated with midazolam, fentanyl, propofol, and succinylcholine. Patient had a cardiac arrest. ROSC achieved after 10 minutes. Probable cause:
    a. Hyperkalemia
    b. Hypokalemia
    c. Hypoglycemia
    d. Hyperglycemia

ANSWERS

1. **Ans. (b)**
   Vincent JL, Fink MP, Moore FA, et al. *Textbook of critical care* (AARC clinical practice guidelines; Capnography during mechanical ventilation). Toronto: Elsevier; 2017. pp. 161, 282.

   Capnography should not be mandated for all patients receiving mechanical ventilator support but indicated for:
   a. Evaluation of end tidal CO_2
   b. Monitoring adequacy of pulmonary, systemic, and coronary blood flow.
   c. Estimation of effective (nonshunted) pulmonary capillary blood flow by a partial rebreathing method.
   d. As an adjunctive tool to screen for pulmonary embolism.
   e. As a monitoring tool for efficacy of CPR

2. **Ans. (d)**
   Pinsky M, Gomez H. Heart lung interactions. In: Vincent JL, Fink MP, Moore F (Eds). *Textbook of critical care.* Toronto: Elsevier; 2017. pp. 320-2.

   Positive pressure inspiration increases ITP and right atrial pressure, decreasing pressure gradient for venous return and RV filling and RV stroke volume.

3. **Ans. (d)**
   Cabello B, Camp F. Non Invasive Positive Pressure Ventilation. In: Vincent JL, Fink MP, Moore FA (Eds). *Textbook of critical care;* Toronto: Elsevier; 2017. pp. 350.
   1. Lower acuity of illness (APACHE Score)
   2. Less air leakage
   3. Improvement of gas exchange, heart rate and respiratory rate within first 2 hours
   4. Ability to cooperate and a higher neurologic score
   5. $PaCO_2$ between 45 and 92 mm Hg
   6. Less air leakage and intact dentition.

4. **Ans. (d)**
   Marrochs S, Walley K. Adjunctive respiratory therapy. In: Vincent JL, Fink MP, Moore FA (Eds). *Textbook of critical care.* Toronto: Elsevier; 2017. pp. 366.
   1. Position of administration device in the circuit
   2. Humidification can decrease aerosol delivery
   3. Drug delivered during inspiratory phase
   4. Larger tidal volumes ensure optimal delivery
   5. Low density gases such as Heliox increase deposition to lower airway
   6. Endotracheal tube size less than 7 mm reduce delivery
   7. Slow inspiratory flow rates increase delivery of nebulized medications

5. **Ans. (d)**
   Vincent JL, Fink MP, Moore FA, et al. *Textbook of critical care* (Ch 65). Toronto: Elsevier; 2017. pp. 434-5.

Rubin LJ. Pulmonary Hypertension. N Engl J Med. 1997;336(2):111-7.

Treatment of pulmonary hypertension:
a. Warfarin, oxygen, diuretics, digoxin, vaccination
b. Prostanoids: Epoprostenol, treprostinil, beraprost, inhaled iloprost
c. Endothelin receptor antagonists: Bosentan, ambrisentan
d. Phosphodiesterase inhibitors: Sildenafil, tadalafil
e. Inhaled nitric oxide

6. **Ans. (a)**

Dorsch J, Dorsch S. Understanding Anesthesia Equipment (Section IV, Monitoring devices). Philadelphia: Lippincott Williams and Wilkins; 2008. pp. 766-8.

The solid loop shows an increase inexpiratory flow, during early part of expiration. The dotted line represents when the double lumen tube is correctly placed. If the bronchial lumen is inserted too deeply, a severe reduction in compliance and tidal volume and diminished inspiratory and expiratory flows will be seen.

7. **Ans. (a)**

Dorsch J, Dorsch S. Understanding Anesthesia Equipment (Section IV, Monitoring devices). Philadelphia: Lippincott Williams and Wilkins; 2008. pp. 765-7.

If there is leak between sensor and the breathing system, pressure volume loop will be normal in shape but will show a decrease in tidal volume and decrease in peak airway pressure. Flow volume loop will show decrease in tidal volume and decrease in peak expiratory flow.

8. **Ans. (d)**

Dorsch J, Dorsch S. Understanding Anesthesia Equipment (Section IV, Monitoring devices, chap 22, gas monitoring). Philadelphia: Lippincott Williams and Wilkins; 2008. pp. 719.

Events that cause an exponential decrease in end tidal CO_2 include sudden hypotension, massive blood loss, circulatory arrest with continued pulmonary ventilation, and pulmonary embolism.

9. **Ans. (c)**

Dorsch J, Dorsch S. Understanding Anesthesia Equipment (Section II Manual Resuscitators). Philadelphia: Lippincott Williams and Wilkins; 2008. pp. 289-90.

The ASTM standard requires that a resuscitator for adults be capable of delivering an inspired oxygen concentration of at least 40% when connected to an oxygen source supplying not more than 15 L/min and at least 85% with oxygen enrichment device supplied by manufacturer.

10. **Ans. (d)**

Dorsch J, Dorsch S. Understanding Anesthesia Equipment (Section 1, gas supply and distribution system), 5th edition. Philadelphia: Lippincott Williams and Wilkins; 2008. pp. 67-70.

Hazards of suctioning:
1. Hypoxemia
2. PEEP loss

CHAPTER 2 Airway Management

3. Increased ICP
4. Risk of nosocomial infection
5. Inadequate suction
6. Trauma

11. **Ans. (a)**
    American College of Surgeons. Initial Assessment and Management (Ch 1). In: ATLS. Chicago: ACS; 2017. pp. 8.

    In trauma, patient's head and neck should not be hyperextended, hyperflexed or rotated to establish and maintain airway.

12. **Ans. (c)**
    O'Connor AR. Radiological review of pneumothorax. BMJ. 2005;330(7506):1493-7.

    Visible visceral pleural edge is seen as a very thin, sharp white line. No lung markings are seen peripheral to this line. The peripheral space is radiolucent compared to adjacent lung.

13. **Ans. (b)**
    American College of Surgeons. Thoracic Trauma (Ch 4). In: ATLS, 9th edition. Chicago: ACS; 2017. pp. 98.

    Initial management of open pneumothorax is accomplished by promptly closing the defect with sterile occlusive dressing large enough to overlap the wound's edges and then taped securely in three sides in order to provide flutter type valve effect. As the patient breathes in, the dressing occludes the wound, preventing air from entering. During exhalation, the open end of the dressing allows air to escape from the pleural space. A chest tube remote from the wound should be placed as soon as possible.

14. **Ans. (b)**
    American College of Surgeons. Trauma in Pregnancy and Intimate partner violence (Ch 12). In: ATLS, 9th edition. Chicago: ACS; 2017. pp. 290.

    Respiratory system changes in pregnancy:
    a. Minute ventilation increases
    b. $PaCO_2$ between 35–40 indicates impending respiratory failure during pregnancy
    c. Oxygen consumption increases
    d. Decreased residual volume

15. **Ans. (c)**
    Vincent WR 3rd, Hatton KW. FAST HUGS BID: updated mnemonic. Crit Care Med. 2009;37(7):2326-7.

    Feeding, analgesia, sedation, thromboprophylaxis, head of the bed elevation, ulcer prophylaxis, glycemic control, spontaneous breathing trial, bowel care, indwelling catheter removal, de-escalation of antibiotics.

16. **Ans. (d)**
    High frequency positive pressure ventilation is indicated on those patients who are hypoxemic or hypercapneic despite adequate and appropriate conventional ventilation.

17. **Ans. (d)**

DW Chang. Weaning from mechanical ventilation. In: Clinical application of mechanical ventilation. New York: CENGAGE Learning Custom Publishing; 2013. pp. 214, 505.

Maximum inspiratory pressure is the amount of negative pressure a patient can generate in 20 sec when inspiring against an occluded measuring device. It is also a measure of ventilatory muscle strength and measure of weaning.

18. **Ans. (c)**

Frerk C, Mitchell VS, McNarry AF, et al; DAS2015 guidelines. Br J Anaesth. 2015;115(6):827-48.
Plan B:
- Maintaining oxygenation, supraglottic airway device insertion.
- Failed intubation should be declared
- The emphasis is on oxygenation via SAD
- Second generation SAD recommended
- A maximum of 3 attempts at SAD insertion
- During rapid sequence induction, cricoid pressure should be removed to facilitate insertion of SAD
- Blind techniques for intubation through a SAD are not recommended.

19. **Ans. (b)**

Chang DW. Airway management in mechanical ventilation (Ch 6). In: Clinical application of mechanical ventilation. New York: CENGAGE Learning Custom Publishing; 2013. pp. 169.

The estimated capillary perfusion pressure in trachea is 30 cm H_2O. If cuff pressure is greater than capillary perfusion pressure, ischemic injury and tissue necrosis may occur.

20. **Ans. (d)**

Chang DW. Airway management in mechanical ventilation (Ch 6). Clinical Application of Mechanical Ventilation. New York: CENGAGE Learning Custom Publishing; 2013. pp. 173.

These conditions impede air flow making ventilation and phonation difficult.

21. **Ans. (d)**

K Nag, Singh DR, Shetti AN, et al. Sugammadex: A revolutionary drug in neuromuscular pharmacology. Anesth Essays Res. 2013;7(3)302-6.

Sugammadex does not bind to plasma proteins.

22. **Ans. (a)**

Gronert GA. Cardiac arrest after succinylcholine: Mortality greater with rhabdomyolysis than receptor upregulation. Anesthesiology. 2001;94(3):523-9.

ACEP US Dept of health and human services, CDCP, June 2009.

Rhabdomyolysis releases potassium. Scoline potentiates hyperkalemia.

Cardiopulmonary Resuscitation

CHAPTER 3

Balkrishna D Nimavat

QUESTIONS

1. Components of high-quality CPR includes all *except*:
   a. Chest compressions of adequate rate
   b. Chest compressions of adequate depth
   c. Full chest recoil between compressions
   d. Excessive ventilation

2. Criteria for not starting CPR includes:
   a. Where attempts to perform CPR would place the rescuer at risk of serious injury
   b. Signs of irreversible death
   c. Valid Do Not Attempt Resuscitation (DNAR) order
   d. All the above

3. Chain of survival in IHCA starts with:
   a. Recognition and activation of emergency response system
   b. Immediate high-quality CPR
   c. Rapid defibrillation
   d. Surveillance and prevention

4. Chain of survival in OHCA is:
   a. Immediate high-quality CPR → Activation of emergency response system → Rapid defibrillation → Basic and advanced EMS → Advanced life support and post-arrest care
   b. Recognition and activation of emergency response system → Immediate high-quality CPR → Rapid defibrillation → Advanced life support and post-arrest care → Surveillance and prevention
   c. Surveillance and prevention → Recognition and activation of emergency response system → Immediate high-quality CPR → Rapid defibrillation → Advanced life support and post-arrest care
   d. Recognition and activation of emergency response system → Immediate high-quality CPR → Rapid defibrillation → Basic and advanced EMS → Advanced life support and post-arrest care

5. Rate of chest compression in adult victims of cardiac arrest:
   a. At least 100/min
   b. Maximum 140/min
   c. 100–120/min
   d. 100–140/min

6. In adult cardiac arrest with an unprotected airway, goal of a chest compression fraction should be at least:
   a. 50%
   b. 60%
   c. 70%
   d. 80%

7. During manual CPR, rescuers should perform chest compressions at a depth of:
   a. At least 2 inches or 5 cm
   b. 5 cm to 6 cm
   c. 5.5 cm to 6.5 cm
   d. 2.5 inches

8. What is true for chest compression/ventilation ratio for adult?
   a. 30:2 with advanced airway
   b. 30:2 without advanced airway
   c. 15:2 without advanced airway
   d. 15:2 with advanced airway

9. Useful clinical findings that are associated with poor neurologic outcome includes all *except*:
   a. Absence of pupillary reflex to light at ≥72 hours after cardiac arrest
   b. Myoclonus during the first 72 hours after cardiac arrest
   c. Absence of the N20 somatosensory evoked potential cortical wave 24 to 72 hours after cardiac arrest or after rewarming
   d. Marked reduction of the gray-white ratio on brain computed tomography within 2 hours after cardiac arrest

10. Identify the false statement:
    a. Vasopressin was removed from the ACLS Cardiac Arrest Algorithm as a vasopressor therapy in recognition of equivalence of effect with other available interventions (e.g. epinephrine)
    b. In nonshockable rhythm, reasonable to administer epinephrine as soon as feasible
    c. For those with a shockable rhythm, there is insufficient evidence to make a recommendation about the optimal timing of epinephrine administration, because defibrillation is a major focus of resuscitation
    d. In OHCA, the combination of intra-arrest vasopressin, epinephrine, and methylprednisolone and post-arrest hydrocortisone improves survival based on 2 RCTs

11. True about postcardiac arrest care includes all *except*:
    a. No superiority of targeted temperature management at 33°C compared with management at 36°C
    b. A prehospital infusion of cold intravenous fluids to initiate hypothermia after OHCA shows no improvement in outcome
    c. All comatose patients with ROSC should have a TTM for at least 72 hours
    d. It is advisable in comatose patients to actively prevent fever

12. Which of the following is false statement?
    a. Amiodarone can be used for VF/pVT that is unresponsive to CPR, defibrillation, and a vasopressor therapy
    b. Magnesium was found to increase rates of ROSC in patient of VF/pVT
    c. Atropine having no therapeutic benefit in PEA and asystole
    d. Routine use of sodium bicarbonate is not recommended in cardiac arrest

13. What is the cutoff for arterial relaxation pressure for improving quality of CPR by optimizing chest compression parameters or giving a vasopressor or both?
    a. 20 mm Hg
    b. 30 mm Hg
    c. 10 mm Hg
    d. 65 mm Hg

14. Central venous oxygen saturation ($ScvO_2$) cut off to improve CPR quality is:
    a. 10%
    b. 20%
    c. 65%
    d. 30%

15. Value of $ETCO_2$ associated with poor ROSC and survival after 20 min of resuscitation is:
    a. 10 mm Hg
    b. 20 mm Hg
    c. 30 mm Hg
    d. 40 mm Hg

16. All are true in situation of cardiac arrest *except*:
    a. If IV access is not available second best choice is IO route
    b. It is advisable to insert central line in patient of cardiac arrest unless contraindicated
    c. Routine measurement of arterial blood gases during CPR has definitive value
    d. If IV or IO access cannot be established, epinephrine, vasopressin, and lidocaine may be administered by the endotracheal route

17. What is wrong statement about special situations of resuscitation?
    a. Naloxone in combination with BLS care for opioid-associated life-threatening emergencies
    b. Intravenous lipid emulsion for treatment of local anesthetic systemic toxicity
    c. For the pregnant woman in cardiac arrest high-quality CPR and relief of aortocaval compression
    d. Use of the Heimlich maneuver for drowning victims

18. The earliest time for prognostication in patients treated with TTM:
    a. 72 hours after cardiac arrest
    b. 24 hours after hypothermia
    c. 24 hours after cardiac arrest
    d. 72 hours after normothermia

19. If there is no ROSC in maternal cardiac arrest/resuscitation efforts for unwitnessed arrest, PMCD should be considered at:
    a. 4 minutes
    b. 8 minutes
    c. 10 minutes
    d. 20 minutes

20. All are true *except*:
    a. The routine use of the impedance threshold device (ITD) as an adjunct to conventional CPR is not recommended
    b. The use of ECPR may be used in selected patients where a reversible cause of cardiac arrest is suspected
    c. The evidence shows benefit with the use of mechanical piston devices for chest compressions versus manual chest compressions in patients with cardiac arrest
    d. The combination of ITD with active compression-decompression CPR is a reasonable alternative to conventional CPR where equipment and properly trained personnel are available

21. What is false about impedance threshold device (ITD) and ACD-CPR?
    a. The impedance threshold device (ITD) is a valve that limits air entry into the lungs during chest recoil between chest compressions
    b. ITD is designed to reduce intrathoracic pressure and enhance venous return to the heart
    c. The ITD and ACD should not be used simultaneously as they counteract each other by effect of venous return
    d. Active compression-decompression CPR (ACD-CPR) is performed with a hand-held device equipped with a suction cup to actively lift the anterior chest during decompression

22. True statement for coronary angiography is:
    a. Emergently for OHCA patients with suspected cardiac etiology and STEMI
    b. Reasonable for select patients after OHCA with suspected cardiac etiology but w/o STE on ECG
    c. Reasonable in postcardiac arrest patients for whom angiography is indicated, regardless of whether is comatose or awake
    d. All the above

23. Identify the true statement for defibrillator.
    a. Biphasic defibrillators were particularly susceptible to waveform modification depending on transthoracic impedance
    b. There are two different designs of biphasic waveform: the biphasic truncated exponential (BTE) and rectilinear biphasic (RLB)
    c. Biphasic waveforms are preferred to monophasic defibrillators for treatment of both atrial and ventricular arrhythmias
    d. All the above

24. **Maximal inspired oxygen concentration should be delivered during phase of:**
    a. CPR
    b. After ROSC
    c. During CPR and ROSC
    d. During CPR but not after ROSC

25. **Higher temperature target (i.e. 36°C) preferred while TTM when patient having:**
    a. Bleeding
    b. Cerebral edema
    c. Seizures
    d. All the above

26. **All are true *except*:**
    a. If victim is in water, wipe out the chest before applying AED
    b. If victim has implanted pacemaker or defibrillator, AED should be placed on it
    c. If patient has transdermal patch remove it before applying pad of AED
    d. If patient having hairy chest AED having difficulty in analyzing the rhythm

27. **All are true statement *except*:**
    a. Defibrillation stuns the heart and thus terminates all electrical activity
    b. Interval from collapse to defibrillation is most important determinants of survival in cardiac arrest patient
    c. AED is not better than manual defibrillator for rhythm interpretation and thus increase interruption in chest compression
    d. Chance of survival reduce per minute about 7% to 10% when bystanders perform CPR

ANSWERS

1. **Ans. (d)**
   2015 American Heart Association Guidelines Update for Cardiopulmonary Resuscitation and Emergency Cardiovascular Care. Circulation. 2015;132(18 Suppl 2):s317.
   - High quality CPR improves survival in cardiac arrest patient.
   - There are 5 components of it: Adequate rate of compression, adequate depth of compression, allow chest recoil, minimal interruption and avoid excessive ventilation.

2. **Ans. (d)**
   2015 American Heart Association Guidelines Update for Cardiopulmonary Resuscitation and Emergency Cardiovascular Care. Circulation. 2015;132(18 Suppl 2):s384.
   - It is advisable to avoid or withhold CPR in situation where there is risk to rescuer like fire or risk of spreading or exposure of infectious diseases.
   - It is futile in cases where there are signs of irreversible death like rigor mortis, dependent lividity, and decapitation.
   - Not attempting CPR is quite mutual in case of DNAR order.

3. **Ans. (d)**
   2015 American Heart Association Guidelines Update for Cardiopulmonary Resuscitation and Emergency Cardiovascular Care. Circulation. 2015;132(18 Suppl 2):s398
   - Sequence of chain of survival in IHCA mentioned like this:
     - Its start with surveillance and prevention followed by, activation of emergency services, start CPR, defibrillation as soon as it arrives (if shockable rhythm) and advance life support care and post-arrest care including TTM.

4. **Ans. (d)**
   2015 American Heart Association Guidelines Update for Cardiopulmonary Resuscitation and Emergency Cardiovascular Care. Circulation. 2015;132(18 Suppl 2):s398

5. **Ans. (c)**
   1. 2015 American Heart Association Guidelines Update for Cardiopulmonary Resuscitation and Emergency Cardiovascular Care. Circulation. 2015;132(18 Suppl 2):s318.
   2. Idris AH, Guffey D, Dunderheaded TP, et al. Relationship between chest compression rates and outcomes from cardiac arrest. Circulation. 2012;125(24):3004-12.
   - According to newer 2015 guideline, rate of compression should be 100 to 120/min.[1]
   - Reason behind putting upper border is due to one large study that shows that increase rate associated with decrease depth of compression.[2]

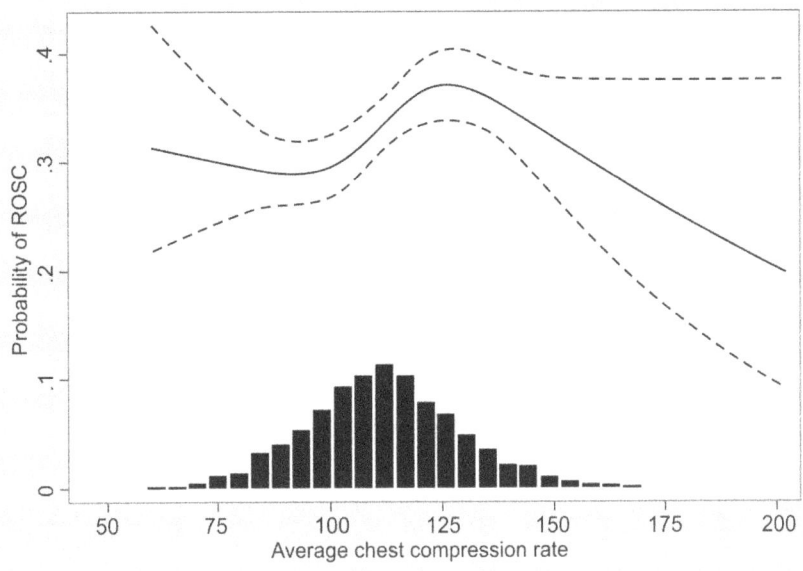

6. Ans. (b)

2015 American Heart Association Guidelines Update for Cardiopulmonary Resuscitation and Emergency Cardiovascular Care. Circulation. 2015;132(18 Suppl 2):s318, s420

- Definition of chest compression fraction is a proportion of time that compressions are performed during cardiac arrest.
- Purpose of putting at least 60% chest compression fraction is to decrease interruption and thus optimize coronary perfusion and blood flow.

7. Ans. (b)

2015 American Heart Association Guidelines Update for Cardiopulmonary Resuscitation and Emergency Cardiovascular Care. Circulation. 2015;132(18 Suppl 2):s318.

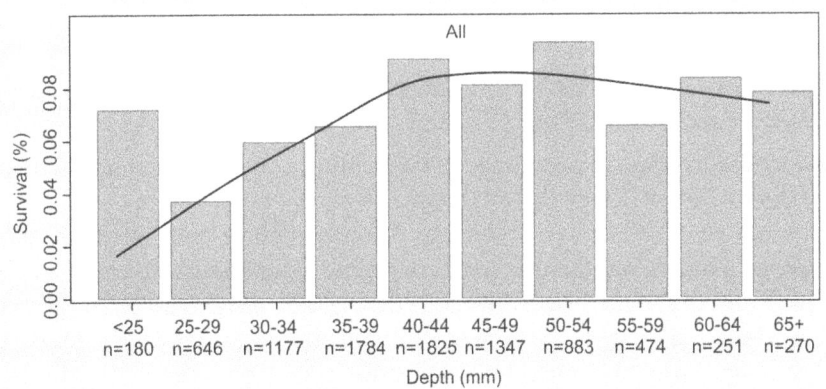

- Depth of chest compression should be at least 2 inches or 5 cm for effective pumping and should not beyond 2.4 inches or 6 cm to prevent potential harm.
- Adding upper limit is based on study that shows injuries are more common with depth of >6 cm compared to 5-6 cm.

8. Ans. (b)

   2015 American Heart Association Guidelines Update for Cardiopulmonary Resuscitation and Emergency Cardiovascular Care. Circulation. 2015;132(18 Suppl 2):s318.

   - When patient airway is not secured, ratio of chest compression to breathing will be 30:2
   - As soon as advanced airway is inserted, chest compression should be continued irrespective to breathing without interruption. Rate of breathing will be 10/min (1 breath every 6 sec).
   - 15:2 is the ratio for pediatric patient when 2 rescuers are available.

9. Ans. (b)

   2015 American Heart Association Guidelines Update for Cardiopulmonary Resuscitation and Emergency Cardiovascular Care. Circulation. 2015;132(18 Suppl 2):s321, s471.

   Findings that are associated with poor neurologic outcome include:
   - *Clinical based*:
     - Absence of pupillary reflex to light at ≥72 hours after cardiac arrest.
     - Presence of status myoclonus during the first 72 hours after cardiac arrest.
     - *Investigation based*: The absence of the N20 somatosensory evoked potential cortical wave 24–72 hours after cardiac arrest or after rewarming.
     - *Imaging based*: Marked reduction of the gray-white ratio on CT brain obtained within 2 hours after cardiac arrest.
     - Extensive restriction of diffusion on MRI brain at 2–6 days after cardiac arrest.
     - *EEG based*: Persistent absence of EEG reactivity to external stimuli at 72 hours after cardiac arrest. Persistent burst suppression or intractable status epilepticus on EEG after rewarming.
     - Absent motor movements, extensor posturing or myoclonus should not be used alone for predicting outcome.

10. Ans. (d)

    2015 American Heart Association Guidelines Update for Cardiopulmonary Resuscitation and Emergency Cardiovascular Care. Circulation. 2015;132(18 Suppl 2):s319-s320, s451, s453.

    - Vasopressin offers no advantage as a substitute or in combination with epinephrine in cardiac arrest (Class IIb, LOE B-R).
    - A randomized control trial, done by Mentzelopoulos et al., gives conclusion that among patients with cardiac arrest requiring vasopressors, combined vasopressin-epinephrine and methylprednisolone during CPR and stress-dose hydrocortisone in postresuscitation shock, compared with epinephrine/saline placebo, shows improved survival to hospital discharge with favorable neurological status. Trial was conducted for in-hospital patients.

- In OHCA, use of steroids during CPR is of uncertain benefit (Class IIb, LOE C-LD).
- For nonshockable rhythm, epinephrine should be administered as soon as feasible (Class IIb, LOE C-LD).
- For shockable rhythm, there is insufficient evidence to make a recommendation as to the optimal timing of epinephrine. As in this case, there is major role of defibrillation.

11. **Ans. (c)**
2015 American Heart Association Guidelines Update for Cardiopulmonary Resuscitation and Emergency Cardiovascular Care. Circulation. 2015;132(18 Suppl 2):s321, s467, s468.
- In comatose (i.e. lack of meaningful response to verbal commands) adult patients with ROSC after cardiac arrest should have TTM (Class I, LOE B-R for VF/pVT OHCA; Class I, LOE C-EO for non-VF/pVT (i.e. nonshockable) and in-hospital cardiac arrest).
- Maintaining a constant temperature between 32°C and 36°C during TTM (Class I, LOE B-R).
- After achieving target temperature, it is advisable to maintain it for 24 hours (Class IIa, LOE C-EO), not for 72 hours.

12. **Ans. (b)**
Antiarrhythmic Drugs during and Immediately after Cardiac Arrest, Part 7: Adult Advanced Cardiovascular Life Support, 2015 American Heart Association Guidelines Update for Cardiopulmonary Resuscitation and Emergency Cardiovascular care. Circulation. 2015;132(18 Suppl 2):s449, s450, s459.
- Amiodarone may be considered for VF/pVT that is unresponsive to CPR, defibrillation, and a vasopressor therapy (Class IIb, LOE B-R).
- The routine use of magnesium for VF/pVT is not recommended in adult patients (Class III: No Benefit, LOE B-R).
- Routine use of atropine during PEA or asystole is unlikely to have a therapeutic benefit (Class IIb, LOE B).
- Routine use of sodium bicarbonate is not recommended in cardiac arrest (Class III, LOE B).
- Routine administration of calcium for treatment of in-hospital and out-of-hospital cardiac arrest is not recommended (Class III, LOE B).
- Atropine is the first-line drug for acute symptomatic bradycardia (Class IIa, LOE B).

13. **Ans. (a)**
Part 7: Adult Advanced Cardiovascular Life Support, 2015 American Heart Association Guidelines Update for Cardiopulmonary Resuscitation and Emergency Cardiovascular Care. Circulation. 2015;132(18 Suppl 2):s459.
- If the coronary perfusion pressure/arterial relaxation "diastolic" pressure is <20 mm Hg, it is suggestive of improvement in quality of CPR by optimizing chest compression parameters or giving vasopressor or both (Class IIb, LOE C).

14. **Ans. (d)**
    Part 7: Adult Advanced Cardiovascular Life Support, 2015 American Heart Association Guidelines Update for Cardiopulmonary Resuscitation and Emergency Cardiovascular Care. Circulation. 2015;132(18 Suppl 2):s459.
    - If $ScvO_2$ is <30%, it is reasonable to consider trying to improve the quality of CPR by optimizing chest compression parameters (Class IIb, LOE C).

15. **Ans. (a)**
    Part 7: Adult Advanced Cardiovascular Life Support, 2015 American Heart Association Guidelines Update for Cardiopulmonary Resuscitation and Emergency Cardiovascular Care. Circulation. 2015;132(18 Suppl 2):s459.
    - In intubated patients, failure to achieve an $ETCO_2$ of greater than 10 mm Hg by waveform capnography after 20 minutes of CPR may be considered as one of the components to end resuscitation efforts but should not be used alone. (Class IIb, LOE C-LD)

16. **Ans. (c)**
    Part 7: Adult Advanced Cardiovascular Life Support, 2015 American Heart Association Guidelines Update for Cardiopulmonary Resuscitation and Emergency Cardiovascular Care. Circulation. 2015;132(18 Suppl 2):s459.
    - Routine measurement of arterial blood gases during CPR should not be carried about and has uncertain value (Class IIb, LOE C).
    - It is reasonable for providers to establish IO access if IV access is not readily available (Class IIa, LOE C).
    - The appropriately trained provider may consider placement of a central line (internal jugular or subclavian) during cardiac arrest, unless there are contraindications (Class IIb, LOE C).
    - If IV or IO access cannot be established, epinephrine, vasopressin, and lidocaine may be administered by the endotracheal route (Class IIb, LOE B).

17. **Ans. (d)**
    2015 American Heart Association Guidelines Update for Cardiopulmonary Resuscitation and Emergency Cardiovascular Care. Circulation. 2015;132(18 Suppl 2):s510, s511, s513.
    - Priorities for the pregnant woman in cardiac arrest are provision of high-quality CPR and relief of aortocaval compression (Class I, LOC LD).
    - Abdominal thrusts or the Heimlich maneuver for drowning victims is not recommended (Class III, LOE C).
    - It may be reasonable to administer ILE, concomitant with standard resuscitative care, to patients with local anesthetic systemic toxicity and particularly to patients who have neurotoxicity or cardiac arrest due to bupivacaine toxicity (Class IIb, LOE C-EO).
    - Empiric administration of IM or IN naloxone to all unresponsive opioid associated life-threatening emergency patients may be reasonable as an adjunct to standard first aid and non–healthcare provider BLS protocols (Class IIb, LOE C-EO).

Chapter 3 Cardiopulmonary Resuscitation

18. **Ans. (d)**
    2015 American Heart Association Guidelines Update for Cardiopulmonary Resuscitation and Emergency Cardiovascular Care. Circulation. 2015;132(18 Suppl 2):s475.
    - The earliest time for prognostication using clinical examination in patients treated with TTM is 72 hours after normothermia (Class IIb, LOE C-EO).
    - Earliest time to prognosticate a poor neurologic outcome using clinical examination in patients not treated with TTM is 72 hours after cardiac arrest (Class I, LOE B-NR).
    - This time until prognostication can be even longer than 72 hours after cardiac arrest if the residual effect of sedation or paralysis confounds the clinical examination (Class IIa, LOE C-LD).

19. **Ans. (a)**
    2015 American Heart Association Guidelines Update for Cardiopulmonary Resuscitation and Emergency Cardiovascular Care. Circulation. 2015;132(18 Suppl 2):s510.
    - PMCD should be considered at 4 minutes after onset of maternal cardiac arrest or resuscitative efforts (for the unwitnessed arrest) if there is no ROSC (Class IIa, LOE C-EO).

20. **Ans. (c)**
    2015 American Heart Association Guidelines Update for Cardiopulmonary Resuscitation and Emergency Cardiovascular Care. Circulation. 2015;132(18 Suppl 2):s441.
    - The routine use of the ITD as an adjunct during conventional CPR is not recommended (Class III: No Benefit, LOE A).
    - No support to routine use of ACD-CPR + ITD as an alternative to conventional CPR. The combination may be a reasonable alternative in settings with available equipment and properly trained personnel (Class IIb, LOE C-LD).
    - The evidence does not demonstrate a benefit with the use of mechanical piston devices for chest compressions versus manual chest compressions in patients with cardiac arrest. Manual chest compressions remain the standard of care for the treatment of cardiac arrest, but mechanical chest compressions using a piston device may be consider as alternative for use by properly trained personnel (Class IIb, LOE B-R).
    - There is insufficient evidence to recommend the routine use of ECPR for patients with cardiac arrest. It may be considered for select patients for whom the suspected etiology of the cardiac arrest is potentially reversible during a limited period of mechanical cardiorespiratory support (Class IIb, LOE C-LD).

21. **Ans. (c)**
    Part 6: CPR Techniques. Circulation. 2005;112:IV-48.
    - The impedance threshold device (ITD) is a valve that limits air entry into the lungs during chest recoil between chest compressions. It is designed to reduce intrathoracic pressure and enhance venous return to the heart.
    - Active compression-decompression CPR (ACD-CPR) is performed with a hand-held device equipped with a suction cup to actively lift the anterior chest during decompression. It is thought that decreasing intrathoracic pressure during the decompression phase enhances venous return to the heart.

ITD devices

Chest wall recoil

Influx of air is prevented, enhancing the vacuum in the chest

Spontaneous breathing

Air will enter if patient creates at least 10 cm H_2O^+ pressure with respiratory effort

ACD-CPR optimizes chest wall recoil

Conventional CPR

ACD-CPR

- The ITD and ACD device act synergistically to enhance venous return during active decompression.

22. **Ans. (d)**

   2015 American Heart Association Guidelines Update for Cardiopulmonary Resuscitation and Emergency Cardiovascular Care. Circulation. 2015;132(18 Suppl 2):s466.
   - Coronary angiography should be performed emergently (rather than later in the hospital stay or not at all) for OHCA patients with suspected cardiac etiology of arrest and ST elevation on ECG (Class I, LOE B-NR).
   - Emergency coronary angiography is reasonable for select (e.g. electrically or hemodynamically unstable) adult patients who are comatose after OHCA of suspected cardiac origin but without ST elevation on ECG (Class IIa, LOE B-NR).
   - Coronary angiography is reasonable in postcardiac arrest patients for whom coronary angiography is indicated regardless of whether the patient is comatose or awake (Class IIa, LOE C-LD).

23. **Ans. (c)**
    1. *2015 American Heart Association Guidelines Update for Cardiopulmonary Resuscitation and Emergency Cardiovascular Care. Circulation. 2015;132(18 Suppl 2):s448.*
    2. *CD Deakin, Nolan JP, Sunde K, et al. European Resuscitation Council Guidelines for Resuscitation 2010 Section 3. Electrical therapies: automated external defibrillators, defibrillation, cardioversion and pacing. Resuscitation. 2010;81:1293-304.*
    - Biphasic waveforms are of three different designs: biphasic truncated exponential (BTE), rectilinear biphasic (RLB), and pulsed biphasic waveforms.[1]
    - Defibrillators (using BTE, RLB, or monophasic waveforms) are recommended to treat atrial and ventricular arrhythmias (Class I, LOE B-NR).[1]
    - Based on their greater success in arrhythmia termination, defibrillators using biphasic waveforms (BTE or RLB) are preferred to monophasic defibrillators for treatment of both atrial and ventricular arrhythmias (Class IIa, LOE B-R).[1]
    - Biphasic defibrillators compensate for the wide variations in transthoracic impedance by electronically adjusting the waveform magnitude and duration to ensure optimal current delivery to the myocardium, irrespective of the patient's size. Thus, least affected by thoracic impedance compared to monophasic defibrillators.[2]

24. **Ans. (d)**
    2015 American Heart Association Guidelines Update for Cardiopulmonary Resuscitation and Emergency Cardiovascular Care. Circulation. 2015;132(18 Suppl 2):s319, s445.
    - It is advisable to use maximal feasible inspired oxygen during CPR but this recommendation applies only while CPR is ongoing and does not apply after ROSC.
    - When supplementary oxygen is available, it may be reasonable to use the maximal feasible inspired oxygen concentration during CPR (Class IIb, LOE C-EO).
    - There are detrimental effects of hyperoxia in the immediate postcardiac arrest period and it is the reason behind avoiding high oxygen supplementation after ROSC.

25. **Ans. (a)**
    2015 American Heart Association Guidelines Update for Cardiopulmonary Resuscitation and Emergency Cardiovascular Care. Circulation. 2015;132(18 Suppl 2):s467.
    - Higher temperatures might be preferred in patients for whom lower temperatures leads to complications (e.g. bleeding), and lower temperatures might be preferred when patients have clinical features that are worsened at higher temperatures (e.g. seizures, cerebral edema).

26. **Ans. (b)**
    American Heart Association. Life is why book for BLS. pp. 39.
    - If victim has hairy chest, AED pads stick to the hair not to the chest leads to difficulty in analyzing the rhythm.
    - Water is conductor of electricity. So for the victim in the water should be wiped out first before applying AED pads.

- In patient of implanted pacemaker or defibrillator if AED pads put on them, they block the delivery of shock.
- Similar things apply to transdermal patch where it is advisable to remove it before applying pads.

27. **Ans. (d)**

    American Heart Association. Life is why book for ACLS. pp. 96-7.
    - AHA does not recommend use of AED when manual defibrillator available and provider is skillful to interpret the rhythm.
    - Reason behind this is that AED takes prolonged time to analyze the rhythm and thus prolonged interruption in chest compression.
    - Sudden cardiac arrest decreases chance of survival by 7–10%/min if no CPR given and 3–4%/min decline when CPR given by bystander.

CHAPTER 4

Shock and Resuscitation

PALEPU B GOPAL

QUESTIONS: SHOCK

1. A 25-year-old man is brought to the emergency department after being submerged in a lake for "a minute or two". He had been water skiing when he lost control and "wiped out" and then was lying face down in the water without moving. He was not breathing when his friends pulled him out of the water but he regained spontaneous respirations after they performed cardiopulmonary resuscitation (CPR). On examination, he is somnolent, but breathing spontaneously with a SpO_2 of 95% on room air and making purposeful movements. The next most important step in management is:
   a. IV antibiotics
   b. Rapid sequence intubation
   c. IV dexamethasone
   d. Cervical spine films

2. A 70-year-old man presented to hospital with community-acquired pneumonia. He weighed 70 kg. His Hb was 12 g/dL, his SaO_2 was 93%, and he was clinically dehydrated with blood pressure 95/60 mm Hg. Which of the following will increase oxygen delivery to his tissues by the greatest degree?
   a. Antibiotics
   b. Fluid challenges
   c. Oxygen therapy
   d. Transfusion 1 unit red cells

3. A 65-year-old woman presents to the emergency room (ER) with signs and symptoms of digitalis toxicity, ventricular tachycardia, and digoxin level of 8.5 ng per mL. She is treated with digitalis antibody fragment therapy and the cardiac rhythm is now sinus. A repeat digoxin level, after the fragments are given, is 12 ng per mL. Which of the following is the most appropriate next step in management?
   a. No acute therapy
   b. Cardioversion at 50 J
   c. Procainamide 1 g IV
   d. Potassium chloride 40 mEq IV

4. A 26-year-old woman is brought to the emergency department after a motor vehicle accident in which she was thrown from the vehicle. Initial evaluation reveals a confused patient with multiple scalp wounds and vital signs of HR 144 beats/min, BP 75/50 mm Hg.

After intubation and fluid resuscitation, initial plain films reveal clear lungs but an obvious pelvic fracture. Diagnostic peritoneal lavage (DPL) reveals a grossly positive tap (aspiration). Which of the following is the next step in management?
   a. Abdominal CT to better determine the need for laparotomy
   b. Pelvic angiography
   c. Thoracotomy with cross-clamping of the aorta
   d. Exploratory laparotomy

5. Regarding cardiac arrest secondary to hypothermia, which one of the following statements is true?
   a. Defibrillation should only be attempted when temperature is >30°C
   b. Temperature of gas delivered to facemask or endotracheal tube (ETT) as well as IV fluids should be warmed to 40°C
   c. Endotracheal intubation should be delayed due to myocardial irritability and subsequent predisposition to VF
   d. Adrenaline dose should be reduced due to decreased drug metabolism and potential toxicity

6. A 30-week-pregnant female is suffering from cardiac arrest. Which one of the following statements is true?
   a. Aortocaval decompression is best achieved with a left lateral tilt maneuver compared with manual displacement of the uterus to the left
   b. Strong evidence exists that aortocaval decompression improves maternal hemodynamics and fetal wellbeing
   c. Perimortem cesarean section performed after 5 minutes of maternal arrest may improve infant survival
   d. Therapeutic hypothermia is proven to be safe and effective in pregnancy after ROSC and is strongly recommended

7. Regarding the use of vasoactive agents in shock, which one of the following statements is false?
   a. Noradrenaline is a potent α-agonist with significant activity at β1-receptors and minimal or no activity at β2-receptors
   b. Adrenaline causes bronchodilatation by acting on α-receptors and causes vasodilatation by acting on β-receptors, hence decreasing leakage of fluids during shock
   c. Isoprenaline is a nonselective β-agonist that causes peripheral vasodilation with subsequent fall in diastolic and mean arterial blood pressure
   d. Dopamine at doses of 5–10 µg/kg/min predominantly acts on α-receptors with a profile similar to noradrenaline

8. "Hypotensive resuscitation" will be the most appropriate for which patient?
   a. A 44-year-old male with a penetrating chest injury
   b. A 30-year-old female with multisite blunt trauma following a road traffic collision with GCS of 15

c. A 55-year-old male with blunt abdominal trauma and severe closed head injury
d. A 22-year-old with a compound femur fracture

9. A 29-year-old, 85-kg, man sustains a grade IV splenic laceration in a motor vehicle collision. He undergoes damage control laparotomy as he is hemodynamically unstable and later on shifted to ICU. On arrival, his BP is 80/40 mm Hg and HR is 125 beats/min. Urine output is 15 mL/hour. After resuscitation with crystalloid and blood products, BP is 117/75 mm Hg, HR is 99 beats/min, and urine output is 100 mL/hour. Lactate level is 5.2 mmol/L, and base deficit is 9 mmol/L. Which one of the following is the most appropriate course of action at this time?
   a. Further aggressive resuscitation should be withheld
   b. His base deficit should be corrected with the administration of sodium bicarbonate
   c. Fibrinogen level has to below 100 mg/dL
   d. A pulmonary artery catheter should be placed to better define his hemodynamics and titrate his resuscitation

10. With respect to adult resuscitation, which statement is incorrect?
    a. Under 24 hours of postcardiac arrest and coma, there are no clinical neurological signs that reliably predict poor outcome
    b. In emergency transcutaneous pacing (TCP), electrical pacing capture occurs when a pacer spike is followed by a wide QRS complex, consistent ST segment, and slurred T wave
    c. In transcutaneous pacing, mechanical capture is achieved with the presence of both an arterial pulse, and blood pressure
    d. In TCP, the pacing output is set at an output that is 10% higher than the threshold of initial mechanical capture

11. For patients undergoing resuscitation after major burns, which is the correct statement?
    a. Due to restriction of head and/or neck involvement, early intubation is very difficult
    b. Suxamethonium can be used safely for intubation
    c. The Parkland formula can be used to predict fluid requirement for the 24-hour period after presentation
    d. Early broad-spectrum antibiotics should be administered as the risk of infection is high in the early phase

12. The correct statement regarding detection of fluid responsiveness is:
    a. Patient's fluid responsiveness can be judged by assessing the clinical status
    b. The reliability of arterial pulse pressure variation in predicting fluid responsiveness in ventilated patients is good
    c. Arterial pulse pressure variation can also be used to assess fluid response in spontaneously breathing patients
    d. Passive leg rising is contraindicated in prediction of fluid response in spontaneously breathing patients

13. The incorrect statement for patients presenting with acute adrenocortical insufficiency (Addisonian crisis) is:

a. They usually present with distributive shock
b. Septicemia-induced Waterhouse–Friderichsen syndrome is not associated with acute adrenal insufficiency
c. Acute steroid withdrawal almost exclusively causes a glucocorticoid deficiency
d. Hypoglycemia, hypokalemia, and hyponatremia are characteristic findings

14. **The true statement regarding FAST scan is:**
    a. It scans five areas to determine the presence of free fluid
    b. This scan can reliably detect fluid collections more than 100–250 mL
    c. Presence of retroperitoneal bleed can be reliably detected with the help of FAST scan
    d. The linear transducer with high frequency and high resolution is the ideal transducer for FAST scan

15. **In the resuscitation of an adult trauma patient, the correct statement is:**
    a. Class III hemorrhagic shock is classified when the blood volume loss is around 15–30%
    b. Pulse pressure remains normal till the exsanguination stage of shock (Class IV)
    c. In the event of failure to secure an IV access, the appropriate sites of intraosseous (IO) access include the sternum, proximal and distal tibia, and proximal humerus
    d. Only adrenaline can be given via the IO route

16. **Which of the following characteristics are best matched in different categories of shock?**
    a. Hypovolemic shock is characterized by a profound reduction in cardiac output and vascular tone very early in the course
    b. Cardiogenic shock is characterized by tachycardia, hypotension, cool peripheries, low mixed venous oxygen saturation (SvO_2), and elevated central venous pressure
    c. Distributive shock is characterized by hypotension, peripheral vasoconstriction, dilated jugular veins, and pulsus paradoxus
    d. Anaphylactic shock is characterized by increased vascular tone, hypovolemia, and low cardiac output state

17. **Which statement is considered as a controversy in the management of septic shock?**
    a. Targeting a mean arterial blood pressure of 80–85 mm Hg compared with 65–70 mm Hg during resuscitation of patients in septic shock does not improve mortality
    b. Albumin replacement in septic shock, in addition to crystalloids, improves overall mortality
    c. High-volume hemofiltration improves hemodynamic profile and mortality in patients with septic shock
    d. Protocol-based early goal-directed therapy (EGDT) with crystalloids in early septic shock results in less fluid being given

18. **Which one of the following is the correct statement regarding fluids used for resuscitation?**
    a. The transvascular exchange of fluid is determined by hydrostatic and oncotic pressures across capillaries and the interstitial space
    b. Fluid resuscitation with chloride-restrictive fluids results in decreased mortality but no difference in the incidence of acute kidney injury

c. The use of hydroxyethyl starch (HES) may be beneficial in early sepsis
d. Albumin use is associated with increased mortality among patients with traumatic brain injury

19. A 45-year-old man is brought to the hospital after a road traffic accident when his motorcycle got struck by another vehicle. At the site of accident, the patient was found 20 feet away from his motorcycle, which was badly damaged. His vital signs include BP of 84/56 mm Hg, HR 125 beats per minute, RR 22 breaths per minute, and pulse oxygenation of 100% on facemask. Which one of the following is the smallest amount of blood loss that produces a decrease in the systolic BP in adults?
    a. Loss of 10% of blood volume
    b. Loss of 15–30% of blood volume
    c. Loss of 30–40% of blood volume
    d. Loss of more than 40% of blood volume

20. A 22-year-old man presents to the emergency department after being ejected from his vehicle following a high-speed motor vehicle collision. Upon arrival, his BP is 85/55 mm Hg and HR is 141 beats per minute. Two large-bore IVs are placed in the antecubital veins and lactated Ringer solution is being administered. After 3 L of crystalloid fluid, the patient's BP is 83/57 mm Hg. Which one of the following statements is most appropriate regarding management of a hypotensive trauma patient who fails to respond to initial volume resuscitation?
    a. Whole blood should be used rather than packed red blood cells (RBCs)
    b. Blood transfusion should begin after 4 L of crystalloid infusion
    c. Type O blood that is Rh-negative should be transfused
    d. Type O blood that is Rh-positive should be transfused

21. A 41-year-old obese man is shifted to ICU for breathing difficulty. The resident doctor in ER has not been able to secure an IV access. After being shifted to ICU, he develops cardiopulmonary arrest with pulseless electrical activity (PEA). CPR is being performed and the patient is intubated. You decided to administer epinephrine to the patient but realized that he does not have IV access. Which one of the following drugs is ineffective when administered through an endotracheal (ET) tube?
    a. Atropine
    b. Lidocaine
    c. Epinephrine
    d. Sodium bicarbonate

22. A 19-year-old man is brought with a stab wound to the right lower abdomen. His temperature is 98.4°F, BP is 130/95 mm Hg, HR is 111 beats per minute, RR is 20 breaths per minute, and oxygen saturation is 98% on room air. He is alert and oriented to person, place, and time. His abdomen is soft and nontender, with normal bowel sounds. He has a 2 cm stab wound with visible subcutaneous fat in his right lower quadrant (RLQ). You initiated the FAST examination. Which type of fluid should you start for his initial resuscitation?

a. 0.9% sodium chloride
b. 10% albumin
c. Type and cross-matched blood
d. Type-specific blood

23. An 82-year-old man with a history of COPD and hypertension presents with shortness of breath and fever. His medications include salbutamol, ipratropium, prednisone, atenolol, and hydrochlorothiazide. His temperature is 102.1°F, BP is 70/40 mm Hg, HR is 110 beats per minute, RR is 24 breaths per minute, and oxygen saturation is 91% on room air. The patient is uncomfortable and mumbling incoherently. On chest examination, you appreciate rales on the left side of his chest. You believe this patient is in septic shock from pneumonia and start IV fluids, broad-spectrum antibiotics, and a dopamine drip. His BP remains at 75/50 mm Hg. Which one of the following is the most appropriate next step in management?
    a. D5 normal saline IV bolus
    b. Phenylephrine IV drip
    c. Hydrocortisone IV
    d. Epinephrine IV drip

24. A 35-year-old woman is admitted to the ICU after a motor vehicle collision. On the 3rd day, she develops fever, hypotension, and generalized body rash. She continues to remain hypotensive even after receiving broad-spectrum antibiotics and 3 liters of crystalloid IV fluids. She is later on started on vasopressors and gets intubated in view of respiratory distress. Regarding the use of pulse pressure variation to help determine if she is volume responsive, which one of the following is correct?
    a. It is accurate, if the patient is taking spontaneous breaths while on mechanical ventilation
    b. It is accurate, if the patient is in atrial fibrillation
    c. It is accurate in patients with left ventricular and right ventricular dysfunction or valvular disorders
    d. A pulse pressure variation more than 13% accurately predicts that the patient will be volume responsive

25. Regarding defibrillation with a manual biphasic defibrillator using pads in patients with cardiac arrest, which one of the following statements is true?
    a. For rescuer safety, chest compressions should briefly be stopped while charging the defibrillator in preparation for delivery of a shock
    b. After delivery of a shock, one should check for the presence or absence of a pulse before restarting chest compressions
    c. Three stacked shocks should initially be delivered in all patients suffering from a ventricular fibrillation (VF) arrest
    d. The default energy level for adults should be set at 200 J for all shocks

26. Regarding the use of vasopressors during cardiac arrest in adults with a shockable rhythm, which one of the following statements is true?

a. It improves return of spontaneous circulation (ROSC) and survival to hospital discharge
b. Vasopressin is associated with a better neurological outcome compared with adrenaline
c. Current evidence suggests that the optimal dose of adrenaline is 1 mg given after the second shock and then every second cycle, if there is no response to defibrillation
d. High-dose adrenaline has not shown improved rates of survival to hospital discharge or neurologic outcome when compared to standard-dose adrenaline

27. The correct statement concerning crystalloid solutions is:
    a. 5% dextrose has a similar osmolality to blood
    b. Hartmann's solution has equal concentrations of Na^+ and Cl^-
    c. Dextrose saline is distributed equally in intracellular fluid (ICF) and extracellular fluid (ECF)
    d. Hartmann's solution is isotonic to blood

28. Which one of the following is the incorrect statement regarding cardiogenic shock?
    a. It is shock due to inability of the heart to maintain the circulation
    b. It is characterized by a low-cardiac output
    c. It is characterized by a low PAOP
    d. It is characterized by a high-systemic vascular resistance

29. Septic shock is characterized by:
    a. Vasoconstriction
    b. A low-cardiac output
    c. A high-systemic vascular resistance
    d. A high-capillary artery occlusion pressure

ANSWERS: SHOCK

1. **Ans. (d)**
   - Trauma in the setting of submersion injuries is usually because of motor vehicle accidents (in which the vehicle crashes into water), or accidents involving diving, boating, or falls from a height into water.
   - Although antibiotics are of use in patients who were submerged in grossly contaminated fluid (e.g. sewage), they have no role in routine fresh or saltwater submersion.
   - Because this patient was involved in a high-speed crash, trauma-related injury should be the next most important issue after ensuring an adequate airway, breathing, and circulation.

2. **Ans. (b)**
   - In many cases, oxygen delivery can be optimized more by giving fluid than by giving oxygen. Hb is delivered to the tissues by the circulation. Each g/dL of Hb carries 1.3 mL of oxygen. Therefore, Hb (g/dL) × oxygen saturation of Hb × 1.3 is the oxygen content of blood.
   - The amount of oxygen delivered per minute depends on the cardiac output.
   - CO = HR × SV, where stroke volume is dependent on preload, contractility, and afterload. So by optimizing the preload, one can increase the oxygen content.

3. **Ans. (a)**
   - The standard serum digoxin assay measures levels of all digoxin in the body, including drug bound to Fab fragments. It is not useful to measure digoxin levels once Fab has been given.
   - Cardioversion may be performed in unstable patients, but is unlikely to be curative in patients with digitalis toxicity.
   - Procainamide may exacerbate dysrhythmias.
   - Potassium chloride can cause life-threatening hyperkalemia.

4. **Ans. (d)**
   - In a hemodynamically unstable patient with a pelvic fracture, a positive aspirate is suggestive of ongoing intraperitoneal hemorrhage and organ injury and is an indication for emergent laparotomy.
   - If the aspirate is negative but the lavage is positive by cell counts, or if the aspirate and lavage are negative, pelvic angiography and stabilization are indicated.
   - A positive diagnostic peritoneal lavage (DPL) by cell count in the setting of a pelvic fracture but a negative aspirate is usually due to retroperitoneal hemorrhage from the pelvic fracture.

5. **Ans. (b)**
   - The current recommendation is that rescuers should attempt defibrillation (up to 3 shocks) without regard for core temperature.
   - Patient should undergo early intubation as it provides effective ventilation with warm, humidified oxygen and isolates the airway to reduce the likelihood of aspiration.

- The optimum rewarming technique is still controversial but warming gas and fluids to 40°C is a simple, safe, and effective method.
- Drug metabolism is markedly reduced at low temperatures, hence, it is recommended to withhold IV medications, if the core temperature is <30°C.

6. Ans. (c)
   - Prognosis for the intact survival of infant is best, if delivery occurs within 5 minutes of maternal arrest; however, if the 5-minute time frame is exceeded, a cesarean section should still be considered.
   - There is no evidence to support that aortocaval decompression improves maternal hemodynamics and fetal wellbeing in pregnant women suffering from cardiac arrest.
   - There is some evidence that manual left uterine displacement is as good as or better than left lateral tilt.
   - There is insufficient evidence to support or refute the use of postcardiac arrest hypothermia.

7. Ans. (d)
   Dopamine's actions are complex and dose-dependent:
   - At low doses (<5 µg/kg/min), it causes vasodilation at vascular D1-receptors in renal, mesenteric, and coronary beds.
   - At doses of 5–10 µg/kg/min, it stimulates cardiac β1-receptors producing inotropic effect.
   - At doses of >10 µg/kg/min, it acts predominantly as an α-agonist.

8. Ans. (a)
   - Hypotensive resuscitation, or permissive hypotension, is advocated in patients with a strong potential for ongoing internal hemorrhage (uncontrolled bleeding) until rapid surgical control of bleeding can be achieved.
   - This approach still remains controversial in the setting of multisite blunt trauma and severe head injury.
   - Traditional fluid resuscitation is recommended for patients with controllable hemorrhage, isolated extremity injuries, and isolated traumatic brain injury.

9. Ans. (c)
   - The optimal fluid resuscitation strategy in trauma is unknown but the most prudent strategy is to combine the entire clinical picture with multiple markers of hypoperfusion while weighing the risk-to-benefit analysis of ongoing fluid and product administration.
   - There is no clear role for a pulmonary artery catheter in this patient.

10. Ans. (d)
    - Patient's neurological status can be commented only after 24 hours of cardiac arrest.
    - The presence of 1 QRS complex after each pacing stimulus suggests but does not confirm the capture. Cardiac capture should be confirmed by detecting the pulse (2-dimensional echocardiography is a good alternative).

- The pacing should be initiated at the maximum current output to ensure that capture is achieved as soon as possible, after which time the current can be gradually reduced to 5–10 mA above the threshold.

11. **Ans. (b)**
    - If intubation is required at an early stage, it is usually technically easy as swelling of the airway has not yet occurred.
    - Succinylcholine is safe in the first 24 hours after a burn—after this time, its use is contraindicated due to the risk of hyperkalemia leading to cardiac arrest, thought to be due to release of potassium from extrajunctional acetylcholine receptors. This can persist up to 1 year post-burn.
    - The Parkland formula (4 mL/kg/% burn) predicts fluid requirement for the first 24 hours after the burn injury (not time of presentation).

12. **Ans. (b)**
    - Clinical evaluation of a patient is a poor and unreliable indicator of fluid need and fluid responsiveness.
    - In ventilated patients, pulse pressure variation or stroke volume variation from arterial waveform analysis can predict fluid responsiveness.
    - In patients who are spontaneously breathing, subsequent changes in intrathoracic pressure make pulse pressure variation analysis difficult.
    - Passive leg raising (PLR) may be useful as an indicator of fluid responsiveness in spontaneously breathing and ventilated patients.

13. **Ans. (b)**
    - Acute adrenocortical insufficiency usually causes distributive shock with relative hypovolemia due to low-systemic vascular resistance secondary to vasodilatation.
    - Waterhouse–Friderichsen syndrome is defined as adrenal gland failure due to bleeding into the adrenal glands, and can occur in fulminant meningococcemia. This is associated with acute adrenocortical insufficiency.

14. **Ans. (b)**
    - The FAST scan is a four-view scan—subcostal, right upper quadrant, left upper quadrant, and suprapubic views.
    - The purpose of bedside ultrasound in trauma is to rapidly identify free fluid (usually blood) and hence guide appropriate management.
    - Volumes of free fluid more than 100–250 mL can be detected by a FAST scan.
    - Increasing the frequency improves image resolution but reduces the degree and accuracy of tissue penetration and hence transducers with high frequency are not ideal for abdominal scanning.

15. **Ans. (c)**
    - Loss of 15–30% blood volume would be Class II hemorrhagic shock. Class III hemorrhagic shock occurs when 30–40% blood volume is lost.
    - Pulse pressure is initially normal in Class I hemorrhage, and decreases with Classes II, III, and IV hemorrhage.

CHAPTER 4 Shock and Resuscitation

- Appropriate sites of intraosseous (IO) access do include the sternum, proximal and distal tibia, and proximal humerus.
- All resuscitation drugs can be given via the IO route.

16. Ans. (b)
    - Hypovolemic shock is characterized by a profound reduction in blood volume with an initial decrease in preload compensated for by an increase in cardiac output and profound vasoconstriction.
    - Cardiogenic shock is characterized by tachycardia, hypotension, low-cardiac output state, low-mixed venous O_2 saturation, high-cardiac filling pressures, and increased systemic vascular resistance.
    - Distributive shock is seen with anaphylaxis, sepsis, and neurogenic shock.
    - Anaphylactic shock is a form of distributive shock associated with decreased vascular tone, deranged blood flow distribution, hypovolemia, and often a high-cardiac output state.

17. Ans. (a)
    - Targeting a MAP of 80–85 mm Hg compared with 65–70 mm Hg during resuscitation of patients in septic shock was found not to improve mortality at either 28 or 90 days.
    - ALBIOS study: Albumin replacement in addition to crystalloids compared to crystalloids alone did not improve the rate of survival at 28 or 90 days in severe sepsis.
    - IVOIRE study found no evidence that high-volume hemofiltration (70 mL/kg/h) for a 96-hour period leads to a reduction in 28-day mortality or improvements in hemodynamic profile or organ function.
    - The PRoCESS, ARISE, and ProMISE studies have found that protocol-based EGDT in septic shock resulted in significantly more crystalloid being given compared to both the protocol-based standard therapy and usual care group.

18. Ans. (d)
    - It is thought that the transvascular exchange of fluid is determined by the endothelial glycocalyx layer, which has been identified on the luminal surface of endothelial cells.
    - The use of chloride-restrictive strategy did not show survival benefit but resulted in decreased incidence of acute kidney injury and also the need for RRT.
    - The use of HES is associated with increased rates of renal replacement therapy and adverse events in the critically ill.
    - In the Saline versus Albumin Fluid Evaluation (SAFE) study, albumin was associated with increased mortality in traumatic brain injured patients.

19. Ans. (c)
    - Class III hemorrhage is characterized by 30–40% blood loss (1,500–2,000 mL). This stage exhibits tachypnea, tachycardia (HR > 120), decrease in systolic BP, delayed capillary refill, decreased urine output, and a change in mental status.

20. Ans. (d)
    - Blood products should be administered, if vital signs transiently improve or remain unstable despite resuscitation with 2–3 L of crystalloid fluid.

- Type-specific blood (e.g. type A, Rh-negative, and unknown antibody) can be provided by most blood banks within 30 minutes and is indicated in unstable patients. If type-specific blood is unavailable, type O packed cells are indicated for patients who are unstable.
- Men should be administered type O, Rh-positive blood.
- To reduce sensitization and future complications, type O, Rh-negative blood is reserved for women of childbearing age.

21. **Ans. (d)**
    - The drugs that can be administered safely and effectively via the endotracheal route include naloxone, atropine, epinephrine, and lidocaine. The endotracheal dosage of a medication should be at least equivalent to the IV route and is usually 2–2.5 times the IV dose administered.

22. **Ans. (a)**
    - Crystalloids such as normal saline (0.9% sodium chloride) or lactated Ringer are the preferred resuscitation fluid.
    - Blood is indicated after 2–3 L of crystalloid infusion and only minimal improvement in vital signs or when the patient has obviously suffered significant blood loss.

23. **Ans. (c)**
    - This patient is in septic shock from pneumonia and also has adrenal crisis.
    - The treatment of adrenal crisis in the face of septic shock is hydrocortisone. Mineralocorticoids, such as fludrocortisone, are not needed. Additional fluids and pressors are appropriate critical care management for sepsis and should be administered after glucocorticoids.

24. **Ans. (d)**
    - A pulse pressure variation of greater than 13% has been verified in the literature to indicate that the patient will likely be volume responsive.
    - However, in order for this to be accurate, the patient must be in sinus rhythm, must not be taking spontaneous breaths, ideally should not be ventilated with very low-tidal volumes, and should not have significant left ventricular or right ventricular dysfunction.

25. **Ans. (d)**
    - The default energy level for adults using a biphasic defibrillator should be set at 200 J for all shocks.
    - ILCOR and the ARC recommend that chest compressions be continued while the defibrillator is charged if using pads.
    - CPR should be restarted immediately after delivering a shock, irrespective of apparent electrical success. A pulse check should not be performed.

26. **Ans. (d)**
    - Current guidelines recommend that the use of vasopressors may be considered in adult cardiac arrest given the evidence that their use favors initial resuscitation with ROSC.

- Three studies and a meta-analysis demonstrated no difference in outcomes (ROSC, survival to discharge, and neurological outcome) with vasopressin compared with adrenaline as first-line pressor in cardiac arrest and the use of either is acceptable.

27. Ans. (c)
    - 5% dextrose has an osmolality of 278 mOsmol/kg, which is less than that of blood at 290 mOsmol/kg.
    - Hartmann's solution has a Na⁺ concentration of 131 mmol/L and Cl- concentration of 111 mmol/L.
    - Hartmann's solution is slightly hypertonic compared to blood, and is distributed in the ECF.
    - Dextrose saline is distributed equally between ICF and ECF. 5% dextrose is distributed throughout total body water.

28. Ans. (c)
    - Cardiogenic shock is characterized by a low-cardiac output, and raised PAOP and SVR.
    - The raised PAOP reflects the elevated left ventricular end-diastolic and left atrial pressures that accompany left ventricular dysfunction.

29. Ans. (c)
    - Cardiac output is usually increased but may be low once metabolic acidosis has supervened.
    - Vasodilatation results in a low SVR.

QUESTIONS: RESUSCITATION

1. During cardiopulmonary resuscitation (CPR), the quality compressions are defined as all of the below, *except*:
    a. Compress the chest at least 5 cm
    b. Compress the chest at the rate of 100–120/min
    c. Minimize interruption in compressions to 20 seconds or less
    d. Switch compressor about every 2 minutes or earlier, if fatigued

2. A suspected acute coronary syndrome (ACS) can be classified into one of the following three classes based on ST-segment deviation in electrocardiogram (ECG), *except*:
    a. ST elevation by 2 mm in two or more leads or new LBBB (STEMI)
    b. ST depression by 0.5 mm or greater or dynamic T-wave inversion with pain (NSTE-ACS)
    c. ST depression and appearance of Q wave in any of the chest leads V1-V6
    d. Normal or nondiagnostic changes in ST-segment or T-wave ECG (low-intermediate-risk ACS)

3. Which of the following is absolute exclusion characteristic in patients with ischemic stroke for fibrinolytic therapy with rtPA?
    a. Arterial puncture at noncompressible site in previous 14 days
    b. Elevated blood pressure (systolic >185 mm Hg or diastolic >110 mm Hg)
    c. Seizure at onset with postictal residual neurological impairment
    d. Major surgery or serious trauma within previous 14 days

4. Which one of the following statements is true in relation to physiological monitoring during CPR?
   a. Persistently low PETCO$_2$ values less than 10 mm Hg during CPR in intubated patients suggest that return of spontaneous circulation (ROSC) is unlikely
   b. In a patient being monitored with intra-arterial catheter, if arterial relaxation (diastolic) pressure is less than 20 mm Hg, it is reasonable to try to improve chest compression and vasopressor therapy
   c. In a patient being monitored with oximetric tipped central venous catheter, if the ScvO$_2$ is less than 30%, it is reasonable to try to improve chest compressions and vasopressor therapy
   d. All of the above statements are true

5. Which one of the following statement is true regarding pharmacological agents utilized during cardiopulmonary resuscitation (CPR)?
   a. Vasopressin offers no advantage as a substitute to epinephrine in cardiac arrest
   b. Epinephrine 1 mg IV is repeated every 5–7 minutes during CPR
   c. Epinephrine is known to increase survival from VF/pulseless VT, if it utilizes during CPR
   d. Amiodarone has not been clinically demonstrated that it improves the rate of ROSC and hospital admission in adults with refractory ventricular fibrillation/pulseless VT

6. Which one of the following statements is true regarding hemorrhagic shock (American College of Surgeons Classification)?
   a. Pulse pressure is increased in Class III shock
   b. Urinary output is usually 5–15 mL/h in Class III shock
   c. Crystalloid + blood resuscitation is recommended in Class II shock
   d. Blood loss is up to 1.5–2 liters in Class II shock

7. Which one of the following statement is not true concerning serum lactate monitoring in shock?
   a. Severity of lactic acidosis directly correlates with the severity of the shock insult
   b. Profound hypoperfusion will always exhibit abnormally high-lactate levels
   c. Patients with significant hepatic dysfunction may manifest higher lactate levels in the absence of anaerobic metabolism
   d. Elevated lactate concentrations predict an increased mortality rate

8. For monitoring preload and fluid responsiveness during resuscitation from shock, which of the following statement(s) is (are) appropriate?
   a. Commonly used preload measures (such as CVP or PAOP or global end-diastolic volume or global end-diastolic area) alone should not be used to guide fluid resuscitation
   b. Using dynamic overstatic variables to predict fluid responsiveness is recommended
   c. Even in fluid-responsive patients, fluid management should be titrated carefully, especially in the presence of elevated intravascular filling pressures or elevated extravascular lung water
   d. All of the above

CHAPTER 4 Shock and Resuscitation

9. Regarding blood and blood product transfusion, the Surviving Sepsis Campaign has stated the following, except:
   a. We recommend that RBC transfusion occurs only when hemoglobin concentration decreases to <7.0 g/dL in adults in the absence of extenuating circumstances, such as myocardial ischemia, severe hypoxemia, or acute hemorrhage
   b. We suggest against the use of fresh frozen plasma to correct clotting abnormalities in the absence of bleeding or planned invasive procedures
   c. We suggest using cryoprecipitate concentrates, if serum fibrinogen levels below 100/ are recorded in a patient with sepsis who has moderate risk of bleeding
   d. We suggest prophylactic platelet transfusion when counts are <10,000/mm^3 (10×10^9/L) in the absence of apparent bleeding and when counts are <20,000/mm^3 (20×10^9/L) if the patient has a significant risk of bleeding

10. "Dynamic changes in arterial waveform-derived variables (i.e. SPV, PPV, and SVV) can predict with a high degree of accuracy in those patients who are likely to respond to a fluid challenge". For this statement to be true, which of the following condition/ conditions should be met?
    a. They should be measured during volume-controlled mechanical ventilation
    b. The tidal volume must be below 6 mL/kg body weight as directed by ARDSNet
    c. The fluid challenge must be in the form of IV bolus of crystalloid only
    d. All of the above

11. In the initial assessment of patients with blunt trauma, all of the following are components of the focused abdominal sonography for trauma (FAST), *except*:
    a. Pericardium
    b. Pleural space
    c. Morison's pouch
    d. Splenorenal space

12. Which one of the following is the correct dose and route of administration of injection adrenaline for the treatment of anaphylactic reaction?
    a. Injection adrenaline 0.3–0.5 mL of 1:1,000 solution subcutaneous
    b. Injection adrenaline 0.3–0.5 mL of 1:1,000 solution intravenous
    c. Injection adrenaline 3.0–5.0 of 1:1,000 solution subcutaneous
    d. None of the above combinations are correct

13. Which one of the following statements is not true regarding fluid resuscitation in shock?
    a. SAFE study reported no difference in the overall risk of death for adults given albumin or saline for intravascular fluid resuscitation in the ICU
    b. The hyperchloremia associated with normal saline resuscitation may increase mortality in critically ill patients
    c. FEAST study in critically ill African children showed increased mortality in children resuscitated with either albumin or 0.9% saline as compared to children who did not receive any fluid bolus

d. ALBIOS study showed improvement in the rate of survival at 28 and 90 days in patients with severe sepsis, when albumin replacement in addition to crystalloids was given, as compared with crystalloids alone.

14. During resuscitation of shock, regarding role of vasopressors and inotropes, which one of the following statements is correct?
    a. The surviving sepsis campaign guidelines recommend norepinephrine as first-line vasopressor in sepsis
    b. Dopamine is preferred agents in patients with cardiogenic shock as it reduces mortality
    c. In VAAST trial, the vasopressin group has shown superior mortality outcome compared to norepinephrine group
    d. The surviving sepsis campaign guidelines recommend phenylephrine as an alternative to vasopressin in norepinephrine (noradrenaline) unresponsive group

15. Which of the following conditions would increase preload, systemic vascular resistance, and heart rate, result in improved hemodynamic stability?
    a. Aortic stenosis
    b. Asymmetric septal hypertrophy (idiopathic hypertrophic subaortic stenosis)
    c. Cardiac tamponade
    d. Mitral regurgitation

16. Which one of the following statements is not true?
    a. In normal conditions, vasopressin is produced in posterior pituitary but can also be synthesized in heart and adrenal gland under stressful conditions
    b. Milrinone is a inotropic agent with potent pulmonary vasodilator property
    c. Levosimendan is recommended only for 24 hours
    d. Phenylephrine causes bradycardia by its direct effect on conducting system of heart

17. Regarding the pulse contour based continuous cardiac output monitor (FloTrac), which one of the following statements is not true?
    a. The cardiac output calculation algorithm of this device is age and weight dependent
    b. The pulse characteristics such as kurtosis and skewness are taken into consideration for estimating cardiac output by this device
    c. Hemodynamic data from this device are reliable in acute liver failure
    d. Atrial fibrillation interferes with functioning of this device

18. Which one of the following statements is appropriate for fluid responsiveness during resuscitation?
    a. Central venous pressure (CVP) is an accurate predictor of fluid responsiveness during resuscitation
    b. The respiratory variation of inferior vena cava (IVC) diameter is reliable indicator for fluid responsiveness even in patients on spontaneous ventilation
    c. Passive leg rising (PLR)-induced changes in arterial pressure are less reliable than simultaneous changes in cardiac output for predicting fluid responsiveness
    d. Preload dependence as evidenced by pulse pressure variation (PPV) is not reliable during mechanical ventilation

CHAPTER 4 Shock and Resuscitation

ANSWERS: RESUSCITATION

1. Ans. (c)
   American Heart Association. (2016). ACLS Provider Manual, 2016. [online] Available from https://ahainstructornetwork.americanheart.org/idc/groups/ahaecc-public/@wcm/@ecc/documents/downloadable/ucm_481402.pdf. [Last accessed June, 2019].

2. Ans. (c)
   American Heart Association. ACLS Provider Manual, 2016. [online] Available from https://ahainstructornetwork.americanheart.org/idc/groups/ahaecc-public/@wcm/@ecc/documents/downloadable/ucm_481402.pdf. [Last accessed June, 2019].

3. Ans. (b)
   American Heart Association. ACLS Provider Manual, 2016. [online] Available from https://ahainstructornetwork.americanheart.org/idc/groups/ahaecc-public/@wcm/@ecc/documents/downloadable/ucm_481402.pdf. [Last accessed June, 2019]..

4. Ans. (d)
   American Heart Association. ACLS Provider Manual, 2016. [online] Available from https://ahainstructornetwork.americanheart.org/idc/groups/ahaecc-public/@wcm/@ecc/documents/downloadable/ucm_481402.pdf. [Last accessed June, 2019].

5. Ans. (a)
   American Heart Association. ACLS Provider Manual, 2016. [online] Available from https://ahainstructornetwork.americanheart.org/idc/groups/ahaecc-public/@wcm/@ecc/documents/downloadable/ucm_481402.pdf. [Last accessed June, 2019].

6. Ans. (b)
   Committee on Trauma of the American College of Surgeons. Advanced Trauma Life Support for Doctors. Chicago: American College of Surgeons; 2008. p. 61.

7. Ans. (b)
   Cheatham ML, Block EFJ, Smith HG, et al. Chapter 157: Shock-An overview. In: Irwin RS, Rippe JM (Eds). Irwin and Rippe's Intensive Care Medicine, 7th edition. Philadelphia: Wolters Kluwer; 2012. pp. 1644-55.

8. Ans. (d)
   Cecconi M, De Backer D, Antonelli M, et al. Consensus on circulatory shock and hemodynamic monitoring. Task force of the European Society of Intensive Care Medicine. Intensive Care Med. 2014;40(12):1795-815.

9. Ans. (c)
   Rhodes A, Evans LE, Alhazzani W, et al. Surviving Sepsis Campaign: International Guidelines for Management of Sepsis and Septic Shock: 2016. Intensive Care Med. 2017;43(3):304-77.

10. **Ans. (a)**
    SAFE Study investigators. A comparison of albumin and saline for fluid resuscitation in the intensive care. N Eng J Med. 2004;350:2247-56.

11. **Ans. (b)**
    Committee on Trauma of the American College of Surgeons. Advanced Trauma Life Support for Doctors. Chicago: American College of Surgeons; 2008. p. 61.

12. **Ans. (a)**
    Acute management of anaphylaxis guidelines ASCIA.

13. **Ans. (d)**
    SAFE Study Investigators. A comparison of albumin and saline for fluid resuscitation in the intensive care. N Eng J Med. 2004;350:2247-56.

    McCluskey SA, Karkouti K, Wijeysundera D, et al. Hyperchloremia after noncardiac surgery is independently associated with increased mortality and morbidity: a propensity-matched cohort study. Anesth Analg. 2013;117(2):412-21.

    Maitland K, Kiguli S, Opoka RO, et al. Mortality after fluid bolus in African Children with severe infection. N Eng J Med. 2011;364:2483-95.

    Caironi P, Tognoni G, Masson S, et al. The Albumin Replacement in Patients with Severe Sepsis or Septic Shock (ALBIOS) Study. N Engl J Med. 370;15:1412-21.

14. **Ans. (a)**
    Kanter J, DeBleux P. Pressors and inotropes. Emerg Med Clin N Am. 2014:32:823-34.

15. **Ans. (c)**
    Khandekar MH, Espinosa RE, Nishimura RA, et al. Pericardial disease: Diagnosis and management. Mayo Clin Proc. 2010;85:572-93.

16. **Ans. (d)**
    Kanter J, DeBleux P. Pressors and inotropes. Emerg Med Clin N Am. 2014:32:823-834.

    Shah P, Cowger JA. Cardiogenic shock. Crit Care Clin. 2014;30:391-412.

17. **Ans. (c)**

18. **Ans. (d)**

CHAPTER 5

Mechanical Ventilation

SACHIN GUPTA, DEEKSHA SINGH TOMAR

QUESTIONS

1. A 66-year-old female is admitted with secondary ARDS and sepsis following emergency bowel resection for mesenteric ischemia. Her height is 165 cm; weight is 101 kg. On lung protective ventilator settings, the following variables are obtained:
   Peak inspiratory pressure (PIP) is 35 cm H_2O
   Plateau pressure (Pplat) is 30 cm H_2O
   Mean airway pressure (Paw) is 20 cm H_2O
   Esophageal balloon pressure (Pes) is 17 cm H_2O
   Transpulmonary pressure (Ptp) is estimated by the formula:
   a. Paw-Pplat
   b. PEEP-Pes
   c. Pplat-Paw
   d. Paw-Pes

2. A 32-year-old man presents to the ICU with acute respiratory distress syndrome (ARDS) caused by urosepsis. He is intubated, started on mechanical ventilation, sedated, and then paralyzed. The ventilator settings are: pressure control-inverse ratio ventilation (PC-IRV) mode with an inspiratory pressure of 25 cm H_2O; respiratory rate (RR), 15 breaths/min; inspiratory time, 2.5 s; FiO_2, 80%; and positive end-expiratory pressure (PEEP), 8 cm H_2O. On these settings, his peak inspiratory pressure (PIP) and plateau pressures (Pp) are 33 cm H_2O, and tidal volume (VT) is 350 mL. Thirty minutes later, he becomes hypotensive, desaturates, and has decreased breath sounds over the left lung. CXR shows a left-sided pneumothorax.
   What changes in ventilator parameters do you expect to find at this time?
   a. PIP, 60 cm H_2O; Pp, 60 cm H_2O; VT, 350 mL;RR, 15 breaths/min
   b. PIP, 60 cm H_2O; Pp, 60 cm H_2O; VT, 200 mL;RR, 15 breaths/min
   c. PIP, 33 cm H_2O; Pp, 33 cm H_2O; VT, 200 mL;RR, 15 breaths/min
   d. PIP, 33 cm H_2O; Pp, 33 cm H_2O; VT, 350 mL;RR, 40 breaths/min

3. A 56-year-old gentleman, a chronic smoker with a k/c/o COPD is admitted to ICU with breathing difficulty and desaturation. After continuous nebulization for 15 minutes, you apply noninvasive ventilation at an initial setting of IPAP of 10 and EPAP of 6 cm H_2O. After half an hour, his saturation does not improve at all.

What will be the change in settings that you would do?
a. Decrease EPAP to 3
b. Decrease IPAP to 6
c. Increase EPAP to 8 and IPAP to 14
d. Increase the respiratory rate
e. Decrease both IPAP and EPAP to 8 and 4 respectively

4. Regarding invasive ventilation of a patient with severe life-threatening asthma, all of the following statements are correct *except*:
a. A tidal volume of 5–6 mL/kg is recommended
b. The ventilator graph should show expiration to be complete before the next breath is delivered
c. Hypercarbia is generally not detrimental except in patients with myocardial dysfunction
d. Pressure control ventilation is considered better than volume control ventilation

5. Regarding the management of acute asthma in adults, which *one* of the following is true?
a. High-inspiratory flow rates are recommended in patients requiring mechanical ventilation
b. Dynamic hyperinflation makes the reading of plateau pressure unreliable in asthmatic patients
c. Poorer outcomes have been shown with the use of noninvasive ventilation (NIV) and so should be avoided
d. Parenteral (IV) salbutamol has no benefit over continuous nebulized salbutamol

6. An adult patient has some spontaneous respiratory efforts and is receiving volume-controlled ventilation with an FIO_2 of 0.40 using a microprocessor ventilator. The source gases to the ventilator fail. According to the ventilator's capabilities, which of the following would the respiratory therapist expect to occur? I. The high airway pressure alarm will sound. II. The low oxygen alarm will sound. III. The ventilator powers off. IV. The safety valve will open:
a. I and III only
b. I and IV only
c. II and III only
d. II and IV only

7. A 40-year-old man gets admitted to ICU with worsening hypoxia secondary to ethanol related severe acute pancreatitis. He was eventually intubated and kept on mechanical ventilation, sedated. His ventilator parameters worsened and so his FiO_2 was escalated to 65% and PEEP increased to 14 cm H_2O. Patient is now on muscle relaxants and his I:E ratio has been adjusted to 1:1. On these settings, his SpO_2 is 83% and plateau pressure is 30 cm H_2O.
Which of the following options would be the most effective next step?

a. Commencing inhaled nitric oxide
   b. Adjusting the PEEP to 20 cm H_2O in line with the ARDS net high PEEP ladder
   c. Placing the patient in the prone position
   d. Inverting the I:E ratio
   e. Commencing high-frequency oscillatory ventilation

8. What is generally thought of as the primary determinant of oxygenation when mechanically ventilated?
   a. Mean airway pressure
   b. PEEP
   c. Inspiratory time
   d. A-a gradient

9. You are taking care of a 34-year old male with status asthmaticus. He is currently intubated and sedated and being treated with continuous salbutamol, steroids, and atracurium and ketamine infusion. His current ventilator settings show a PIP of 36, PEEP of 5, Vt 6 mL/kg, RR of 12, Inspiratory time 1.5, and FiO_2 of 45%. A plateau pressure is measured and is 22. His most recent arterial blood gas reads as pH 7.08, PCO_2-80, PO_2-65 and his $EtCO_2$ reads 50. What would be the most appropriate next step in managing this patient?
   a. Increase the respiratory rate to 16
   b. Initiate inhaled anesthetic agent
   c. Increase the peak pressures to 40 to achieve higher tidal volumes
   d. Decrease the inspiratory time to 1

10. A hemodynamically stable 70-kg, 40-year-old man with adult respiratory distress syndrome is being mechanically ventilated with the following settings:

    Tidal volume - 500 mL, Respiratory rate 12/min, FiO_2 0.80, I:E ratio 1:2, PEEP 5 cm H_2O
    ABG of the patient shows PaO_2 50 mm Hg, $PaCO_2$ 40 mm Hg, and pH 7.42

    Which of the following changes in ventilator settings is most appropriate?
    a. Increase FiO_2
    b. Increase positive end-expiratory pressure
    c. Increase tidal volume
    d. Increase ventilatory rate

11. A 70-year-old female presents to the emergency department with an acute exacerbation of COPD. She is given oxygen by face mask and inhaled b2-agonist and anticholinergic agents. The patient continued to deteriorate with minimal improvement in her respiratory status and was being evaluated for possible NIV therapy. Which of the following findings would make intubation a better choice for this patient?
    a. Worsening respiratory acidosis
    b. Rapidly deteriorating mental status
    c. A PaO_2 of >50 mm Hg on arterial blood gas despite supplemental oxygen therapy
    d. Evidence of respiratory muscle fatigue

12. A mechanically ventilated patient has an increased airflow resistance due to unknown reasons. What should one see on the pressure-volume (P-V) display?
    a. Widening (bowing) of the P-V loop
    b. Narrowing of the P-V loop
    c. Shifting of the P-V slope toward the volume axis
    d. Shifting of the P-V slope toward the pressure axis

13. A postoperative patient is recovering in the intensive care unit on volume-controlled mode. What should be the preset and variable component in this mode of ventilation depending on the compliance and airway resistance characteristics?
    a. Peak inspiratory pressure, tidal volume
    b. Peak inspiratory pressure, peak flow
    c. Tidal volume, peak inspiratory pressure
    d. Tidal volume, peak flow

14. Concerning ventilator associated pneumonia (VAP), the correct statement is:
    a. Selective decontamination of the digestive tract has no effect on VAP rates
    b. VAP is associated with increased morbidity but has no effect on mortality
    c. Lung protective ventilation (6 mL/kg) reduces rates of VAP
    d. VAP is defined as pneumonia occurring after 48 hours of ventilation
    e. Gastric ulcer prophylaxis with PPI increases VAP rates

15. Regarding airway pressure release ventilation (APRV), the correct statement is:
    a. Peak pressures are higher than with BIPAP for a given tidal volume
    b. To prevent patient/ventilator asynchrony, patients should be on neuromuscular blockade
    c. T_{high} is usually a minimum of 4 seconds
    d. Spontaneous breathing is sensed by the ventilator and mandatory breaths synchronized
    e. Hypercapnia is a contraindication to its use

16. For weaning a patient from mechanical ventilation by adopting the T-piece trial, the physiological parameter that predicts successful weaning is:
    a. Vital capacity > 8 mL/kg
    b. Rapid shallow breathing index > 100 second/liter
    c. PaO_2 /FiO_2 > 200 mm Hg
    d. Maximal Inspiratory pressure of –15 cm H_2O
    e. Static lung compliance with inspiratory pressure of 30 cm H_2O giving a tidal volume of > 10 mL/kg

17. A 55-year-old male develops a bronchpleural fistula following a rupture of bulla. He is put on invasive ventilation due to respiratory distress but maintaining adequate tidal volume is difficult to large volume of air leak up to 2.5 L/min.
    Which one of the following would be most effective in achieving adequate ventilation in this patient?

a. Adding PEEP of 7.5 cm of H_2O
b. Decreasing the inflation pressure
c. Increasing the flow rate by 2.5 L/min
d. High frequency jet ventilation
e. Decreasing the respiratory rate

18. Regarding the use of heat and moisture exchange (HME) filters, which is the true statement?
    a. HME only filters latex particles but not viral or bacterial particles
    b. An HME filter that has no bacterial or viral filtration properties should be green in color
    c. According to the manufacturer's instructions, insertion of an HME filter between a patient and a breathing circuit allows that breathing circuit to be used for more than one patient
    d. In general, hydrophobic filters are better than electrostatic ones in the prevention of fluid contamination of anesthetic breathing circuits
    e. Electrostatic filters are better than hydrophobic ones in the prevention of particulate contamination of ventilator breathing circuits

19. Regarding the use of bilevel positive airway pressure (BiPAP) in acute hypercapnic respiratory failure in chronic obstructive pulmonary disease (COPD), adjustment of which one of the following parameters will most effectively reduce PCO_2 levels?
    a. Increase positive end-expiratory pressure (PEEP)
    b. Increase inspiratory positive airway pressure (IPAP)
    c. Increase PEEP and IPAP proportionally
    d. Decrease the timed ventilations when in spontaneous/timed (S/T) mode

20. During controlled ventilation:
    a. Airway pressure generated depends on the compliance and resistance of the respiratory system and circuit
    b. The inspiratory pressure waveform is constant during volume ventilation
    c. In time triggering, breathing frequency is variable and has no set frequency
    d. Triggering is when the ventilator incorrectly cycles to inspiration
    e. Cycling is only used to dictate when the expiratory phase is complete

ANSWERS

1. Ans. (d)
Transpulmonary pressure reflects the pressure gradient across the lung opposing alveolar collapse is measured as the difference between alveolar pressure and intrapleural pressure. Clinically, alveolar pressure is estimated by airway pressure and intrapleural pressure is estimated by esophageal pressure. Conditions leading to elevated intrapleural pressure (abdominal compartment syndrome, alterations in chest wall compliance, obesity) may thus lead to negative transpulmonary pressure and favor alveolar collapse. A pilot trial of transpulmonary pressure-guided ventilator titration to achieve positive transpulmonary pressure in ARDS demonstrated increased oxygenation and respiratory compliance, with a trend towards a mortality difference.

2. Ans. (c)
PC-IRV is performed by setting an inspiratory pressure, inspiratory time with the I/E > 1:1, and RR. In PC mode, the target is pressure (the set inspiratory pressure) and the VT varies depending on the set inspiratory pressure, inspiratory time, airway resistance (patient and ventilator tubing), and compliance of the lung and chest wall. When lung compliance decreases (mucous plugging, pulmonary edema, or pneumothorax in this case), VT goes down, but the selected inspiratory pressure is maintained throughout the cycle. Because this patient is paralyzed, the RR cannot increase. In volume-control mode, the target is flow. When lung compliance decreases, airway pressure increases, maintaining the set VT and flow rates. PC-IRV mode may be used in ARDS when severe hypoxemia and ventilation/perfusion mismatch is present.

3. Ans. (c)
Increasing EPAP and IPAP would increase the pressure support to the patient. EPAP in NIV is a surrogate of PEEP in invasive ventilation. The difference between IPAP and EPAP is pressure support which the patient is receiving through NIV. The minimum difference between IPAP and EPAP should be 4, so just by increasing EPAP to improve hypoxemia will not help. Similarly by increasing IPAP alone, we would increase pressure support which will increase the tidal volume but it would not help in oxygenation.

4. Ans. (d)
Dynamic hyperinflation in a patient with severe asthma can cause barotrauma to the lung and severely compromise venous return to the heart. Generally a ventilator rate of 6-8 breaths/min and a tidal volume of 5-6 mL/kg are recommended. A long expiratory time should be set with an I:E ratio > 1:2. Full expiration before the next breath should be confirmed clinically by observing the patient's chest rise and fall. In addition, this should be confirmed on the ventilator graph. Moderate hypercarbia and acidosis is well tolerated but hypercarbia may be detrimental in patients with myocardial depression. During pressure controlled ventilation, tidal volume may fluctuate and this may cause significant hypoventilation. Therefore, pressure-controlled ventilation may not be the ideal mode and volume-controlled ventilation is usually preferred.

5. **Ans. (a)**

   The principles of ventilation in COPD include small tidal volumes, a long expiratory time, and a slow respiratory rate. The high-inspiratory flow rate is an important component of allowing long expiratory times. Dynamic hyperinflation can be assessed by measuring the plateau airway pressure by occluding the expiratory valve at the end of inspiration and recording the pressure after a 5-second pause. This is the most easily measured estimate of alveolar pressure at the end of inspiration and is affected by the degree of hyperinflation. Ideally this should be maintained at <25 cm H_2O. There is a paucity of randomized trial data regarding the use of NIV in asthma. There are as yet no clear guidelines for the use of NIV in severe asthma. Similarly, there is a paucity of good evidence regarding the use of IV salbutamol. However, IV β–agonists should be considered if there is no response to nebulized bronchodilator therapy.

6. **Ans. (d)**

   The high airway pressure alarm sounds only if the system exceeds the set pressure limit. This is unrelated to source gas delivery. Loss of the oxygen source gas will cause the oxygen pressure alarm to sound and will decrease the FiO_2 delivered. All ventilators require at least a 50 psi gas source. Source gas failure will not affect the electrical operation of the ventilator. In response to source gas failure, the patient can spontaneously breathe through the safety valve.

7. **Ans. (c)**

   Use of the prone position for refractory hypoxemia in acute respiratory distress syndrome (ARDS) has gained favor in recent years. The PROSEVA (Proning Severe ARDS patients) trial managed to demonstrate a statistically significant reduction in death at both 28 and 90 days with 16-hour sessions in the prone position for patients with severe ARDS. As such, use of the prone position is rapidly becoming a standard of care for those patients with a P/F ratio of <150 mm Hg.

8. **Ans. (a)**

   The mean airway pressure is the primary determinant of oxygenation when on mechanical ventilation. Hence, changes that result in increased mean airway pressure generally help to improve oxygenation (i.e. changes in iTime, PEEP or going to HFOV).

9. **Ans. (d)**

   This patient with status asthmaticus has evidence of severe obstructive lung disease, as evidenced by a large peak to plateau pressure gradient (36 – 22 = 14 cm H_2O). He also has a large A-E ($PaCO_2$ - $EtCO_2$) gradient indicating significant dead space, likely as a result of hyperinflation. Due to this high airway resistance, he needs further time for exhalation. This can be achieved in several ways. One would be to decrease the respiratory rate. By decreasing the RR from 12 to 10, you increase the total cycle time from 5 seconds (12 breaths per min = 1 breath per 5 seconds while 10 breaths per min = 1 breath per 6 seconds), and thus the E time would increase from 3.5 seconds (5 – 1.5) to 4.5 seconds. Increasing the respiratory rate, while theoretically improving minute ventilation, would exacerbate the inability to exhale and thus worsen your hypercarbia and acidosis.

In addition, you could decrease the inspiratory time to 1 second, now making expiratory time 5 − 1 = 4 seconds and I:E ratio 1:4. Inhaled anesthetic is a possibility but would likely be used after ventilator adjustments and other adjuvant medications (heliox, terbutaline, magnesium, aminophylline, etc.) had been tried. Increasing the peak pressure risks barotrauma (although mitigated by the high airway resistance since the alveolus only ends up seeing the plateau pressure of 22) while your tidal volumes are likely adequate.

10. **Ans. (b)**
Increasing the tidal volume and respiratory rate will increase the minute ventilation but not correct hypoxemia. Increasing the FiO_2 in a patient whose alveoli are not recruited will result in increase in V/Q mismatching and shunt and will not have effect on PaO_2. By recruiting the alveoli with the application of PEEP will help solve the issue.

11. **Ans. (b)**
This patient meets criteria for some method of assisted ventilation, but a rapidly deteriorating mental status would make her a poor candidate for NIPPV. To review, indications for mechanical ventilation (intubation) in the setting of COPD exacerbation include evidence of respiratory muscle fatigue, worsening respiratory acidosis, deteriorating mental status, and clinically significant hypoxemia despite supplemental oxygen therapy. NIPPV can be used instead of intubation in this situation and has been associated with better outcomes in terms of short-term mortality rates, symptomatic improvement, intubation rates, and length of hospitalization in patients. Contraindications to the use of NIPPV include an uncooperative or obtunded patient, inability to clear airway secretions, hemodynamic instability, respiratory arrest, recent facial or gastroesophageal surgery, burns, poor mask fit, or extreme obesity.

12. **Ans. (a)**
Widening of the PV loop happens whenever there is increased resistance as the lower inflection point shifts as it represents the critical opening pressure of the alveoli. Narrowing of the PV loop is also called as beaking and is due to overdistension. Shifting of the PV loop toward the volume axis means that the compliance is better whereas shifting it toward the pressure axis means that the compliance is decreasing and the lungs are becoming more stiff.

13. **Ans. (c)**
In volume-controlled ventilation, tidal volume is a preset variable and the ventilator delivers this set tidal volume at varying peak inspiratory pressure depending on the resistance and compliance of the respiratory system.

14. **Ans. (e)**
VAP is defined as pneumonia occurring 48 hours or more after intubation. It is associated with increased ventilator days, length of stay and increased attributable mortality of 9%. SDD reduces VAP rates. Lung protective ventilation reduces iatrogenic lung injury but not VAP rates.

15. **Ans. (c)**
    APRV is a ventilator mode using a prolonged high pressure with intermittent release of pressure for tidal ventilation and carbon dioxide clearance. For a given tidal volume peak airway pressure is lower than for a BIPAP ventilator mode. If hypercapnia becomes a problem then T_{high} may need to be shortened. Spontaneous breaths can occur throughout the ventilator cycle.

16. **Ans. (c)**
    Predicting successful weaning is very difficult but physiological parameters associated with successful weaning include a maximum inspiratory pressure of -20 to -25 cm H_2O, vital capacity >10 mL/kg, and static lung compliance with an inspiratory pressure of <30 cm H_2O gives a tidal volume of >8 mL/kg.

17. **Ans. (d)**
    In bronchopleural fistula, bronchus is in direct connection with the pleural cavity, some of the tidal volume is lost into the pleural cavity affecting achievable lung ventilation. Management of a ventilated patient with a bronchopleural fistula is particularly challenging and it is often difficult to wean a patient from the ventilator. High frequency ventilation with small tidal volumes, low airway pressure and a high respiratory rate provides the best chance of ventilating the lungs in these patients if conventional ventilation fails.

18. **Ans. (d)**
    Heat and moisture exchange (HME) filters usually have two functions, one as a heat and moisture exchange and the other as a filter for bacterial and viral particles. Internationally recognized color coding for filters is as follows: HME only = blue; HME + filtration = green; filtration only = yellow. Studies suggest that not all filters are equally effective. In general, hydrophobic filters are better than electrostatic ones in the prevention of both fluid and particulate contamination of the breathing circuits, although manufacturers of both types claim prevention of transmission of all viral and bacterial particles of > 99.95%.

19. **Ans. (b)**
    Increasing IPAP would increase the difference between IPAP and EPAP and hence, the pressure support would increase. This increase would augment the tidal volume generated in each breath and so the minute ventilation will increase and give rise to decrease in PCO_2 levels.

20. **Ans. (a)**
    Airway pressure generated during controlled ventilation depends on the compliance and resistance of the respiratory system and circuit. Inspiratory flow is constant (square wave) during volume-controlled ventilation. In time triggering, breaths are delivered according to a preset frequency. Triggering is when the ventilator detects a drop in airway pressure or flow that occurs when a patient makes a spontaneous breath, instigating the ventilator to deliver a positive pressure inspiratory breath. Volume, time, and flow can be used to cycle the ventilator.

CHAPTER 6

Respiratory System

BALASAHEB PAWAR

QUESTIONS

1. Which of the following is not a feature of life-threatening bronchial asthma?
   a. PEFR < 50% of predicted
   b. Cyanosis
   c. Silent chest
   d. Poor respiratory efforts

2. A 67-year-old female was admitted with swollen and painful right lower limb. On admission, she developed breathlessness and desaturation. She was shifted to ICU, where her BP was found to be 80 systolic. Which of the following statement regarding the immediate management of this patient is true?
   a. *ECG pattern:* S1 Q3 T3 is an indication for thrombolysis
   b. If systemic hypotension is present, thrombolysis is contraindicated
   c. D-dimer is very helpful for diagnosis of PE but only a negative result is of any value
   d. Thrombolysis is first-line treatment in nonmassive PE

3. A 63–year-old patient brought to ER with severe dyspnea, increased cough with sputum production. In ER, his saturation was 72%, he was started on oxygen through face mask, all the following statements regarding O_2 therapy in COPD patient are false, *except*:
   a. Hyperventilation can cause respiratory alkalosis and loss of consciousness is a risk
   b. Sudden increase in arterial oxygen can precipitate diaphragmatic spasm
   c. Decreased arterial oxygen is the stimulus for breathing in a client with COPD
   d. Oxygen administration can trigger reflex bronchospasm

4. A 56-year-old female admitted with 4 days history of acute onset of cough, fever, left side chest pain, and dyspnea. All of the following statements regarding the diagnosis of community acquired pneumonia are true, *except*:
   a. Gram's staining and culture of sputum are positive in more than 80% of cases of pneumococcal pneumonia when a good-quality specimen (> 10 inflammatory cells per epithelial cell) can be obtained before, or within 6–12 hours after, the initiation of antibiotics
   b. Blood cultures are positive in about 70–75% of inpatients with pneumococcal pneumonia
   c. In hematogenous *Staphylococcus aureus* pneumonia, blood cultures are nearly always positive, but they are positive in only about 25% of cases in which inhalation or aspiration is responsible for the CAP
   d. ELISA for *Legionella,* urinary antigen is positive in about 74% of patients with pneumonia caused by *Legionella pneumophila* serotype 1

5. A 62-year-old male diabetic admitted with limb cellulitis sepsis. He was shifted to ICU for breathlessness. He was started on NIV, his chest X-ray showed B/L diffuse infiltrates, his P/F ratio was 160. Due to worsening hypoxia, patient was intubated. All of the following statements regarding the diagnosis of acute respiratory distress syndrome are true, *except*:
   a. A plasma BNP level below 100 pg/mL favors ARDS, but higher levels neither confirm heart failure nor exclude ARDS
   b. Cardiogenic pulmonary edema cannot be excluded on the basis of an echocardiogram, since diastolic dysfunction and volume overload may exist even if the left heart function appears normal
   c. There is ample evidence that there is generally no value to routine right heart catheterization for either the diagnosis or management of ARDS
   d. Flexible bronchoscopy can obtain lower respiratory samples for microscopic analysis and microbiologic culture and should be performed routinely in all ARDS patients

6. Risk factors for poor outcome for CAP are all, *except*:
   a. Age > 65 years
   b. Pleural effusion
   c. Neoplastic illness
   d. Female sex

7. Ultrasonographic findings of pneumothorax are all, *except*:
   a. Absence of lung sliding
   b. Lung point sign
   c. Stratosphere sign
   d. Comet tail artifact

8. Accepted indications for hyperbaric oxygen therapy are all, *except*:
   a. Air or gas embolism
   b. Clostridial myositis/myonecrosis
   c. Intracranial abscess
   d. Inhalational gas associated ARDS

9. CURB-65 includes all, *except*:
   a. Urea
   b. Creatinine
   c. Age
   d. Confusion

10. Factors that increase the $P(a-ET)CO_2$ gradient are all, *except*:
    a. Increased dead space ventilation
    b. Decreased cardiac output
    c. Positive pressure ventilation
    d. Increased pulmonary perfusion

ANSWERS

1. **Ans. (a)**

   As per BTS guidelines for bronchial asthma, following are the features of life-threatening bronchial asthma. It does not include PEFR < 40%.

Life-threatening asthma	Any one of the following in a patient with severe asthma:	
	Clinical signs	*Measurements*
	Altered conscious level	PEF <33% best or predicted
	Exhaustion	SpO_2 <92%
	Arrhythmia	PaO_2 <8 kPa
	Hypotension	"Normal" $PaCO_2$ (4.6–6.0 kPa)
	Cyanosis	
	Silent chest	
	Poor respiratory effort	

2. **Ans. (c)**

   Acute pulmonary embolism (PE) is a common and sometimes fatal disease. PE has a wide variety of presenting features, ranging from no symptoms to shock or sudden death. Electrocardiogram (ECG) abnormalities, although common in patients with suspected PE, are nonspecific. The most common findings are tachycardia and nonspecific ST-segment and T-wave changes (70%). Abnormalities historically considered to be suggestive of PE (S1Q3T3 pattern, right ventricular strain, and new incomplete right bundle branch block) are uncommon (less than 10%). An elevated D-dimer alone is insufficient to make a diagnosis of PE, but can be used to rule out PE. D-dimer testing is best used in conjunction with clinical probability assessment tools. PE is stratified into massive, submassive, and low-risk based upon the presence or absence of hypotension and right ventricular dysfunction or dilation. The initial approach should focus upon restoring perfusion with intravenous fluid resuscitation and vasopressor support (if needed), as well as oxygen supplementation and airway stabilization with intubation and mechanical ventilation (if needed).

3. **Ans. (c)**

   Austin MA et al, Effect of high flow oxygen on mortality in chronic obstructive pulmonary disease patients in prehospital setting: randomized controlled trial.

   It is essential to administer oxygen to patients with significant hypoxemia to avoid the life-threatening complications of a low arterial oxygen tension (PaO_2). Similarly hypoxic COPD should receive O_2. But COPD patients, who have chronically elevated $PaCO_2$ levels, survive on hypoxic drive for breathing. Because of the risk of prompting worsened hypercapnia with excess supplemental oxygen, administration of supplemental oxygen should target a pulse oxygen saturation (SpO_2) of 88–92% or an arterial oxygen tension (PaO_2) of approximately 60–70 mm Hg. In two small randomized trials, titrating supplemental oxygen to SpO_2 88–92% resulted in a lower mortality compared with high flow (nontitrated) oxygen.

4. **Ans. (b)**
Microscopic examination of pulmonary secretions may provide immediate information about possible causative organisms. Results on Gram's staining and culture of sputum are positive in more than 80% of cases of pneumococcal pneumonia when a good-quality specimen (>10 inflammatory cells per epithelial cell) can be obtained before, or within 6–12 hours after, the initiation of antibiotics. The yield diminishes with increasing time after antibiotics have been initiated and with decreasing quality of the sputum sample. Nebulization with hypertonic saline (so-called induced sputum) may increase the likelihood of obtaining a valid sample.

Blood cultures are positive in about 20–25% of inpatients with pneumococcal pneumonia but in fewer cases of pneumonia caused by *Haemophilus influenzae* or *Pseudomonas aeruginosa* and only rarely in cases caused by *Moraxella catarrhalis*. In hematogenous *Staph. aureus* pneumonia, blood cultures are nearly always positive, but they are positive in only about 25% of cases in which inhalation or aspiration is responsible for the CAP. ELISA for legionella urinary antigen is positive in about 74% of patients with pneumonia caused by *Legionella pneumophila* serotype 1, with increased sensitivity in more severe disease.

5. **Ans. (d)**
A plasma BNP level below 100 pg/mL favors ARDS, but higher levels neither confirm heart failure nor exclude ARDS. This derives from an observational study of patients with ARDS (n = 33) or cardiogenic pulmonary edema (n = 21). The study found that a plasma BNP level less than 100 pg/mL identified ARDS with a sensitivity, specificity, positive predictive value, and negative predictive value of 27%, 95%, 90%, and 44%, respectively. Many clinicians use transthoracic echocardiography as the first-line diagnostic test, if cardiogenic pulmonary edema cannot be excluded by clinical evaluation and measurement of the BNP level. While severe aortic or mitral valve dysfunction, severe diastolic dysfunction, or a severely reduced left ventricular ejection fraction favors cardiogenic pulmonary edema, the latter is insufficient to confirm primary cardiogenic pulmonary edema because some precipitants of ARDS (e.g. septic shock) can cause an acute, severe cardiomyopathy that develops concomitantly with ARDS. In addition, cardiogenic pulmonary edema cannot be excluded on the basis of an echocardiogram, since diastolic dysfunction and volume overload may exist even if the left heart function appears normal. There is ample evidence that there is generally no value to routine right heart catheterization for either the diagnosis or management of ARDS. However, pulmonary artery catheterization may be considered if primary cardiogenic pulmonary edema cannot be excluded on the basis of the clinical evaluation, plasma BNP measurement, and echocardiogram. Flexible bronchoscopy can obtain lower respiratory samples for microscopic analysis and microbiologic culture, if the noninvasive techniques are unsuccessful. It can also identify abnormalities that may not be detected with noninvasive sampling. Therefore, flexible bronchoscopy is a reasonable next step whenever noninvasive sampling is nondiagnostic.

6. **Ans. (d)**
   Risk factors for a poor outcome from community-acquired pneumonia are age >65 years, hyponatremia, pleural effusion, neoplastic illness, male sex, neurologic illness, respiratory rate >30/min, tachycardia >125/min, systolic BP <90 and diastolic BP <60 mm Hg, and confusion.

7. **Ans. (d)**
   Lung sonography has rapidly emerged as a reliable technique in the evaluation of various thoracic diseases. One important, well-established application is the diagnosis of a pneumothorax. Prompt and accurate diagnosis of a pneumothorax in the management of a critical patient can prevent the progression into a life-threatening situation. Sonographic signs, including "lung sliding", "B-lines", or "comet tail artifacts", A-lines", and "the lung point sign" can help in the diagnosis of a pneumothorax.

8. **Ans. (d)**
   Accepted indications for HBOT are: air or gas embolism, carbon monoxide poisoning, decompression sickness, clostridial myonecrosis, crush injury and other forms of traumatic ischemia, enhanced healing of problematic wounds, including diabetic wounds, severe anemia, actinomycotic brain abscess, necrotizing soft tissue infections, refractory osteomyelitis, and radiation necrosis of soft tissue and bone.

9. **Ans. (b)**

   1 point given for each of:
   - Confusion
   - Urea (>7 mmol/L)
   - Respiratory rate (≥30/min)
   - BP (SBP <90 mm Hg or DBP ≤60 mm Hg)
   - Age (≥ 65 years)

Risk class	Mortality (%)	Recommended site of care
0	0.7	Outpatient
1	2.1	Outpatient
2	9.2	Short hospital stay/supervised outpatient
3	14.5	Hospital, assess for ICU
4	40	Hospital, assess for ICU
5	57	Hospital, assess for ICU

10. **Ans. (d)**
    P (a-ET)CO_2 gradient as an index of alveolar dead space. Under normal circumstances, the $PETCO_2$ (the CO_2 recorded at the end of the breath which represents PCO_2 from alveoli which empty last) is lower than $PaCO_2$ (average of all alveoli) by 2–5 mm Hg, in adults. The (a-ET)PCO_2 gradient is due to the V/Q mismatch in the lungs (alveolar dead space) as a result of temporal, spatial, and alveolar mixing defects. In healthy children, the (a-ET)PCO_2 gradient is smaller (-0.65–3 mm Hg) than in adults. This is due to a better

V/Q matching, and hence a lower alveolar dead space in children than in the adults. The (a-ET)PCO_2/$PaCO_2$ fraction is a measure of alveolar dead space, and changes in alveolar dead space correlate well with changes in (a-ET)PCO_2. An increase in (a-ET)PCO_2 suggests an increase in dead space ventilation. Hence (a-ET)PCO_2 is an indirect estimate of V/Q mismatching of the lung.

Reduction in cardiac output and pulmonary blood flow result in a decrease in $PETCO_2$ and an increase in (a-ET)PCO_2. Increases in cardiac output and pulmonary blood flow result in better perfusion of the alveoli and a rises in $PETCO_2$.

CHAPTER 7

Hemodynamic Monitoring

HARISH MM, SUHAIL S SIDDIQUI, JACOB GEORGE PULINILKUNNATHIL, SUDHINDRA P KANAVEHALLI

QUESTIONS

1. A 28-year-old male patient without any comorbid conditions admitted to ICU with history of fever and breathing difficulty. On evaluation his respiratory rate 39/min, blood pressure 118/66 mm Hg, temperature 101°F. P/F ratio was 150, initially tried on noninvasive ventilation and because he worsened clinically, he got intubated and started on mechanical ventilation as per ARDSNET protocol. In the meantime his blood pressure dropped to 84/46 mm Hg, he was inserted with invasive lines and initiated on FloTrac® monitor. His SVV-16%, SV 66 mL/beat, CO 2.6 L/min. Based on the clinical scenario which of the following is the further management option in terms of hemodynamic support?
   a. Because SVV is more than 10% patient is likely to be fluid responsive, hence will give fluid challenge
   b. SVV value is not a reliable indicator of fluid responsiveness in the current scenario
   c. Since the patient is having low cardiac output, he needs to be started on Dobutamine
   d. Will check the IVC diameter to assess the fluid responsiveness

2. In relation to passive leg rising (PLR) test, which of the following is *correct*?
   a. To start with patient should be started from supine position
   b. PLR is unreliable in patients with spontaneous breathing
   c. It is mandatory to have real time cardiac output monitoring, while assessing fluid responsiveness
   d. Transthoracic ECHO is the best way to assess fluid responsiveness, as it is noninvasive and easy to perform

3. A 44-year-old lady admitted with history of fever, burning micturition. On evaluation her urine shows 20–30 pus cells with total counts of 18,000 with more than 70% of neutrophils. Clinical diagnosis of urosepsis was made in the due course of management, her BP dropped to 86/43 mm Hg. After initial bolus of 1.5 L of crystalloids her blood gas shows lactate of 4 mmol/L. She is on minimal sedation and ventilated in pressure support mode. On re-examination she is confused, BP is 85/35 mm Hg, HR is 115 bpm (sinus tachycardia), SpO_2 is 95% on 60% oxygen. Because of persistent shock even with on-going resuscitation, decision was taken to initiate advanced hemodynamic monitoring. Which among the following is the best to predict fluid responsiveness at this clinical scenario?

a. Measuring the central venous pressure and continue to fluid bolus till it becomes more than 14 cm H_2O
b. Insertion of a pulmonary artery catheter and pulmonary artery occlusion pressure measurement
c. Measuring the inferior vena cava using echocardiography
d. Response of esophageal Doppler to passive leg raising

4. A 36-year-old male shifted to ICU from the ward with history of fever and breathing difficulty, on evaluation he was confused, blood pressure 86/46 mm Hg, heart rate 126 beats/minute, 90% saturation on 6 L of oxygen with respiratory rate of 36 per minute and was also having perianal discharging sinus. He was initiated on high flow nasal oxygen and given initial fluid bolus of 1.5 liter. In view of clinical deterioration invasive lines are taken, in relation to his further fluid management which of the following is false?
    a. Fluid responsiveness is frequently defined as an increase in CVP (≥15% from baseline) with a fluid challenge
    b. Fluid challenge: Give 500 mL of crystalloid (or 250 mL colloid) over 10–15 minutes and observe effect
    c. A patient whose stroke volume increases following a fluid challenge is on the ascending limb of the Frank-Starling (FS) curve
    d. A marked rise in CVP with fluid challenge indicates a failing ventricle

5. A 65-year-old-male chronic smoker presented to ICU with acute onset of chest pain and sweating, his ECG showed significant ST segment elevation across anterior leads with positive troponin. While on the therapy he collapsed suddenly with hypotension, his echocardiography suggested severe mitral valve rupture with mitral regurgitation. As a hemodynamic mechanical support intra-aortic balloon pump (IABP) was initiated. Which among the following is not correct in relation to IABP?
    a. Systolic blood pressure usually decreases during IABP use
    b. The balloon inflates immediately following the dicrotic notch on the arterial waveform
    c. The balloon deflates during isovolumetric contraction of the left ventricle
    d. IABP insertion is absolutely contraindicated in patients with bleeding manifestation

6. A 58-year-old man was posted for elective major abdominal surgery. As part of intraoperative hemodynamic monitoring, he was initiated on esophageal Doppler. Initial esophageal Doppler measurements include a flow time corrected (FTc) of 260 ms, which rises to 320 ms following a 500 mL fluid challenge and his peak velocity value is 115 cm/second. In relation to his readings what is the further line of fluid management?
    a. A low FTc always indicates more fluid is required
    b. This patient has compromised cardiac contractility
    c. FTc is a marker of afterload and preload in this patient
    d. Dobutamine should be started at this point as to improve the vital organ perfusion

7. When any patient is started on esophageal Doppler following assumptions are made when determining stroke volume *except*?
    a. 70% of total cardiac output passes the probe
    b. The ascending aorta runs parallel to the esophagus

c. The diameter of the aorta is constant throughout systole
d. The values of stroke volume remains constant irrespective of the position of esophageal Doppler probe, as the chances of error are less

8. Following are the parameters of a patient in shock (transpulmonary thermodilution: volume view) while on controlled ventilation with 8 mL/kg tidal volume and with sinus rhythm. Extravascular lung water (EVLW) 2 mL/kg, global end diastolic volume (GEDV) 350 mL/kg, stroke volume variability (SVV) 18%, stroke volume index (SVI) 65 mL/b/m². What is the further line of management in relation to fluid?
   a. As the patient is having good stroke volume index no further fluid administration is required
   b. Given value of EVLW suggest patient is not having any extravasation hence still more fluid can be given
   c. As the value of GEDV suggest volume depletion, with SVV more than 15% he is a right candidate for further fluid administration
   d. At this point he does not require any fluid therapy irrespective of the values of volume view

9. In relation to measurement of cardiac output by thermodilution technique which of the following is true?
   a. A pulmonary artery catheter is the mandatory requirement
   b. Tricuspid regurgitation will always underestimate the cardiac output
   c. Volume of the injectate will make difference cardiac output measurement
   d. Tricuspid regurgitation will always overestimate the cardiac output

10. A 58-year-old male came with acute onset of chest pain, he was diagnosed with severe anterior wall myocardial infarction, with on-going medical therapy he was floated with pulmonary artery catheter. In this particular scenario which of the following condition will not overestimate pulmonary artery occlusion pressure (PAOP) as compared to left ventricular end-diastolic pressure (LVEDP)?
    a. Mitral stenosis
    b. Mitral regurgitation
    c. Massive pulmonary embolism
    d. Catheter tip in West zone III

11. In relation to the working principle of invasive blood pressure measurement, which of the following is true?
    a. The catheter connecting the arterial cannula to the transducer should be short, stiff, and narrow to reduce resonance
    b. Bubbles and clots cause under damping
    c. The resonant frequency of the system should be less than 10Hz
    d. The primary harmonic of the system is 1–2 Hz

12. When we measure cardiac output using arterial pressure wave in a patient who is on positive pressure ventilation, which of the following statement is true?
    a. Pulse pressure variation (PPV) is better indicator than systolic pressure variation (SPV) in terms of predicting fluid responsiveness

b. Pulse pressure is directly proportional to stroke volume in all the clinical conditions without any errors
c. The maximum fall in systolic pressure coincides temporally with the peak inspiratory pressure
d. The cardiac output measured using arterial pressure waveform is a reliable guide to fluid therapy in all the clinical conditions

13. A 40-year-old man presents with fever, cough with expectoration and shortness of breath. On examination his room air SpO_2 was 75%. ABG showed PaO_2 of 45, $PaCO_2$ of 31. His BP was 90/60 mm Hg. Auscultation revealed crackles bilaterally and CXR showed infiltrates bilaterally. His screening echo revealed good cardiac function with normal sized chambers with EF 60% and collapsing IVC. A diagnosis of ARDS was made and patient was managed with HFNC with FiO_2 of 65% after which his SpO_2 picked up to 92%. Which of the following is true regarding hemodynamic management in this patient?
    a. Dynamic indices of fluid responsiveness like pulse pressure variation is more accurate than other methods
    b. IVC collapsing >55% during expiration and resuming size during inspiration is a good indicator of hypovolemia
    c. PLR test is the best method to assess fluid responsiveness
    d. High lactates will invariably tell that patient needs fluid resuscitation

14. Which of the following best defines septic shock in terms of hemodynamic assessment?
    a. Preserved ejection fraction (EF) with low cardiac output (CO) with normal to increased systemic vascular resistance (SVR)
    b. Normal to low EF with normal to high CO with normal to low SVR
    c. Elevated EF with high cardiac output with normal to high SVR
    d. Low EF with normal to low CO and normal to low SVR

15. Which of the following is/are true in relation to mini fluid challenge test?
    a. Giving 100 mL of crystalloid over 1 minute
    b. Giving 100 mL of colloid over 1 minute
    c. Test is easy to perform with good practicality at the bedside
    d. It can be considered positive even when there is rise in CVP after giving fluid, hence does not require real time cardiac output monitoring

16. Which of the following is most correct regarding central venous oxygen saturation ($ScvO_2$) and mixed venous oxygen saturation (SvO_2)?
    a. In normal individuals SvO_2 is less than $ScvO_2$
    b. Changes in the SvO_2 will reflect changes in the cardiac output, if hemoglobin, arterial oxygen saturation (SaO_2) and oxygen uptake (VO_2) remains constant
    c. The relation between $ScvO_2$ and SvO_2 will remain constant in all the clinical status
    d. Currently robust data available to positively suggest using $ScvO_2$ and SvO_2 as target for fluid resuscitation

17. A 28-year-old male came with history of fever and breathing difficulty since 2 days, he was already partially treated in other hospital on outpatient basis. In the ER his BP was 82/46 mm Hg, heart rate 134 beats/minute, ABG showing severe metabolic acidosis with lactate of 5.4 mol/L. In relation to his hemodynamic monitoring and initial resuscitation, which of the following is true?
    a. Patient should be checked for fluid responsiveness before administering fluid bonus
    b. A rise in lactate in sepsis and septic shock is always due to tissue hypoperfusion
    c. Studies showed that targeting lactate as resuscitation marker is superior to targeting central venous oxygen saturation
    d. Vasopressors should be started when patient is on ongoing fluid resuscitation when he is not able to maintain mean arterial pressure

18. Which of the following is true regarding hemodynamic monitoring tools?
    a. The CVP and PAOP parallel each other closely in patients with EF >50%.
    b. PAOP is a better predictor of myocardial performance than LV end diastolic volume (LVEOV)
    c. An inverse correlation has been demonstrated between CO and SvO_2
    d. Cardiac filling pressures appears to be a reliable indicator of preload than intravascular lung volume

19. Which of the following is false regarding $Pv\text{-}aCO_2$ (partial pressure difference of venoarterial carbon dioxide) gap?
    a. It is determined by the conjunction of macro- and/or microvascular blood flow, the total CO_2 production (both aerobic and anaerobic), and the complex relationship between CO_2 partial pressures and CO_2 blood contents (Haldane effect)
    b. $Pv\text{-}aCO_2$ should be considered as a marker of tissue perfusion and tissue hypoxia
    c. An increased $Pv\text{-}aCO_2$ usually suggests a "low" or "insufficient" cardiac output. However, during severe inflammatory conditions, alterations in functional capillary density and heterogeneity of microvascular blood flow could also account for venous CO_2 accumulation
    d. An elevated $Pv\text{-}aCO_2$ should encourage clinicians to optimize the cardiac output, especially when lactate levels are increased and clinical signs of hypoperfusion are present

20. In relation to cardiac output monitoring in critically ill patients, which of the following is false?
    a. "Normal" cardiac output value among critically ill patients is 2.5–5 L/minute
    b. Determining whether or not a cardiac output is adequate for a patient must include an assessment of tissue perfusion and the presence of compensatory mechanisms
    c. Recent data suggest that normalizing cardiac output to supraphysiological level increased the mortality among critically ill patients
    d. If cardiac output is inadequate, treatments can be aimed at one or more of its four determinants depending on the specific underlying causes and patient status: preload, afterload, myocardial contractility, and heart rate

Chapter 7 Hemodynamic Monitoring

21. In relation to end expiratory occlusion test, which of the following is correct?
    a. To consider the test to be positive there should be increase in stroke volume or cardiac output by about >15% from the baseline
    b. The time required to achieve positive result with end expiratory occlusion test will be at least 5 seconds
    c. Percentage change in the pulse contour is a better predictor of fluid response when we do end expiratory occlusion test
    d. Patient should be paralyzed and should not have any spontaneous breathing efforts while doing the test

22. In terms of hemodynamic manifestation of septic which of the following will not fit?
    a. Hypovolemia is always absolute in septic shock
    b. Sepsis induced cardiomyopathy may be primary or secondary
    c. Inadequate oxygen extraction due to intracellular (probably mitochondrial) abnormalities
    d. Septic shock will manifest most commonly with cardiac output and compromised systolic function

23. A 28-year 60 kg female, with type 1 diabetes mellitus met with an accident and sustained injury to her forearm. Initial management was of little benefit and she developed fever after 2 days with pus discharge. Next day she presented to accident and emergency department and on examination there: PR: 130/min, regular, BP: 104/50 mm Hg, Oral temperature: 103 F, RR: 28/min, peripheries were cold to touch and she is disoriented. ABG showed: Metabolic acidosis with raised lactates (lactates: 5). All of the following statement about the case are true *except*:
    a. Raised lactates are usually the biochemical marker of tissue dysoxia
    b. Absence of hypotension precludes diagnosis of shock
    c. Urine output monitoring is required in the case
    d. Cold peripheries and disorientation are suggestive of shock in this patient

24. The above mentioned patient was given 2 liters of Ringer's lactate and broad spectrum intravenous antibiotics. However, her clinical condition deteriorated and she got intubated and was started on controlled mechanical ventilation [Volume control mode, Tidal volume (Vt): 6 mL/kg of predicted body weight (PBW), Respiratory rate (RR): 24/min, PEEP: 8 FiO_2: 50%]. An arterial line and central line was inserted and urinary catheterization was also done, monitors showed sinus tachycardia, CVP of 12, PPV (pulse pressure variation) of 18%. Her urine output dropped to 10 mL per hour for 2 hours, and the ABG showed lactates of 4 mmol/L. Identify the true statement for the case:
    a. Dopamine is the first choice of vasopressor in such cases as it will increase urine output by acting on dopaminergic receptors
    b. High CVP precludes fluid resuscitation
    c. Dobutamine should be started to bring the lactates down
    d. Fluid resuscitation should be continued in view of high PPV

25. A 60-year male, a case of intracranial space occupying lesion (ICSOL) is scheduled for surgery. However, he had to be taken for emergency craniotomy due to neurological deterioration. Intraoperative IV fluids, blood and blood products adequately replaced and patient was brought to the ICU with endotracheal tube on controlled mechanical ventilation [Volume control mode, Tidal volume (Vt): 6 mL/kg of predicted body weight, Respiratory rate (RR): 24/min, PEEP: 8 FiO_2: 50%]. After 6 hours patient became hypotensive and dropped his urine output to 15 mL/hr, Lactates: 4.5 mmol/L, pupils bilaterally equal and reacting to light. Monitor showed PR: 120/min, regular, BP: 90/40 mm Hg, CVP: 13 cm H_2O, PPV: 8%. To decide on giving fluid for resuscitation, which is the correct statement pertaining to the case?
    a. PPV of 8 precludes volume infusion
    b. Passive leg raising (PLR) test should be done
    c. Tidal volume challenge is the test of choice to decide fluid resuscitation in this case
    d. CVP of 13 precludes volume expansion

26. All of the statements are true about pulmonary vascular permeability index (PVPI) *except*:
    a. Is a parameter given by PICCO/Volume view monitor
    b. Normal value is 1–3
    c. Is useful to differentiate type of pulmonary edema permeability versus hydrostatic
    d. Is ratio of pulmonary blood volume (PBV) to extravascular lung water (EVLW)

27. A 72-year-old 70 kg male patient with no medical comorbidities is admitted to the ICU after extended right hepatectomy. Intraoperative losses have been adequately replaced, and he is currently on controlled ventilation with arterial line in place. Vitals: PR: 110 breaths/min, BP: 110/60 MAP: 77 urine output 50 mL/hr. Two hours later the monitor showed the following vitals: PR: 120/min, BP: 94/55 MAP: 68. His urine output: 40 mL/hr, ABG: pH: 7.34, PCO_2: 48 mm Hg, PO_2: 68 on 40% FiO_2, HCO_3: 23, Lactate 0.76 mmol/L, PPV: 20, abdominal drains: minimal serosanguinous fluid. Which one is correct statement regarding management?
    a. Fluid boluses should be given as the patient is fluid responsive
    b. Noradrenaline should be started
    c. Wait and watch
    d. Transfuse blood

28. A 54-year-old male known case of COPD on treatment admitted to ICU with increased cough, with fever, yellowish sputum. On examination: P/R: 124 breaths/min, regular, BP: 120/80 mm Hg, RR: 32/min Chest: B/L rhonchi with left lower zone crepts. 2D echocardiography is not showing any left or right ventricular defect. ABG: pH: 7.36, PO_2: 70 on O_2 mask with 10 lpm O_2, PCO_2: 74, HCO_3: 33, lactate: 3. Started on nebulization with beta 2 agonist, antibiotics and noninvasive ventilation, however did not improve hence intubated and protective lung ventilation started. Currently PR: 160 breaths/min, regular, BP: 100/50 mm Hg, after 1.5 liter crystalloid BP did not improve and started on noradrenaline infusion at 0.3 mcg/kg/min to maintain a MAP of 70, lactates increasing, UOP decreasing: 30-20-15 mL/hr PICCO inserted, CI: 4 GEDV: 450, ELWI: 6, PVPI: 3, SVV: 16. What should be done?

a. Volume expansion should be done
   b. Wait and watch as cardiac index is normal
   c. Dobutamine should be started
   d. Tidal volume challenge

29. Patient worsened and developed atrial fibrillation with fast ventricular rate noradrenaline minimally increased. Now CI: 6, GEDV: 780, ELWI: 5, PVPI: 2, SVV: 10. Urine output improved and now it is 20–30 mL/hr. Current vitals: PR: 165 breaths/min, irregularly, irregular, how will you assess fluid responsiveness in this patient?
   a. Patient is not fluid responsive as SVV is 10
   b. Do PLR to assess fluid responsiveness
   c. Do tidal volume challenge (TVC) test
   d. As the ELWI is in normal range we can give fluids without assessment for fluid responsiveness

30. In the abovementioned patient dyselectolytemia corrected, acidosis improved, now PR: 120 breaths/min normal sinus rhythm, lactates normalizing, noradrenaline reduced to 0.05 mcg/kg/min, urine output now 40–50 mL/hour, however 2D echocardiography now shows poor left ventricular ejection function likely septic cardiomyopathy. Line of management:
   a. Add dobutamine
   b. Wait and watch
   c. Add levosimendan
   d. Digoxin

31. Dynamic measures of fluid responsiveness based on heart lung interactions (e.g. SVV, PPV, SPV) have limitations of validity in all *except*:
   a. Spontaneous breathing
   b. Raised intra-abdominal pressure
   c. Compliant lungs
   d. Bronchopleural fistula with more than 50% volume leak

32. Pick the correct combination:
   a. *Septic shock:* Cardiac output high, systemic vascular resistance high, neck veins full
   b. *Cardiogenic shock:* Cardiac output low, systemic vascular resistance high, neck veins full
   c. *Obstructive shock* secondary to acute pulmonary embolus: Cardiac output high, systemic vascular resistance high, neck veins full
   d. *Hypovolemic shock:* Cardiac output low, systemic vascular resistance high, neck veins full

33. Lactate clearance can be used as a marker for adequacy of fluid resuscitation in all *except* in present of:
   a. Epinephrine infusion
   b. Dobutamine infusion
   c. Dopamine infusion
   d. Vasopressin infusion

34. A 36-year-old male, a known asthmatic on irregular treatment presents to casualty with acute onset breathing difficulty of 3 hours duration, after exposure to industrial smoke. In the casualty, the patient is conscious, oriented, having a heart rate of 115 beats/minute, blood pressure 150/100 mm Hg, respiratory rate of 40/minute and is afebrile. He denies history of fever or any other symptoms. An ABG taken in the emergency room reads as follows: pH 7.42, PCO_2 – 30 mm Hg, PO_2 – 56 mm of Hg, HCO_3 – 20 mEq/L, lactate 2.4 mmol/L (on room air). He was started on continuous nebulization with salbutamol with high flow oxygen and stat dose of intravenous hydrocortisone. After 1 hour, the patient symptoms have reduced and he feels better. The air entry is equal bilaterally and the wheeze although present has reduced in severity. Repeat ABG values are—pH 7.30, PCO_2 – 30 mm Hg, PO_2 – 156 mm Hg, HCO_3 – 17 mEq/L, lactate 5 mmol/L (on 4 L/min oxygen via nasal canula). Which of the following correctly describes the patient's clinical setting?
    a. Patient is having sepsis as he is having tachypnea and elevated lactates
    b. Patient is in severe shock and needs intubation as the lactate levels have almost doubled
    c. Patient needs further evaluation and fluid resuscitation as the lactate levels are worsening
    d. Patient needs observation only and no further intervention as he seems to be improving

35. A 32-year-old male, is shifted to ICU after a damage control surgery for blunt abdominal trauma on mechanical ventilation. He has undergone fluid resuscitation with 2 liters of crystalloids, massive transfusion as per protocol (4 packed cells, 4 PRBC, and 1 SDP) and 1 liter of 5% albumin. He has currently undergone a splenectomy, ligation of the splenic artery and a branch of the pancreatico-splenic artery. The abdomen was not closed and is planned for definitive surgery with abdominal closure once the intensivist gives a clearance. In the ICU, the patient is having cold clammy extremities, heart rate of 136 beats/minute (sinus rhythm), arterial blood pressure reading 99/70 mm Hg, supported with noradrenaline 0.5 mcg/kg/min, and the urine output for the past 3 hours have been 5 mL/hr. Laboratory values and ABG taken on ICU admission reads as follows: pH 7.24, PCO_2 – 43 mm Hg, PO_2 – 72 mm Hg, HCO_3 – 10 mEq/L, lactate 10 mmol/L, S. Sodium – 143 mmol/L, S. chloride – 118 mmol/L, Albumin – 2.4 g/L (on ACVC mode with TV of 6 mL/kg, PEEP 12, FiO_2 – 0.6 and respiratory rate of 14/minute). Which of the following correctly describes the patient's clinical setting?
    a. The patient is in circulatory shock as the lactates are high and other features of tissue hypoperfusion are obvious
    b. Fluids cannot be administered further as the FiO_2 requirement is already 0.6 with a PEEP of 12
    c. The patient is having a BP of 99/70 - Map of 80. Hence shock is unlikely and noradrenaline can be reduced
    d. Patient has already received adequate fluids. Further fluid requirement should be administered after assessment of fluid status by the IVC diameter on ultrasound

36. In this patient transfusion-related acute lung injury (TRALI) is suspected although fluid overload and pulmonary edema cannot be ruled out. How can you better differentiate ARDS from pulmonary edema in this patient?
    a. Low global end diastolic volume
    b. PVPI >3
    c. USG lung—number of B lines
    d. Chest X-ray

37. A 54-year-old male, case of pyelonephritis and septic shock is admitted to the ICU. As protocol, he was given 30 mL/kg of crystalloids over 3 hours and norepinephrine has been started at 0.05 mcg/kg/min. He was intubated in view of worsening shock and respiratory distress and is on tidal volume 8 mL/kg, sedated and paralyzed. The lung compliance measured is 36 L/cm H_2O. Overnight he received multiple fluid boluses but the vasopressor requirement increased and he developed atrial fibrillation. The intensivist on duty wants to confirm fluid responsiveness before further administration of fluids. Which method will you suggest?
    a. Pulse pressure variation >10%
    b. IVC distensibility >13–18%
    c. Change in pulse pressure during a passive leg raising maneuver by 15%
    d. Tidal volume challenge test

38. A 32-year-old male, is shifted to ICU after a damage control surgery for blunt abdominal trauma on mechanical ventilation. He has undergone fluid resuscitation with 2 liters of crystalloids, massive transfusion as per protocol (4 packed cells, 4 PRBC, and 1 SDP) and 1 liter of 5% albumin. He has currently undergone a splenectomy, ligation of the splenic artery and a branch of the pancreatico-splenic artery. The abdomen was not closed and is planned for definitive surgery with abdominal closure once the intensivist gives a clearance. A fluid challenge was given and the patient was deemed fluid responsive. However, the CVP rose from 5 cm H_2O to 9 cm H_2O. Which of the following is correct regarding CVP measurement in this patient?
    a. The applied PEEP has to be subtracted from the value of CVP to know the real CVP
    b. Apply a PEEP of Zero and measure CVP/disconnect the ventilator and measure CVP
    c. Continue following the trends in CVP trace rather than an absolute value
    d. Irrespective of the PEEP, a CVP of 8 is high and the patient needs diuretics

39. A 72-year-old male, known case of hypertension, old inferior wall MI presents to the casualty in breathing difficulty and circulatory shock. Clinical examination was suggestive of pulmonary edema and it was decided to apply noninvasive ventilation to aid the failing left ventricle. With the application of positive pressure ventilation in a controlled way, what happens to the transmural pressure of left ventricle?
    a. Increases
    b. Decreases
    c. Remains same as ventilation affects only right side and not left side of the heart
    d. Cannot be predicted

40. A 68-year-old male, hypertensive on treatment is shifted to ICU after an exploratory laparotomy for perforation peritonitis. On examination, his extremities are cold, and he is having a tachycardia of 130 bpm, hypotensive (BP 80/35 mm Hg). Operating room notes show a urine output of 50 mL over the past 4 hours. The esophageal Doppler probe is inserted and vales obtained are as follows—corrected flow time 200 ms, peak velocity 90 cm/s, stroke volume 80 mL. Which of the following statements is *true* regarding this patient?
    a. Corrected flow time is a marker of preload
    a. Values are suggestive of impaired cardiac function
    b. Patient is in fluid overload and required diuretics
    c. Other causes of hypotension including obstructive shock needs to be ruled out

41. A 55-year-old male, post PTCA for inferior wall myocardial infarction, with moderate LV function and RV dysfunction is admitted with pneumonia and shock. In view of the complex clinical scenario, a PA catheter is inserted and the values obtained are as follows—CI - 3.4L/min/m², RAP - 14 mm Hg, PASP - 45 mm Hg, PADP - 18 mm Hg, PAOP - 22 mm Hg. What is the inference from the values?
    a. This is suggestive of cardiogenic shock - patient needs dobutamine
    b. This is suggestive of pulmonary embolism and patient needs thrombolysis
    c. These values are suggestive of pulmonary hypertension, probably due to diseased lung states
    d. No comments can be made and no interventions can be done based upon the above values

42. A 33-year-old female, is admitted to the ICU with a diagnosis of scrub typhus. She is currently intubated and ventilated and is requiring noradrenaline at the rate 0.3 mcg/kg/min for maintaining a MAP of 65. The ABG taken shows a pH of 7.2, with a PO_2 of 88 on FiO_2 80, PCO_2 of 41 and lactate of 4. Simultaneous central venous ample shows pH of 7.19 with SaO_2 of 68, PCO_2 of 51. Which of the following is a correct interpretation of the hemodynamics of this patient?
    a. The $SCVO_2$ is normal, hence it is assumed that oxygen delivery is adequate and currently no interventions need to be done
    b. This patient might benefit from further optimization of cardiac output and oxygen delivery
    c. Manipulating microcirculation in this patient is of no benefit in view of already high $SCVO_2$
    d. Monitoring $SCVO_2$ is of no use as early goal-directed therapy has not been found to have any benefit

43. Regarding arterial pressure-based cardiac output (APCO), which of the following statements are correct?
    a. Arterial pressure-based cardiac output (APCO) is a calibrated system and works on the principle of transpulmonary thermodilution
    b. The values provided by arterial pressure-based cardiac output (APCO) is highly accurate and reliable in patients with septic shock

c. Arterial pressure-based cardiac output (APCO) monitoring requires a central venous line and a central arterial line
d. Arterial pressure-based cardiac output (APCO) is operator independent

44. A 26-year-old male presented to the casualty with breathing difficulty of 1-hour duration which started immediately after he landed in the airport after an 18-hour flight. He was wheeled into emergency department. The vitals noted in the emergency department are—a heart rate of 130 beats/minute, respiratory rate 30/minute, blood pressure – 88/60 mm Hg, and saturation of 76% on room air. The ECG showed sinus tachycardia with a right axis deviation and bedside echo showed severe RV dysfunction with moderate tricuspid regurgitation. A diagnosis of pulmonary embolism was made and the patient was shifted to the ICU for anticoagulation and rescue thrombolysis. In the ICU the respiratory distress worsened and the patient was intubated. He was started on volume control ventilation of 6 mL/kg tidal volume and PEEP 5 with FiO_2 50%. An arterial line was transduced which showed a PPV of 24%. In view of borderline blood pressure, and a raised PPV, the ICU resident decides to transfuse 500 mL of crystalloids. Which of the following statements are correct?
    a. A PPV of 24% irrespective of low tidal volume is suggestive of fluid responsiveness
    b. This patient should undergo tidal volume challenge test to assess for fluid responsiveness
    c. The PPV in this patient is falsely high and large volume fluids should not be administered.
    d. The magnitude of PPV is very high and at least 1 liter of fluid should be administered

ANSWERS

1. **Ans. (b)**

   In terms of predicting fluid responsiveness SVV is better indicator than IVC, but patient should satisfy certain prerequisites like—(1) he should not have spontaneous breathing; (2) he should be on minimal tidal volume of 8 mL/kg; and (3) he should not have any arrhythmias.

   Above patient is initiated on ARDSNET protocol as he is having moderate to severe ARDS, which means he is on not more than 6 mL/kg of tidal volume. Hence low tidal volume is not sufficient to give the cardiopulmonary interaction to give changes in stroke volume, so the reliability of SVV in predicting the fluid responsiveness will be poor.

   Using IVC diameter alone may not be a good predictor of fluid responsiveness, because if we measure single reading of IVC diameter it is as good as that of CVP. But if we measure its collapsibility or distensibility then we can predict the fluid responsiveness in a reliable way.

2. **Ans. (c)**

   PLR should be started from semirecombinant position, and then only it is possible to challenge the system in an adequate way, as it leads to autotransfusion of at least 300 mL of volume from splanchnic and mesenteric circulation. The PLR is reliable even in spontaneously breathing patients, as the fluid challenge not affected by the cardiopulmonary interaction. The sustainability of PLR is very short, i.e. about 60-90 seconds, hence a real time cardiac output monitoring is essential. Cardiac output can be calculated by using transthoracic method, but it is more cumbersome, subjective and time consuming. Hence a real time monitoring is essential to pick up the changes in cardiac output in the first 60-90 seconds only.

3. **Ans. (d)**

   Antonelli M, Levy M, Andrews PJ, et al. Haemodynamic monitoring in shock and implications for management. Intensive Care Med. 2007;33:575-90.

   Barbier C, Loubieres Y, Schmit C, et al. Respiratory changes in inferior vena cava diameter are helpful in predicting fluid responsiveness in ventilated septic patients. Intensive Care Med. 2004;30:1740-6.

   Measuring CVP is not a reliable indicator of fluid responsiveness, as the value of CVP is affected by many confounding factors like intrapleural, intra-abdominal pressures and valvular abnormalities. Again measuring the CVP in an optimal way (at the end of diastole and end of expiration) is very difficult. Pulmonary artery occlusion pressure has been shown to be a poor predictor of volume-responsiveness, as this will also affected by many confounding factors like CVP.

   IVC diameter measurement should be tagged to respiratory cycle, single value is not use full in the clinical setting. Ideally, we need to measure the percentage of variation in relation to inspiration and expiration again in relation to weather patient is on spontaneous or controlled ventilation.

Passive leg raising autotransfuses about 300 mL of blood into the central circulation. If stroke volume increases significantly (>10% as measured by esophageal Doppler), this indicates preload-responsiveness. Even though readings of esophageal Doppler are positional dependent, among the available options measuring change in stroke volume in a real time manner using esophageal Doppler is the appropriate answer.

4. **Ans. (a)**

   Monnet X, Marik PE, Teboul JL. Prediction of fluid responsiveness: an update. Ann Intensive Care. 2016;6:111.

   Monnet X, Pinsky MR. Predicting the determinants of volume responsiveness. Intensive Care Med. 2015;41:354-6.

   For all practical purposes, globally accepted definition of fluid responsiveness is increase in stroke volume or cardiac output by about 10–15% from the baseline after giving adequate fluid challenge, as defined by Paul Marik giving crystalloid of 500 mL or colloid of 250 mL over a period of 10–15 minutes is essential to challenge the system with adequate volume. It is very important to give value to both volume and time of fluid infusion.

   Rise in CVP after giving fluid challenge is not an ideal indicator of fluid responsiveness, as the rise may be just because of transmitted pressure from pleura or peritoneum or may be from valvular dysfunction. In the same time rise of CVP disproportionately in response to fluid challenge can be used as safety limit to stop the fluid challenge and it may indicate inability of the left side of the ventricle to pump out the fluid administered.

   This also suggests that patient is in the flatter portion of the Frank–Starling curve, further administration of fluid may lead to extravasation. As long as the patient is in the ascending portion of the starling curve there will be corresponding increase in stroke volume in response preload challenge.

5. **Ans. (d)**

   Staniatis SJ, Spandoni SM. 1997. Getting to the heart of IABP Therapy. RN. 1997;60(1): 38-43.

   The concepts of Intra-aortic balloon pumping. Datascope clinical support services. Fairfield: Datascope Medical Co. Ltd.; 1999.

   The balloon inflates during diastole, beginning with the closure of the aortic valve (marked by the dicrotic notch on the arterial pressure waveform). It deflates during isovolumetric contraction sufficiently before ejection to allow diastolic pressure to fall to a lower level, this reduces afterload and reduces cardiac work and myocardial oxygen consumption.

   Systolic and diastolic blood pressures usually decrease slightly with IABP use, but the augmented diastolic pressure (the peak pressure produced during IABP inflation in diastole) is higher to increase coronary perfusion (Fig. 1).

   Only absolute contraindication for IABP insertion is severe aortic insufficiency. Coagulopathy, peripheral vascular disease, and aortic aneurysm make a relative contraindication.

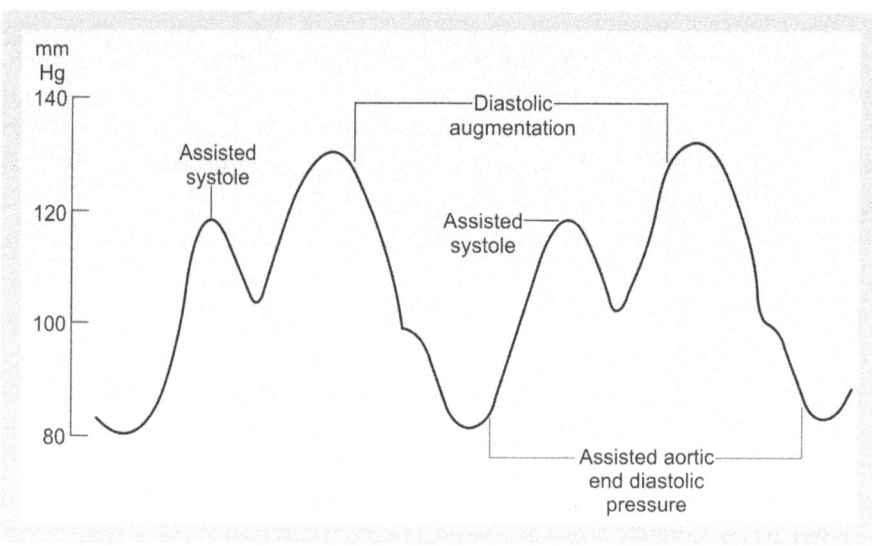

Fig. 1: Working principle of IABP 1:1 frequency.

6. **Ans. (c)**

Dark PM, Singer M. The validity of transesophageal Doppler ultrasonography as a measure of cardiac output in critically ill adults. Intensive Care Med. 2004;30(11):2060-6.

Valtier B, Cholley BP, Belot JP, et al. Noninvasive monitoring of cardiac output in critically ill patients using transesophageal Doppler. Am J Respir Crit Care Med. 1998;158(1):77-83.

Two parameters are important when patient is on esophageal Doppler. One is corrected (systolic) flow time (FTc) which indicates afterload (normal = 0.33–0.36 s), another peak velocity (PV) which indicates contractility with normal range of values which are age related (20 years 90–120 cm/sec, 90 years 30–60 cm/sec). FTc value is inversely related to afterload (a low FTc indicates a high afterload).

Since hypovolemia causes an increase in systemic vascular resistance, FTc is also an indirect marker of preload and is often used for this purpose (which decreases in hypovolemia, because of compensatory increase in peripheral vascular resistance).

However, other conditions such as obstructive shock, cardiac failure, and vasopressor therapy may similarly increase afterload (reducing FTc) despite adequate or excessive preload.

Although an FTc of ~340 ms is considered "normal", this should not be a target of fluid therapy. As with all forms of cardiac output monitoring, trends are more important than single reading. Esophageal Doppler also gives value of stroke volume, if a fluid bolus produces an increase in FTc and a significant (>10%) increase in stroke volume, this suggests that patient is volume responsive and more volume is required.

If there is little or no change, giving further fluid may be harmful. The above patient showed response in increasing FTc after fluid bolus if this is going to be associated with corresponding increase in stroke volume, patient is considered fluid responsive. Since he is having normal peak velocity his cardiac contractility looks good and no need to add Dobutamine when patient is having good contractility to improve tissue perfusion. He basically needs to be monitored with repeated trends of FTc and stroke volume with on-going fluid challenge if persistently having signs and symptoms of decreased perfusion.

7. **Ans. (a)**

   Dark PM, Singer M. The validity of transesophageal Doppler ultrasonography as a measure of cardiac output in critically ill adults. Intensive Care Med. 2004;30(11):2060-6.

   Valtier B, Cholley BP, Belot JP, et al. Noninvasive monitoring of cardiac output in critically ill patients using transesophageal Doppler. Am J Respir Crit Care Med. 1998;158(1):77-83.

   Several assumptions are made in determining cardiac output. It is assumed that 70% of the total stroke volume (SV) enters the descending aorta (therefore total SV = measured SV/0.7). The descending aorta is assumed to run parallel to the esophagus (a divergence of just 10° can cause an error of ~20–30%), hence proper positioning of the probe is very important.

   SV is obtained by multiplying the velocity time integral (VTI) by aortic cross-sectional area, which is assumed to remain constant throughout systole. It is also assumed for this calculation that all red blood cells are moving at maximum velocity. The hematocrit has no bearing on stroke volume determination.

   For the above reasons using esophageal Doppler is a good modality of hemodynamic monitoring in operation theater as most of the patients will be under anesthesia, hence accurate positioning can be achieved.

8. **Ans. (d)**

   Michard F, Teboul J. Predicting fluid responsiveness in ICU patients. Chest. 2002;121: 2000-8.

   Isakow W, Schuster DP. Extravascular lung water measurements and hemodynamic monitoring in the critically ill: bedside alternatives to the pulmonary artery catheter. Am J Physiol Lung Cell Mol Physiol. 2006;291:L1118-31.

   Magder S. Fluid status and fluid responsiveness. Curr Opin Crit Care. 2010;16:289-96.

   Patient's GEDV is less than the normal values (650–800 mL/kg) which suggest he is preload deficit and his SVV is more with satisfactory prerequisite conditions for its reliability to tell that he might respond to fluid therapy. Again low value of EVLW (normal is 3–7 mL/kg) indicates that he is in the safety zone as there is no extravasation. Overall above patient's volume view values fit into preload deficiency with predicted responsive to fluid challenge in a positive way. But patient does not have any signs of hypoperfusion as he is having normal urine output and normal lactate level, as long as the patient is in well perfused status it is not indicted to give fluid just based on the monitoring parameters.

   At any given point of time normal heart is also fluid responsive, then it does not mean all of us require fluid therapy. As long as we do not have any signs and symptoms of poor perfusion we do not require any fluid therapy. To give fluid patient should be preload deficit, he should have manifestations of hypoperfusion and along with he should be preload responsive.

9. **Ans. (c)**

Morgan TJ. Haemodynamic monitoring. In: Bersten AD, Soni N (Eds). Oh's Intensive Care Manual, 5th edition. Edinburgh: Butterworth- Heinemann; 2003.

Only pulmonary thermodilution requires pulmonary artery catheter, transpulmonary thermodilution techniques do not require a pulmonary artery catheter, but do require a central line and an arterial cannula. In case volume view or PiCCO monitoring we inject the cold saline through the central line (internal jugular vein) and will measure at the femoral artery. As compared to PA catheter where we measure cardiac output at the tip of PA, in case of volume view or PiCCO we measure at the femoral artery.

According to the Stewart-Hamilton equation, cardiac output is inversely proportional to the area under the time-temperature curve. A small volume of injectate will tend to overestimate cardiac output since it will thermally equilibrate rapidly with the surrounding environment and generate only a small temperature-time peak. The ideal volume should be at least 15–20 mL.

Another parameter which have impact is the temperature of the injectate, cold injectate should be ice-cold; the closer the temperature is to blood temperature, the less precise the measurement.

In patients who are having tricuspid regurgitation (TR) cardiac output value depends upon innate contractility of the heart. Patients with good contractility will have good cardiac output and those with poor contractility will have low cardiac output. Hence the temperature curve in relation to time depends upon the innate cardiac contractility than the tricuspid regurgitation itself.

10. **Ans. (d)**

Robin E, Costecalde M, Lebuffe G, et al. Clinical relevance of data from the pulmonary artery catheter. Crit Care. 2006;10(Suppl 3):S3.

In certain conditions PAOP may not give clear idea about left ventricular end diastolic pressure, suppose above patient had any of the complications like mitral stenosis, mitral regurgitation or massive pulmonary embolism PAOP will be more than LVEDP.

In mitral stenosis, left atrial pressure is elevated (where a large A-wave will be present) hence it obviously elevates PAOP. In mitral regurgitation, the regurgitant jet of blood will increase mean left atrial pressure also. Any cause of increased pulmonary vascular resistance increases the PAOP-left ventricular end-diastolic pressure gradient that applies to massive pulmonary embolism also.

When we place PA catheter, the catheter tip should be in the West zone III, then only it measure pulmonary artery pressure. If the catheter tip is in West zones I or II, a continuous column of fluid in continuity with the left atrium will not be present throughout the respiratory cycle, since alveolar pressure will exceed pulmonary venous pressure. In this case PAOP will exceed diastolic pulmonary artery pressure, and will overestimate LVEDP.

11. **Ans. (d)**

Stoker MR. Principles of pressure transducers, resonance, damping and frequency response. Anaesth Intens Care. 2004;5(11):371-5.

Two frequencies are important when patient is on invasive arterial pressure monitoring—one is primary harmonic, which is in reference to patients and other is natural frequency, which is in relation to transducer system. Primary harmonic is the lowest frequency that can be used to describe the arterial pressure trace. For arterial blood pressure measurement the normal range is 60–120 beats per minute (i.e. the primary harmonic is 1–2 Hz).

The resonant (or natural) frequency of a measuring system is that frequency at which the undamped transducer system oscillates with maximal amplitude. If the resonant frequency is within the clinical range of input frequencies, excessive oscillation (resonance) will occur, with overestimation of systolic and underestimation of diastolic pressures. The resonant frequency should be at least 10 times the fundamental frequency (or primary harmonic).

Lots of patient and system related factors can cause dampening. One reason is connecting tube length, this should be short, stiff and wide to ensure that the resonant frequency is above the clinically encountered range.

Damping is the process whereby some of the energy of the oscillations produced within the measuring system is absorbed, thus reducing their amplitude. It means how fast the system comes to rest. The transducer system is little bit overdamped. A certain amount of damping is desirable to minimize excessive oscillation. Bubbles, clots, and kinks may cause excessive damping of the signal however.

12. **Ans. (a)**
Lamia B, Chemla D, Richard C, et al. Clinical review: interpretation of arterial pressure wave in shock states. Crit Care. 2005;9:601-6.

Pulse pressure is directly proportional to stroke volume, and inversely related to the compliance of the arterial tree. Changes in pulse pressure across the respiratory cycle therefore reflect changes in stroke volume.

But in elderly patients slight change in pulse pressure will cause an exaggerated change in cardiac output, hence in elderly patients with atherosclerosis the reliability of PPV is questioned. A change in pulse pressure (DPP) >13% in a mechanically ventilated patient is a sensitive and specific indicator of a positive response to a fluid challenge.

PPV is definitely superior than SPV as the former will take into consideration of both systolic and diastolic blood pressure, also in SPV a part of the variation is due to factors other than stroke volume changes such as the cyclic direct effects of intrathoracic pressure on the thoracic aorta wall. As part of heart lung interaction in a patient who is on positive pressure ventilation during inspiration there is a brief increase in intrathoracic pressure, which will squeeze the left atrium and will empty into left ventricle, hence there will be increase in left ventricular preload. In the same time there will be reduction of transaortic pressure which means the afterload of left ventricle. The fall in systolic pressure (i.e. cardiac output) comes a few heartbeats later as the effects of reduced right heart preload are transmitted to the left heart; this coincides temporally with expiration.

Another important point we have to remember is the cardiac output which we measure by using arterial waveform is the mimic of tone and compliance of arterial tree, hence at the extremes of tone the reliability of cardiac output is questioned. When patient is on high dose of vasopressors reliability is questioned as it tells about the tone of vessel than giving an idea about the real cardiac output.

13. **Ans. (c)**
    Pinsky MR. Functional hemodynamic monitoring. Interns Care Med. 2002;28:386.

    Dynamic indices of preload assessment, like PPV/SVV etc., cannot be used here as the patient is spontaneously breathing. Prerequisites for using dynamic indices are as follows: mechanical ventilation (no spontaneous respiration), tidal volume 8 mL/kg, good right and left heart function, no arrhythmias and also in severe vasoconstriction status. False positive results are obtained in right ventricular dysfunction.

    IVC collapses during inspiration (not expiration) and resumes size during expiration in spontaneously breathing patients. The opposite happens during mechanical ventilation. IVC collapsibility of >55% indicates hypervolemia in spontaneously breathing patients and variability >15% indicates volume depletion in controlled ventilation. But still current available data favoring the reliability of IVC variation as volume responsiveness is poor.

    PLR can be used to assess fluid responsiveness even when patient is having arrhythmias or is spontaneously breathing. PLR with any real time cardiac output assessment like transthoracic Doppler aortic flow, PiCCO (pulse contour cardiac output) or volume view can give a very good assessment of fluid responsiveness.

    Lactate may not be just a marker of hypoperfusion alone. It just tells about production and clearance. Mechanisms other than impaired tissue oxygenation may cause an increase in blood lactate, including an activation of glycolysis, a reduction in pyruvate dehydrogenase activity, or liver failure.

14. **Ans. (b)**

    Septic shock is one of the major causes of distributive shock, where systolic will be normal to high and diastolic will be low with decreased SVR. The reason for low SVR is because of peripheral vasodilatation caused by inflammatory mediators, hence they present with wide pulse pressure. Sepsis is one of the causes for hyperdynamic circulation hence they usually have normal to high cardiac output, but they tend to have normal to low EF as they tend to have sepsis induced cardiomyopathy which will present with global hypokinesia with dilated cardiomyopathy.

    Hence most common presentation of septic shock is normal to low EF with normal to high CO and normal to low SVR.

15. **Ans. (d)**
    Biais M, de Courson H, Lanchon R, et al. Mini-fluid Challenge of 100 ml of Crystalloid Predicts Fluid Responsiveness in the Operating Room. Anesthesiology. 2017:127:450-6.
    Mallat J, Meddour M, Durville E, et al. Decrease in pulse pressure and stroke volume variations after mini-fluid challenge accurately predicts fluid responsiveness. Br J Anaesth. 2015;115(3):347-9.
    Toscani L, Aya HD, Antonakaki D, et al. What is the impact of the fluid challenge technique on diagnosis of fluid responsiveness? A systematic review and meta-analysis. Crit Care. 2017;21:207.

Mini fluid challenge has been defined in two ways—one in ICU as giving 100 mL of colloid over 1 minute and the same volume has been tried using crystalloid among surgical patients. Hence both the options *a* and *b* are correct.

Even though the test looks easy its practical applicability is minimal, because we need a real time cardiac output monitoring and that monitor should be highly sensitive to pick up the changes in cardiac output which induced by the minimal amount of fluid (100 mL).

16. **Ans. (b)**

    Marx G, Reinhart K. Venous oximetry. Curr Opin Crit Care. 2006;12(3):263-8.
    Rivers E, Nguyen B, Havstad S, et al. Early goal-directed therapy in the treatment of severe sepsis and septic shock. N Engl J Med. 2001;345(19):1368-77.
    Yu H, Chi D, Wang S, et al. Effect of early goal-directed therapy on mortality in patients with severe sepsis or septic shock: a meta-analysis of randomised controlled trials. BMJ Open. 2016;6:e008330.

    A true mixed venous sample (called SvO_2) is drawn from the tip of the pulmonary artery catheter, and include all of the venous blood returning from the head and arms (via superior vena cava), the gut and lower extremities (via the inferior vena cava) and the coronary veins (via the coronary sinus). Mixed venous oxygen saturation (SvO_2) can help to determine whether the cardiac output and oxygen delivery is high enough to meet a patient's needs. It can be very useful if measured before and after changes are made to cardiac medications or mechanical ventilation, particularly in unstable patients. Normal SvO_2 is 60–80%.

    If the SvO_2 is low (<60%), it means either that oxygen delivery is reduced (decreased Hb, hypoxia or decreased cardiac output), or that oxygen consumption is increased (shivering, hyperthermia or seizures).

    The value of mixed venous saturation correlates directly with cardiac output if other variables remain constant.

    In healthy individuals, SvO_2 is 3–5% higher than $ScvO_2$ because the lower body extracts less oxygen than the upper body making the inferior vena cava saturation higher. The primary cause is that the kidneys and liver receive a high proportion of cardiac output but oxygen consumption is low relative to delivery.

    In shock, this relationship changes and the $ScvO_2$ may exceed SvO_2 values by up to 8%. This is because in shock states, splanchnic and renal circulation fall followed by an increase in O_2 extraction in these tissues. In septic shock, regional O_2 consumption of the gastrointestinal tract increases. On the other hand, flow to the heart and brain is maintained. Hence the relationship between mixed and central venous oxygen saturation is not reliable. Currently three major trails (PROCESS, PROMISE, ARISE) showed that $ScvO_2$ is a less reliable guide for resuscitation in critically ill patients.

17. **Ans. (d)**

    Jones AE1, Shapiro NI, Trzeciak S, et al. Lactate clearance vs central venous oxygen saturation as goals of early sepsis therapy: a randomized clinical trial. JAMA. 2010;303(8):739-46.

Gomez H, Kellum JA. Lactate in sepsis. JAMA. 2015;313(2):194-5.

Levy MM, Evans LE, Rhodes A. The Surviving Sepsis Campaign Bundle: 2018 update. Intensive Care Med. 2018;44:925.

Above patient is a young without any comorbid conditions, also patient is in shock with background of high lactate. In this condition initial approach should be to give fluid resuscitation but not to challenge the system, when a patient is having manifestation of septic shock obviously it is very important to give fluid resuscitation than to challenge his system. It is very important in the initial hour when the patient is in ER.

In patients with septic shock the rise in lactate is not because of hypoperfusion but it is mainly because of mismatch between production and clearance of lactate. In sepsis there will be overproduction of lactate because of catecholamine surge, also there will be inhibition of pyruvate dehydrogenase enzyme, which is essential for moving pyruvate into Krebs cycle.

There are multiple theories proposed behind the lactate production in sepsis, hence lactate in sepsis may not be always because of end organ hypoperfusion.

None of the major studies showed any difference in outcome benefit either we use lactate or central venous oxygen saturation as target for resuscitation. But some studies showed if there is lactate clearance of about 10% in an hour after starting resuscitation, the resuscitation is in the way of success.

Current guidelines suggest when patient is not able to maintain adequate mean arterial pressure with ongoing fluid resuscitation we can start hand in hand vasopressors to preserve end organ perfusion, so one should not wait too much time on low mean arterial pressure without initiating on vasopressors.

18. **Ans. (a)**

Toy EC, Suarez M, Liu TH. Hemodynamic monitoring: Case files. Crit. Care. 2016;48-57.

The CVP and PAOP parallel to each other closely in patients with EF >50%. In EF <40%, the correlation between the CVP and PAOP decreases due to changes in myocardial compliance caused by myocardial hypertrophy or a stiff LV.

Two-dimensional echocardiography provides significant information including left ventricular cavity size, fractional shortening, and abnormalities in regional wall motion. Two-dimensional colored echocardiography enables a quantification of shunts, CO, and provides a noninvasive assessment of concomitant valvular disease. TTE end diastolic volume (LVEOV) is a better predictor of myocardial performance than PAOP. Echocardiography is the first diagnostic method which should be used in hemodynamic instability especially when suspicion of aortic dissection, endocarditis, or pulmonary embolism.

A linear correlation has been demonstrated between the CO and SVO_2. SVO_2 reflects the overall oxygen reserve of the whole body. However, a normal SVO_2 value does not rule out an impaired oxygen supply to individual organs. $SVO_2 = (SAO_2 - VO)/(1.39 \times Hb \times CO)$. With decrease in CO/Hb, SVO_2 decreases. Depressed left ventricular performance increases hydrostatic pressure in the pulmonary circulation, influencing fluid flux across a damaged pulmonary microvascular membrane. Extravascular lung water (EVLW) can be measured at the bedside using a double-dye technique with indocyanine green. Intrathoracic blood volume appears to be a more reliable indicator of preload than cardiac filling pressure.

19. **Ans. (b)**
Mekontso-Dessap A, Castelain V, Anguel N, et al. Combination of venoarterial PCO$_2$ difference with arteriovenous O$_2$ content difference to detect anaerobic metabolism in patients. Intensive Care Med. 2002;28(3):272-7.
Ospina-Tascón GA, Umaña M, Bermúdez W, et al. Combination of arterial lactate levels and venous-arterial CO$_2$ to arterial-venous O$_2$ content difference ratio as markers of resuscitation in patients with septic shock. Intensive Care Med. 2015;41(5):796-805.

Physiology determining venous CO$_2$ increases is complex. However, Pv-aCO$_2$ globally reflects blood flow alterations at both macro- and microvascular levels, more than tissue dysoxia. Meanwhile, an elevated Cv-aCO$_2$/Ca-vO$_2$ ratio could reflect anaerobic metabolism, and it could add important prognostic information in patients with shock. Despite the physiological bases of such monitoring CO$_2$-derived variables, its clinical utility during resuscitation in shock remains to be proved in future experimental and clinical studies. Tissue-to-arterial and venous-to-arterial CO$_2$ differences should be considered as markers of tissue perfusion rather than indicators of tissue hypoxia. Concomitance of high Pv-aCO$_2$ (>6.0 mm Hg) and low SvO$_2$ levels usually reflects low cardiac output in both inflammatory and noninflammatory conditions.

Under aerobic conditions, further efforts to increase the cardiac output in order to prevent the possible onset of tissue hypoxia in the presence of a high Pv-aCO$_2$ remain controversial.

An increased venous-arterial carbon dioxide to arterial-venous oxygen content difference ratio (Cv-aCO$_2$/Ca-vO$_2$) could reflect the presence of anaerobic metabolism. There is some experimental evidence that high Cv-aCO$_2$/Ca-vO$_2$ ratio can be reversed by resuscitation maneuvers, at least during early stages of shock.

A high Cv-aCO$_2$/Ca-vO$_2$ ratio could offer additional prognostic information in septic shock. Whether Cv-aCO$_2$/Ca-vO$_2$ ratio could anticipate lactate increase during early stages of shock remains to be elucidated.

20. **Ans. (a)**
Vincent JL. Understanding cardiac output. Crit Care. 2008;12:174.
Tavazzi G, Kontogeorgis A, Guarracino F, et al. Heart rate modification of cardiac output following cardiac surgery: the importance of cardiac time intervals. Crit Care Med. 2017;45:e782-8.

Among critically ill patients there is nothing called normal cardiac output, cardiac output is a relative phenomenon. Any cardiac output value can be inadequate or excessive depending on the specific conditions of the individual at the time of measurement. Hence concept of matching cardiac output in ICU is a relative phenomenon, which depends on demand of a particular patient in relation to his ongoing illness.

Finally adjusting anything to improve cardiac output should involve either to improve preload, afterload, contractility, and heart rate. Indirectly we have to give fluids/blood or start inotropic agents or start vasopressors or some agents which increases heart rate. Many of the studies which increased the cardiac output supranormally to achieve improved tissue perfusion does not showed any additional outcome benefit, instead some studies showed increased mortality.

21. **Ans. (c)**

    Monge Garcia MI, Gil Cano A, Gracia Romero M, et al. Noninvasive assessment of fluid responsiveness by changes in partial end-tidal CO_2 pressure during a passive leg-raising maneuver. Ann Intensive Care. 2012;2:9.

    The ideal way of doing end expiratory occlusion test is by giving the occlusion for at least 15 seconds which should allow the increase in cardiac preload to cross the pulmonary circulation and pass on the left side. Duration of 5 sec is insufficient. It has been shown that if cardiac output measured by the pulse contour analysis increased by more than 5% at the end of a 15 sec end-expiratory occlusion (EEO), the cardiac output response to a subsequent volume expansion is very likely.

    Change in cardiac output or stroke volume is not a reliable parameter to tell about the positivity of the test. If cardiac output is measured continuously, as for example with the analysis of the contour of the pulse wave, the test has the advantage of being very simple to achieve. Changes in cardiac output must be measured continuously and in real time. But also, the technique must be precise enough to detect changes of a few percent only. From this point of view, pulse contour analysis is perfectly adapted. Nevertheless, it requires an arterial catheter, or alternatively, a noninvasive system that estimates blood pressure in a continuous and noninvasive way.

22. **Ans. (a)**

    Liu YC, Yu MM, Shou ST, et al. Sepsis-induced cardiomyopathy: mechanisms and treatments. Front Immunol. 2017;8:1021.
    A review of sepsis-induced cardiomyopathy. J Intens Care. 2015 3:48.

    Septic shock is one subtype of shock that can manifest many types of hemodynamic variability. Being a distributive type of shock the hypovolemia may be because of absolute or relative, may not be always absolute. Relative hypovolemia is basically because of peripheral vasodilatation. Septic patients can have myocardial dysfunction which can lead to dilated cardiomyopathy and global hypokinesia, rarely it can have isolated left or right-sided dysfunction. If cardiac dysfunction developed before initiation of vasopressors we label it as primary and if it is after starting the vasopressors it is called secondary cardiomyopathy.

    In sepsis the problem is in oxygen uptake and utilization not the oxygen delivery, hence the measures which taken to improve cardiac output and oxygen delivery not showed any outcome benefit.

    The utilization of oxygen is directed toward the cytokine surge and not to the ATP production. Septic shock is the subtype of shock where there will be low ejection fraction with compromised contractility and good cardiac output, this is the part of manifestation of sepsis induced cardiomyopathy.

Chapter 7 Hemodynamic Monitoring

23. **Ans. (b)**

    Cecconi M, De Backer D, Antonelli M, et al. Consensus on circulatory shock and hemodynamic monitoring. Task Force of the European Society of Intensive Care Medicine. Intensive Care Med. 2014;40:1795-815.

    The diagnosis of acute circulatory failure is based on a combination of clinical, hemodynamic and biochemical signs. The clinical signs of shock typically include arterial hypotension (although this is not always present), associated with signs of altered tissue perfusion, visualized through the three "windows" of the body: the peripheral window (skin that is cold, clammy and pale or discolored the renal window (decreased urine output: <0.5 mL/kg/h); the neurologic window (altered mental characterized by obtundation, disorientation and confusion). The presence of low blood pressure should not be a prerequisite for defining shock as compensatory mechanisms may preserve blood pressure through vasoconstriction, while tissue perfusion and oxygenation are already decreased significantly.

24. **Ans. (d)**

    Rhodes A, Evans L, Alhazzani W, et al. Surviving sepsis campaign: International guidelines for management of sepsis and septic shock: 2016. Intens Care Med. 2017;43:304-77.

    Bellomo R, Chapman M, Finfer S, et al. Low-dose dopamine in patients with early renal dysfunction: a placebo-controlled randomised trial. Australian and New Zealand Intensive Care Society (ANZICS) Clinical Trials Group. Lancet. 2000;356:2139-43.

    De Backer D, Vincent JL. Should we measure the central venous pressure to guide fluid management? Ten answers to 10 questions. Crit Care. 2018;22:43.

    It looks like a case of septic shock secondary to skin and soft tissue infection. Noradrenaline is the first choice of vasopressors. Dopamine is a differential vasoactive agent which increases urine output but without any effect on renal outcome or mortality. The guidelines recommend against using low-dose dopamine for renal protection. The recent guidelines on septic shock resuscitation suggest using dobutamine in patients who show evidence of persistent hypoperfusion despite adequate fluid loading and the use of vasopressor agents. However, in this patient the PPV is high which is suggestive of fluid responsiveness. Hence, fluid resuscitation should be done with careful monitoring for any adverse effects of fluid resuscitation and further addition of dobutamine or vasopressin should be done after optimizing fluid status. In the patient CVP is high, however it is a marker of preload and has very poor efficacy in predicting if the patient will respond to fluid or not.

25. **Ans. (c)**

    Myatra SN, Prabu NR, Divatia JV, et al. The changes in pulse pressure variation or stroke volume variation after a "tidal volume challenge" reliably predict fluid responsiveness during low tidal volume ventilation. Crit Care Med. 2017;45:415-21.

    Myatra SN, Monnet X, Teboul JL. Use of tidal volume challenge to improve the reliability of pulse pressure variation. Crit Care. 2017;21:60.

    Monnet X, Teboul JL: Passive leg raising. Intensive Care Med. 2008;34:659-63.

The patient has hypotension along with sign of hypoperfusion (low urine output, raised lactates). It may seem that the patient is not fluid responsive as PPV is only 8%, however, PPV should be interpreted with caution as this patient is being ventilated with protective lung volumes (tidal volume 6 mL/kg of PBW). Hence, in this case PPV of 8% does not preclude fluid responsiveness. To assess for fluid responsiveness, we can either give a fluid challenge exogenously or by passive leg raising (PLR) which is reversible and endogenous. In this case being a postoperative neurosurgical patient with concerns of raised intracranial pressure PLR maneuver will not be a good choice. Tidal volume challenge (TVC) is a test which has proven efficacy in unmasking the fluid responsive versus fluid not responsive patient if they are being ventilated with tidal volumes < 8 mL/kg. TVC is a simple test to do and does not require any patient position change. In this maneuver, tidal volume is increased from 6 to 8 mL/kg of predicted body weight (PBW), the absolute change in PPV and SVV (ΔPPV6–8 and ΔSVV6–8) reliably predicts fluid responsiveness with cutoff values of 3.5% and 2.5%, respectively, whereas PVV and SVV at Vt 6 mL/kg PBW do not. Option (d) is automatically ruled out (see explanation of question 24).

26. **Ans. (d)**

    Monnet X, Anguel N, Osman D, et al. *Assessing pulmonary permeability by transpulmonary thermodilution allows differentiation of hydrostatic pulmonary edema from ALI/ARDS.* Intensive Care Med. 2007;33:448-53.

    Litton E, Morgan M. *The PiCCO monitor: A review.* Anaesth Intensive Care. 2012;40:393-409.

    Pulmonary vascular permeability index (PVPI) is a useful parameter given by cardiac output monitors using transpulmonary thermodilution methods (PICCO and volume view). It is derived from the ratio of EVLW to pulmonary blood volume. In cases of permeability related pulmonary edema (like ARDS), there is increase in EVLW with no or little change in pulmonary blood volume. Hence, PVPI increases above normal range of 1–3, on the contrary, in hydrostatic pulmonary edema there is increase in EVLW and also in pulmonary blood volume thus the value of PVPI essentially remains within or near normal. In patients with raised EVLW, PVPI may help in differentiating between these two types of pulmonary edema.

27. **Ans. (c)**

    Marik PE. *Fluid responsiveness and the six guiding principles of fluid resuscitation.* Crit Care Med. 2016;44:1920-2.

    Cecconi M, De Backer D, Antonelli M, Beale R, Bakker J, Hofer C, et al. *Consensus on circulatory shock and hemodynamic monitoring. Task Force of the European Society of Intensive Care Medicine.* Intensive Care Med. 2014;40:1795-815.

    The patient has become hypotensive, however, the hypotension is not causing hypoperfusion. His urine output has decreased however it is still >0.5 mL/kg/hour, which seems adequate for him, lactates are within normal limit, there is no evidence of bleed on examining the drain and in such cases absence of hypoperfusion, presence of hypotension alone and/or in presence of fluid responsiveness does not warrant fluid resuscitation.

Chapter 7 Hemodynamic Monitoring

28. **Ans. (a)**

    Myatra SN, Monnet X, Teboul JL. Use of tidal volume challenge to improve the reliability of pulse pressure variation. Crit Care. 2017;21:60.

    The patient is in septic shock secondary to left sided pneumonia with underlying COPD and more importantly there is normal biventricular function. Despite being on protective lung ventilation his SVV is high and hence in this case it is not mandatory to do tidal volume challenge test. Also, the patient's GEDV is lower which is though a volumetric marker of reduced preload is also substantiating the need of fluid resuscitation.

29. **Ans. (b)**

    Myatra SN, Monnet X, Teboul JL. Use of tidal volume challenge to improve the reliability of pulse pressure variation. Crit Care. 2017;21:60.
    Myatra SN, Prabu NR, Divatia JV, et al. The changes in pulse pressure variation or stroke volume variation after a "tidal volume challenge" reliably predict fluid responsiveness during low tidal volume ventilation. Crit Care Med. 2017;45:415-21.

    Patient is on protective lung ventilation (Vt = 6 mL/kg of PBW), it seems tempting to use TVC, however validity of SVV/PPV/SPV vanishes in cases of arrythmia, spontaneous breathing and several other contraindications to interpret fluid responsiveness. However, passive leg raising test can be reliably interpreted and can identify fluid responders, if patient is fluid responder, he can be given fluid resuscitation. Fluid is considered as drug and should be administered only after verifying the indication, in prescribed dosage and not to be given blindly.

30. **Ans. (b)**

    Rhodes A, Evans L, Alhazzani W, et al. Surviving sepsis campaign: International guidelines for management of sepsis and septic shock: 2016. Intensive Care Med. 2017;43:304-77.

    Myocardial dysfunction consequent to infection occurs in a subset of patients with septic shock, but cardiac output is usually preserved by ventricular dilation, tachycardia, and reduced vascular resistance. Some portion of these patients may have diminished cardiac reserve, and may not be able to achieve a cardiac output adequate to support oxygen delivery. Decreased ejection fraction may not necessarily indicate inadequate cardiac output. Concomitant measurement of cardiac output along with a measure of the adequacy of perfusion is preferable. In the case above hypoperfusion is not evident hence wait and watch would be the best strategy unless hypoperfusion is there which may require inotropic support.

31. **Ans. (c)**

    Monnet X, Marik PE, Teboul JL. Prediction of fluid responsiveness: an update. Ann Intensive Care. 2016;6:111.

    The major conditions where the PPV and SVV are unreliable include spontaneous breathing and cardiac arrhythmias. In the case of ARDS, the low tidal volume mechanical ventilation is done, which reduces the amplitude of the change in intrathoracic pressure that causes the PPV and SVV, similarly a bronchopleural fistula causing a tidal volume leak of >50% will also amount to low tidal volume ventilation even if the patient is being ventilated with conventional tidal volume. Also the low lung compliance prevents use of PPV and SVV since it reduces the transmission of alveolar pressures to intravascular and cardiac compartments. Other conditions which limit the accuracy of PPV and SVV are raised intra-abdominal pressure, open chest and right heart failure.

32. **Ans. (b)**

Hall JB, Schmidt GA, Kress JP. Principles of critical care, 4th edition. New York: McGraw Hill Education; 2015.
Webb A, Angus DC, Finfer S, et al. Oxford textbook of critical care, 2nd edition. New York: Oxford University Press; 2016.

Various shock types can be differentiated based on their hemodynamic variables of cardiac output (CO), neck veins (akin to cardiac filling pressures) and systemic vascular resistance (SVR). All the types of shock present with decreased cardiac output except for septic shock where CO may be high. All types of shock present with increased SVR except distributive (septic) shock where neck veins are full due to cardiac. Neck veins are collapsed in patients presenting with distributive shock and hypovolemic shock, however they are distended in the other two forms of shock. These characteristics can be used to differentiate between various forms of shocks.

33. **Ans. (a)**

Rhodes A, Evans L, Alhazzani W, et al. Surviving sepsis campaign: International guidelines for management of sepsis and septic shock: 2016. Intensive Care Med. 2017;43:304-77.

Epinephrine may increase aerobic lactate production via stimulation of skeletal muscle β2-adrenergic receptors and thus may preclude the use of lactate clearance to guide resuscitation. There is no data suggestive of hyperlactatemia with dobutamine, dopamine or vasopressin.

34. **Ans. (d)**

Vink EE, Bakker J. Practical use of lactate levels in the intensive care. J Intens Care Med. 2017;33(3):159-65.

Hyperlactatemia (levels more than 4 mmol/L) in critical ill patients is considered to be associated with an increased morbidity and mortality (approximately 50% mortality in patients with shock) and is thereby considered to be a prognostic marker. However, the other etiologies of hyperlactatemia should also be considered, viz. seizures, drugs (metformin, nucleoside reverse transcriptase inhibitors, adrenergic drugs), inborn errors of metabolism, liver dysfunction, thiamine deficiency, malignancies such as lymphoma, carbo monoxide poisoning, severe anemia, pheochromocytoma, etc. in this patient, there is no signs of organ dysfunction or infection. Hence it is unlikely that the patient is having sepsis and hyperlactatemia might be secondary to salbutamol nebulization itself. The arterial blood gas is improving with improvement in alveolar–arterial gradient also. Hence this patient needs observation only and no further intervention.

35. **Ans. (a)**

Vincent JL, Weil MH. Fluid challenge revisited. Crit Care Med. 2006;34(5):1333-7.
Vincent JL, DeBacker D. Circulatory Shock. N Engl J Med. 2013;369:1726-34.

Mikkelsen ME, Christie JD, Lanken PN, et al. *The adult respiratory distress syndrome cognitive outcomes study: long-term neuropsychological function in survivors of acute lung injury. Am J Respir Crit Care Med. 2012;185:1307-15.*

Shock—the clinical manifestation of circulatory failure is diagnosed based on clinical, hemodynamic, and biochemical signs. This patient is having features of shock and tissue hypoperfusion such as cold clammy extremities, tachycardia, narrow pulse pressure, and persistent oliguria. The hyperlactatemia might reflect the hypoperfusion state partly (as an underlying congestive liver damage cannot be ruled out in the current scenario). In these patients, circulation and tissue hypoperfusion has to be optimized. Although the patient has received aggressive intravenous fluids, it cannot be deemed adequate unless further assessment regarding tissue hypoperfusion, fluid status, fluid responsiveness, and fluid tolerance is made. A fluid challenge may be considered and if he is a fluid responder, guarded fluids may be administered. A high requirement of FiO_2 is not a contraindication for further fluids although caution needs to be exercised. Fluid restriction and deresuscitation takes priority only after salvaging the patient and after attaining hemodynamic stability. Once hemodynamic stability is attained, aggressive attempts to reduce the positive fluid balance has to be made (deresuscitation). The FACTT trial that looked into a conservative fluid balance in ARDS patients enrolled patients after stabilization. Although the patients had fewer ventilator free days the cognitive dysfunction in the conservative group is of real concern. Inferior vena cava diameter per se is a marker of preload and is a poor marker of fluid responsiveness. The validity of IVC diameter in patients with an open abdomen has not been adequately studied. Hence other parameters should be chosen to decide on fluid administration in this patient.

36. **Ans. (b)**

Tagami T, Ong MEH. Extravascular lung water measurements in acute respiratory distress syndrome: why, how, and when? Curr Opin Crit Care. 2018;24(3):209-15.

Jozwiak M, Teboul JL, Monnet X. Extravascular lung water in critical care: recent advances and clinical applications. Ann Intensive Care. 2015;5(1):38.

In general, patients with high extravascular lung water index more than 7–10 suggests pulmonary edema (EVLWI >7–10). Whether that is due to increased permeability or increased hydrostatic force needs to be differentiated as the management differs in both. A PVPI of less than 2 represents normal pulmonary permeability while a PVPI >3 suggests an increased permeability of pulmonary capillaries. Although an increased permeability of the pulmonary vessels is the hallmark of ARDS, it has to be remembered that it may not be the only cause of accumulation of raised EVLW in ARDS. Patients with poor cardiac function can simultaneously have leaky pulmonary vessels also and both values need to be taken into consideration in the appropriate clinical context. Extravascular lung water may be overestimated after lung resection surgeries, and overestimated or underestimated depending upon the positive end-expiratory pressure applied or may be underestimated in cases of heterogeneous lung injury. PVPI is indirectly calculated parameter and is derived from the GEDVI. PVPI can be overestimated in case the venous access is in the femoral veins due to the extra blood volume of inferior vena cava that participates in the calculation of transpulmonary thermodilution.

37. **Ans. (b)**

Cavallaro F, Sandroni C, Antonelli M. Functional hemodynamic monitoring and dynamic indices of fluid responsiveness. Minerva Anestesiol. 2008;74(4):123-35.

Dynamic indices that evaluate fluid responsiveness can be classified into three groups— (1) indices determined by the cyclic variations in stroke volume induced by the cyclic changes in intrathoracic pressure during positive pressure ventilation, e.g. PPV SVV; (2) indices determined by mechanical ventilation but not dependent on the cyclic variations of stroke volume, e.g. the vena cava diameter; (3) indices that are based on preload-redistribution maneuvers, independent from the standard mechanical ventilation, e.g. passive leg raising.

The variables of group 1 depend on heart lung interactions, and require a tidal volume of at least 8 mL/kg, and lung compliance at least 30 L/cm H_2O and normal sinus rhythm).

The use of IVC variability in ICU is also limited by all the limitations of group 1 and also has other pre-requisites such as absence of intra-abdominal hypertension, active breathing, etc. However it is not affected by arrythmia.

All these limitations are overcome by the 3rd group if they directly estimate the changes in cardiac output and stroke volume secondary to by a transient increase in venous return.

The change in pulse pressure during a PLR to diagnose fluid responsive states is not sensitive enough and hence not advocated. Tidal volume challenge test has the same limitations of PPV and SVV except that it overcomes the limitation of low tidal volume and lung protective ventilation. Hence IVC variability is the best option among the choices.

38. **Ans. (c)**

Magder S. Central venous pressure: a useful but not so simple measurement. Crit Care Med. 2006;34(8), 2224-7.

The CVP is measured in relation to the atmospheric pressure whereas in reality the heart is surrounded by pleural pressure. Assuming the pleural pressure to be almost zero at the end of expiration, CVP is measured at the end of expiration in spontaneously breathing patients. However, in patients on positive pressure ventilation with PEEP, the transmural central venous pressure will always be higher. The degree of peep transmitted to the CVP depends on the lung compliance and there is no easy method to measure the exact transmural CVP. Disconnection of mechanical ventilation or using a zero PEEP for measuring CVP is not advocated as it causes loss of recruited lung and worsens lung injury. An arbitrary number cannot be subtracted for every PEEP as the net PEEP that is transmitted depends on the lung compliance. However, in clinical practice, the absolute value of CVP is probably of not that importance and it is the hemodynamic response to a change in central venous pressure that is important. Hence *answer c* is the correct option. Static measures of CVP do not tell anything regarding fluid status and fluid responsiveness of a patient as there are numerous other factors associated with it.

39. **Ans. (b)**

Shekerdemian L, Bohn D. Cardiovascular effects of mechanical ventilation. Arch Childhood. 1999;80:475-80.

Transmural pressure—it is the pressure difference between the pressure within a closed chamber or vessel and the pressure surrounding it. During positive pressure ventilation, as the pleural pressure remains positive, the difference of the LV chamber pressure minus the pleural pressure – (transmural pressure of LV) will reduce. This will help in reducing the afterload of the heat and thereby the work of the left side of heart.

40. **Ans. (a)**

Prentice D, Sona C. Oesophageal Doppler monitoring for hemodynamic assessment. Crit Care Nursing Clin North Am. 2006;18(2):189-93.

Singer M. Oesophageal Doppler. Curr Opin Crit Care. 2009;15:244-8.

Normal value is 0.33–0.36 second. A flow time corrected (FTc) <330 ms is usually suggestive of hypovolemia although a raised afterload or poor contractility can also cause reduced FTc. In the presence of normal peak velocity, a reduced FTc is suggestive of hypovolemia.

Peak velocity – indicates contractility – normal value depends on age and range varies from 90 m/s to 120 cm/s in young adults and in elderly it is 30–60 cm/s.

Reduced waveform base with a reduced waveform height (peak velocity is suggestive of increased afterload.

The various values obtained with an esophageal Doppler in various clinical scenarios are as follows:

- *Hypovolemic shock:* Reduced cardiac output, reduced FTc, reduced waveform base, normal peak velocity (unless in cases of severe hypovolemia where peak velocity also might reduce).
- *Cardiogenic shock:* Reduced cardiac output, reduced FTc, markedly reduced peak velocity (rounded waves on esophageal Doppler).
- *Distributive shock:* Cardiac output increased, FTc increased, peak velocity normal or increased.
- *Obstructive shock:* Reduced cardiac output, reduced FTC, reduced peak velocity.

41. **Ans. (d)**

Sturgess DJ, Watts RP. Hemodynamic monitoring. In: Bersten AD, Handy JM (Eds). Oh's intensive care manual, 8th edition. New York: Elsevier; 2017.

The pulmonary catheter or transpulmonary thermodilution is the preferred method of cardiac output monitoring in patients with complex problems. When the pulmonary artery is correctly wedged, it gives a rough estimate of the left ventricular filling pressures. The pulmonary artery diastolic pressures are usually higher than the wedge pressures because the diastolic pressure also accounts for the resistance to flow in the pulmonary circulation. When the flow is abolished (wedging) there is a pressure drop of approximately 5 mm Hg as we record the wedge pressure. Thus, measuring the PADP can be used as a surrogate for wedge pressure, thereby abolishing the need for repeated wedging. Here the values show a PADP that is *lower* than the PAWP which is unrealistic. These reading errors may be due to the errors in floating the PA catheter or during the measurement of the actual pressures. These errors suggest that the whole set of values are better considered invalid and not to be acted upon.

42. **Ans. (b)**

    Vallet B, Pinsky MR, Cecconi M. Resuscitation of patients with septic shock: please "mind the gap"! Intensive Care Med. 2013;39:1653-5.

    Mallat J, Lemyze M, Tronchon L, et al. Use of venous-to-arterial carbon dioxide tension difference to guide resuscitation therapy in septic shock. World J Crit Care Med. 2016;5:47-56.

    The given values suggest severe hypoxemia ad hyperlactatemia suggesting tissue hypoxia or a DO_2/VO_2 mismatch. Although the venous sample shows a normal venous saturation, the A-VCO_2 gap of more than 6 suggests that the hemodynamic status and tissue oxygen delivery can be further optimized by optimizing cardiac output. The ratio of $AVCO_2/C(a-v)O_2$ ratio of 1.4 identifies the presence of anaerobic metabolism and global tissue hypoxia.

43. **Ans. (d)**

    Alhashemi J, Cecconi M, Hofer C. Cardiac output monitoring: an integrative perspective. Crit Care. 2011;15:214.

    Camporota L, Beale R. Pitfalls in hemodynamic monitoring based on the arterial pressure waveform. Crit Care. 2010;14:124.

    FloTrac® is a method of estimating cardiac output that works on the principle of pulse contour analysis. It works on the principle that the pulse pressure of the patient is directly proportional to stroke volume. The system measures the mean arterial pressure (MAP) and also the standard deviation of the pressure (σ_{AP}) around the MAP. The algorithm repeatedly analyzes data points of the pressure trace at 100 Hz and σ_{AP} is then adjusted for variables such the pulse rate, arterial compliance, vascular tone, skewness and kurtosis (symmetry of the arterial waveform, distinctness of the waveform) and calculates the cardiac output.

    It does not require any new arterial lines and is easy to install on the preexisting arterial line. It is an uncalibrated system, needs no external calibration, and is operator independent. However, the system is not validated in extreme vasoconstricted or vasodilated systems, especially in ICU population.

44. **Ans. (c)**

    Mahjoub Y, Pila C, Friggeri A, et al. Assessing fluid responsiveness in critically ill patients: false-positive pulse pressure variation is detected by Doppler echocardiographic evaluation of the right ventricle. Crit Care Med. 2009;37:2570-5.

    Kim YK, Shin WJ, Song JG, et al. Effect of right ventricular dysfunction on dynamic preload indices to predict a decrease in cardiac output after inferior vena cava clamping during liver transplantation. Transplant Proc. 2010;42:2585-9.

Huai-wu He, Da-wei Liu. The pitfall of pulse pressure variation in the cardiac dysfunction condition. Crit. Care. 2015;19(1):1.

This patient has right ventricular dysfunction due to acute pulmonary embolism. In patients with right ventricular (RV) dysfunction, the increase of the RV afterload and decrease of the RV stroke volume that is normally seen is further accentuated and his will result in a false positive high PPV value. This high PPV is in fact due to the accentuated increase in afterload rather than fluid responsiveness. The evaluation of RV function is thus important while using PPV for predicting fluid responsiveness. Similarly, in patients with severe left ventricular (LV) dysfunction, the positive pressure ventilation facilitates LV ejection due to a reduction in the transmural pressure and afterload reduction. This is manifested as an amplified response of the delta up fraction of pulse pressure variation which would again result in a false-positive PPV. Hence echocardiographic assessment of biventricular function is important before relying on PPV solely as a marker of fluid responsiveness.

CHAPTER 8

Infection Control

RIPENMEET SALHOTRA, SUPRADIP GHOSH

QUESTIONS

1. Your hospital is celebrating infection control week. You have been assigned to teach the importance of hand hygiene to hospital staff. Which of the following statement regarding hand hygiene is incorrect?
   a. Hands should be washed with soap and water when visibly dirtier soiled with blood/body fluids
   b. Alcohol-based hand rubs can be used when hands are not visibly dirty
   c. During surgical hand preparation, all hand jewelry, nail polish, and artificial nails should be removed
   d. There is no need to practice hand hygiene whenever gloves are removed

2. A young patient is admitted to your ICU with 3 days of fever and running nose followed by dyspnea and dry cough. He has bilateral infiltrates on chest X-ray. A nasal swab taken for H1N1 PCR is positive. Which of the following statement is incorrect regarding infection control with regards to this patient?
   a. A separate room is desirable but not necessary
   b. Patient transport in hospital should be minimized
   c. H1N1 is spread via droplet transmission
   d. Special air handling and ventilation are required to prevent its spread

3. All statements are true about droplet transmission, *except*:
   a. It is technically a form of contact transmission
   b. It typically occurs when the droplet size is less than 5 µm
   c. Healthcare personnel must wear a mask, if within one meter of patient
   d. *Neisseria meningitidis* spreads via droplet transmission

4. Airborne transmission occurs by dissemination of either airborne droplet nuclei or small particles in the respirable size range containing infectious agents that remain infective over time and distance. Infectious agents to which this applies include all, *except*:
   a. *Mycobacterium tuberculosis*
   b. Varicella zoster
   c. Rubella (Measles)
   d. *Mycoplasma pneumoniae*

5. A 25-year-old male was admitted with cough, fever, and malaise for 2 weeks. Examination of sputum smear shows AFB (acid fast bacilli). Isolation precautions required to prevent transmission of tuberculosis to other patients and healthcare personnel include all, *except*:
   a. He should be nursed in a private room with private bathroom
   b. Air flow should be in the direction from hall into the room (negative air pressure)
   c. Air in his room should be changed at least three times per hour
   d. Door of his room must be kept closed

6. The patient in of pulmonary tuberculosis (sputum positive) is started on antitubercular treatment and seems clinically better. Criteria for discontinuation of isolation precautions for MTB is/are:
   a. Patient has three consecutive negative AFB sputum smears collected at least 8 hours apart
   b. Patient has received standard ATT for at least 2 weeks
   c. Patient has demonstrated clinical improvement
   d. All of the above must be present to discontinue isolation precautions

7. Transmission of *Mycobacterium tuberculosis* is linked to close contact with infectious TB patients during following procedures:
   a. Bronchoscopy
   b. Open abscess irrigation
   c. Autopsy
   d. All of the above

8. A patient of COPD on mechanical ventilation for type 2 respiratory failure develops new onset fever associated with thick tracheal secretions and a new infiltrate on chest X-ray. A BAL culture grew *Acinetobacter baumannii* which was resistant to carbapenems (CRAB). Evidence-based recommendations on measures for the prevention and control of CRAB in intensive care unit include:
   a. Patient should be physically separated from noncolonized or noninfected patients using single room isolation or cohorting patients with the same resistant pathogen
   b. Compliance with enhanced and more frequent environmental cleaning protocols of the immediate surrounding area (that is, the "patient zone") should be ensured
   c. Hypochlorite is an acceptable solution for environmental cleaning for control of CRAB
   d. All of the above

9. Incorrect statement regarding cleaning of "housekeeping surfaces" in intensive care units is:
   a. "High touch surfaces" require cleaning and disinfection at least daily and more frequently
   b. "Low touch surfaces" require cleaning on a regular basis but less frequently
   c. "Terminal cleaning" is done only after death of a patient
   d. MRSA, VRE, *Acinetobacter baumannii, C. difficile,* and *Norovirus* can survive inpatient environment for prolonged periods

10. An elderly male in ICU for pneumonia and respiratory failure develops diarrhea associated with new onset fever and leukocytosis. A stool sample is positive for *C. difficile* toxin. Incorrect statement regarding infection control of Clostridium difficile infection (CDI) in hospitals is:
    a. Preferably placed in single rooms with separate toilets
    b. Healthcare personnel must wear gloves and gown while caring for patients with CDI
    c. Contact precautions should be started only after laboratory confirmation of CDI
    d. Handwashing with soap and water has better efficacy of spore removal than performing hand hygiene with alcohol-based hand rubs

11. How long shall isolation (contact precautions) be continued for a patient of *C. difficile* infection?
    a. Till 7 days of treatment with oral vancomycin
    b. Till 10 days of treatment with oral vancomycin
    c. At least till 48 hours after diarrhea has resolved
    d. Should continue till discharge in all patients

12. A 38-year-old female with stage 2A breast cancer is admitted with history of fever since a day. She was found hypotensive in the emergency and shifted to ICU. She had completed three cycles of chemotherapy 7 days prior. Her absolute neutrophil counts are 350 cells/uL. Precautions to be taken to prevent healthcare associated infection include all, *except*:
    a. Hand hygiene should be meticulously followed by those caring for her
    b. Standard precautions should be followed by healthcare personnel caring her
    c. She should be placed in a positive pressure room with > 12 air changes per hour and HEPA filtration of incoming air
    d. Plants and dried or fresh flowers should not be allowed in her room or vicinity

13. A 28-year-old male patient of TBI develops fever while in ICU. Pan cultures (blood, tracheal aspirates, and urine) are sent. Meanwhile a urine microscopy report shows absence of pyuria. Correct statement regarding pyuria in a catheterized patient is:
    a. Pyuria is diagnostic of CAUTI
    b. Pyuria accompanying a bacterial growth of ≥ 10^5 cfu/mL in a catheterized urine sample is an indication for antimicrobial treatment
    c. Absence of pyuria in a symptomatic patient suggests a diagnosis other than CAUTI
    d. None of the above

14. A 65-year-old patient of advanced cirrhosis on mechanical ventilation for hepatic encephalopathy is running new onset fever. No obvious source of infection is identifiable. The attending intensivist suspects CAUTI. Correct statement regarding CAUTI is:
    a. Presence of odorous or cloudy urine in a catheterized patient is an indication for urine culture
    b. CAUTI is defined as growth of ≥10^3 cfu/mL of ≥ 1 bacterial species in a catheterized urine sample with signs and symptoms compatible with UTI and no other identified source of infection

    c. Specimen of urine for culture can be obtained from collection bag, if sampling port is not available
    d. If the urinary catheter is removed its tip should be sent for culture

15. A patient in your ICU develops sudden decrease in urine output. The doctor on duty suspects obstructed catheter and advices the nurse to flush it with saline. Which of the following statement is correct regarding management of suspected catheter obstruction?
    a. Catheter should be irrigated with saline to open
    b. Catheter should be changed with a new one
    c. A bladder ultrasound should be performed and irrigation or change should be avoided unless retention is present
    d. None of the above

16. Which of the following interventions is/are effective in reducing CAUTI?
    a. Screening and treatment of CA-ASB (catheter-associated asymptomatic bacteriuria)
    b. Securing catheter to patient's lower extremity to prevent traction
    c. Antimicrobial coated (silver alloy/antibiotic) urinary catheters
    d. All of the above

17. Residual gastric volume is measured periodically while a patient is on enteral nutrition. Which of the following statements, regarding this strategy for prevention of VAP is correct?
    a. It has shown to reduce the rates of VAP
    b. Percentage of target calorie intake is similar whether feeding is provided based on residual gastric volume measurement or not
    c. There is no difference in VAP rates whether feeding is provided based on residual gastric volume measurement or not
    d. None of the above

18. You have been approached by a representative of a medical equipment manufacturer. He claims that endotracheal tube with new improved cuffs can prevent VAP in your ICU. True regarding evidence on newer cuff designs and material for prevention of VAP include:
    a. *In vitro* and observational studies suggested reduced microaspiration and VAP rates using tracheal tubes with tapered cuffs
    b. *In vitro* and observational studies suggested reduced microaspiration and VAP rates using tracheal tubes with polyurethane cuffs as compared to PVC cuffs
    c. A recent RCT found no significant impact of using tapered cuffs on incidence of microaspiration or VAP
    d. All of the above

19. According to National Health Safety Network definition of ventilator-associated event (VAE), in a patient who is on mechanical ventilation for more than 48 hours with stable ventilatory requirements, ventilator-associated condition (VAC) is defined as:

a. An increase in daily minimum FiO$_2$ requirement of ≥ 0.2
   b. Purulent respiratory secretions or a positive culture of endotracheal aspirate
   c. Purulent respiratory secretions and a positive culture of endotracheal aspirate
   d. Fever, leukocytosis, and change in antibiotics

20. **Novel endotracheal tubes with subglottic secretion drainage ports have been introduced in your ICU because of concerns about rising VAP rates. Correct statement regarding this strategy to prevent VAP is:**
    a. These endotracheal tubes have drainage port below the cuff to suck out subglottic secretions
    b. Recommended only in patients expected to require greater than 48–72 hours of mechanical ventilation
    c. Patients who are admitted to ICU intubated with traditional ETT should be extubated to insert an endotracheal tube with subglottic secretion drainage
    d. None of the above

21. **Risk of surgical site infections (SSIs) depends on:**
    a. Type of operating procedure
    b. ASA score of patient
    c. Duration of surgery
    d. All of the above

22. **While examining a patient during rounds in ICU, you notice that the transparent dressing of CVC is soiled with blood. Which of the following statements is incorrect?**
    a. Dressing of this patient should be replaced with a new one after following hand hygiene
    b. Gauge dressing is preferred over transparent dressing when exit site is bloody
    c. Routine replacement (even when not soiled or loose) is recommended every 2 days for gauge dressing and every 7 days for transparent dressings
    d. Routine replacement of CVC dressing is not recommended and should only be replaced when soiled, loosened, or damp

23. **An elderly female is admitted to ICU postbilateral total knee arthroplasty (TKA). She was given injection cefazolin before incision as antimicrobial prophylaxis. Which of the following is true?**
    a. Give no further dose of injection cefazolin
    b. Continue injection cefazolin for 24 hours after procedure
    c. Continue injection cefazolin for 3 days after procedure
    d. Duration of dosing will depend on whether a drain is *in situ* or not

24. **A young patient of trauma has a central venous catheter *in situ* since 3 days. He develops new onset fever and leukocytosis. There are no signs and symptoms suggestive of a site of infection. The central line insertion site has no discharge and there is no induration. Paired blood cultures (one from CVC and one from peripheral vein) grow *Staphylococcus* aureus (from both sets) and differential time to positivity is 3 hours. Patient has:**

a. Central line-associated bloodstream infection (CLABSI)
b. Catheter-related bloodstream infection (CRBSI)
c. Both the terms are same
d. Given data is not enough to differentiate the two

25. Which of the following have not proven effective in prevention of ventilator-associated pneumonia?
    a. Use of kinetic beds
    b. Stress ulcer prophylaxis
    c. Closed tracheal suctioning system
    d. All of the above

26. Which of the following intervention is recommended to prevent CRBSI?
    a. Tubing used to infuse lipid containing solutions must be changed every 4–6 hours
    b. Tubing used to infuse propofol must be changed every 24 hours
    c. Exchange over guidewire can be done to replace a nontunneled catheter, if infection is suspected
    d. Prepare skin with a >0.5% chlorhexidine preparation with alcohol before central venous catheter and peripheral arterial catheter insertion and during dressing changes

27. Correct sequence of donning of personal protective equipment (PPE) from first to last is:
    a. Wear mask, wear eye protection, wash hands, put on apron, wear gloves
    b. Wash hands, put on apron, put on mask, wear eye protection, don gloves
    c. Put on apron, put on mask, wear eye protection, wash hands, don gloves
    d. None of the above

28. Sharps injury may be defined as an incident where the skin is punctured by an instrument or object that is contaminated with high-risk body fluids. High-risk body fluids and tissues include all, *except*:
    a. Blood
    b. Cerebrospinal fluid
    c. Peritoneal fluid
    d. Urine

ANSWERS

1. **Ans. (d)**
   WHO guidelines on hand hygiene in healthcare: A summary, 2014.

2. **Ans. (d)**
   Siegel JD, Rhinehart E, Jackson M, et al; the Healthcare Infection Control Practices Advisory Committee. 2007 Guideline for Isolation Precautions: Preventing Transmission of Infectious Agents in Healthcare Settings. Am J Infect Control. 2007;35(10 suppl 2):S65-164.
   - Influenza (including H1N1) is spread via "droplet transmission".
   - A separate room if available must be assigned to the patient but is not absolutely necessary.
   - Organisms transmitted by the droplet route do not remain infective over long distances, and therefore do not require special air handling and ventilation.

3. **Ans. (b)**
   Siegel JD, Rhinehart E, Jackson M, et al; the Healthcare Infection Control Practices Advisory Committee. 2007 Guideline for Isolation Precautions: Preventing Transmission of Infectious Agents in Healthcare Settings. Am J Infect Control. 2007;35(10 suppl 2):S65-164.
   - Droplet transmission is technically a form of contact transmission. Droplets traditionally have been defined as being >5 µm in size.
   - The maximum distance for droplet transmission is currently unresolved. Historically, the area of defined risk has been a distance of ≤3 feet around the patient and is based on epidemiologic and simulated studies of selected infections.
   - Examples of infectious agents that are transmitted via the droplet route include *Bordetella pertussis*, influenza virus, adenovirus, rhinovirus, SARS-associated corona virus, group A *Streptococcus*, and *Neisseria meningitidis*.

4. **Ans. (d)**
   Mycobacterium tuberculosis, varicella zoster virus, and rubella virus spread via airborne transmission. In contrast *Mycoplasma pneumoniae* spreads via droplet transmission.

5. **Ans. (c)**
   Centers for Disease Control and Prevention. Guidelines for Preventing the Transmission of Mycobacterium tuberculosis in Health-Care Settings, 2005. MMWR 2005;54(No. RR-17).

   Mycobacterium tuberculosis spreads via airborne transmission and special AII (airborne infection isolation) precautions are required to prevent its spread. These include nursing in a private room with negative air pressure maintained. A minimum of 6–12 ACH (air changes per hour) are recommended. In addition healthcare personnel entering their room must wear at least N95 disposable respirators.

6. **Ans. (d)**
   Centers for Disease Control and Prevention. Guidelines for Preventing the Transmission of Mycobacterium tuberculosis in Health-Care Settings, 2005. MMWR 2005;54(No. RR-17).

Three consecutive sputum smears negative to AFB along with demonstrated clinical improvement with minimum 2 weeks of ATT is required to consider discontinuation of isolation precautions. This is not true for patients harboring MDR TB in whom isolation should be continued throughout the hospital stay.

7. **Ans. (d)**

   Centers for Disease Control and Prevention. Guidelines for Preventing the Transmission of Mycobacterium tuberculosis in Health-Care Settings, 2005. MMWR 2005;54(No. RR-17).

   Procedures that involve instrumentation of the lower respiratory tract or induction of sputum can increase the likelihood that droplet nuclei will be expelled into the air. These procedures include endotracheal intubation, suctioning, diagnostic sputum induction, and aerosol treatments (bronchoscopy and laryngoscopy). Gastric aspiration and nasogastric tube placement can also induce cough in certain patients. Other procedures that can generate aerosols include irrigating TB abscesses, and performing autopsies on cadavers with untreated TB disease.

8. **Ans. (d)**

   WHO Guidelines for the prevention and control of carbapenem-resistant Enterobacteriaceae, Acinetobacter baumannii, and Pseudomonas aeruginosa in healthcare facilities. Geneva: World Health Organization; 2017.

   - The "patient zone" contains the patient and his/her immediate surroundings. Typically, this includes all inanimate surfaces that are touched by or in direct physical contact with the patient, such as the bed rails, bedside table, bed linen, infusion tubing, bedpans, urinals, and other medical equipment.
   - Several studies have used hypochlorite [generally a concentration of 1,000 parts per million (ppm)] as an agent to undertake environmental cleaning for CRAB though the optimal agent has not yet been defined.

9. **Ans. (c)**
   - Housekeeping surfaces in a hospital can be divided into two groups:
     1. High touch surfaces life side rails, tray table, room door knob, etc. have frequent hand contact and require frequent cleaning and disinfection.
     2. Low touch areas like floors and ceilings require less frequent cleaning.
   - Terminal cleaning refers to all methods used for disinfection of either a room or a patient zone between occupying patients (e.g. after patient discharge).

10. **Ans. (c)**

    Clinical Practice Guidelines for Clostridium difficile Infection (CDI) 2018.

    - Patients with suspected CDI should be placed on preemptive contact precautions pending the *C. difficile* test results, if test results cannot be obtained on the same day.
    - Though hand hygiene before and after contact of a patient with CDI and after removing gloves can be done with either soap and water or an alcohol-based hand hygiene product there is increased efficacy of spore removal with soap and water.

11. **Ans. (c)**
    Contact precautions should be continued for at least 48 hours after diarrhea has resolved. Prolong contact precautions until discharge is required only if CDI rates remain high despite implementation of standard infection control measures against CDI.

12. **Ans. (c)**
    The patient is suffering from febrile neutropenia. A "protective environment" with AII (airborne infection isolation) is required for allogeneic HSCT (hematopoietic stem cell transplant) patients to minimize fungal spore counts in air to reduce risk of invasive environmental fungal infections. This protective environment includes HEPA filtration for incoming air, positive room air pressure, and > 12 ACH (air changes per hour). However, this practice has not shown any benefit in other immunocompromised patients including postchemotherapy neutropenic patients.

    Standard precautions (not contact precautions) should be practiced while dealing with immunocompromised patients unless indicated by specific infections (e.g. MDRO and CDI).

    Potted plants in vicinity of these patients have been associated with invasive fungal infections, hence should be avoided.

13. **Ans. (c)**
    - Pyuria or pyuria accompanying significant bacteriuria is not diagnostic of CAUTI and henceforth not an indication for antibiotic treatment.
    - The diagnosis of CAUTI requires significant bacteriuria in a catheterized patient with signs and symptoms compatible with UTI and no other identified source of infection.
    - However, absence of pyuria in a symptomatic patient suggests a diagnosis other than CAUTI.

14. **Ans. (b)**
    Hooton TM, Bradley SF, Cardenas DD, et al. Diagnosis, prevention, and treatment of catheter-associated urinary tract infection in adults: 2009 International Clinical Practice guidelines from the Infectious Diseases Society of America. Clin Infect Dis. 2010;50: 625-63.
    - Odorous or cloudy urine is often considered as a sign of infection. However, not all individuals with UTI have an unpleasant odor to their urine, and not all urine with an unpleasant odor is indicative of bacteriuria.
    - It is recommended that specimens should be obtained by sampling through the sampling port using aseptic technique or, if a port is not present, puncturing the catheter tubing with a needle and syringe. Culture specimens should not be obtained from the drainage bag.

15. **Ans. (c)**
    Irrigation of or changing the urinary catheter may introduce infection into the patient's urinary tract and hence should be avoided unless retention is confirmed on ultrasound of bladder.

16. **Ans. (b)**

 Hooton TM, Bradley SF, Cardenas DD, et al. Diagnosis, prevention, and treatment of catheter-associated urinary tract infection in adults: 2009 International Clinical Practice guidelines from the Infectious Diseases Society of America. Clin Infect Dis. 2010;50:625-63.

 Sampathkumar P. Reducing catheter-associated urinary tract infections in the ICU. Curr Opin Crit Care. 2017;23(5):372-7.

17. **Ans. (c)**

 Reignier J, Mercier E, Le Gouge A, et al. Effect of not monitoring residual gastric volume on risk of ventilator-associated pneumonia in adults receiving mechanical ventilation: a randomized controlled trial. JAMA. 2013;309:249-56.

 Klompas M, Branson R, Eichenwald E, et al. Strategies to Prevent Ventilator-Associated Pneumonia in Acute Care Hospitals: 2014 Update. Infect Control Hosp Epidemiol. 2014;35(8):915-36.

 A recent multicenter RCT was performed in adult patients requiring invasive mechanical ventilation and compared absence of residual gastric volume monitoring versus measurement of gastric volume every 6 hours. VAP rate was similar in both groups. In addition, the proportion of patients receiving 100% of their target calorie intake was higher in the group in which monitoring was not done, suggesting that this measurement should not be performed.

18. **Ans. (d)**

 Klompas M, Branson R, Eichenwald E, et al. Strategies to Prevent Ventilator-Associated Pneumonia in Acute Care Hospitals: 2014 Update. Infect Control Hosp Epidemiol. 2014;35(8):915-36.

 Philippart F, Gaudry S, Quinquis L, et al. Randomized intubation with polyurethane or conical cuffs to prevent pneumonia in ventilated patients. Am J Respir Crit Care Med. 2015;191:637-45.

 Jaillette E, Girault C, Brunin G, et al. Impact of tapered-cuff tracheal tube on microaspiration of gastric contents in intubated critically ill patients: a multicenter cluster-randomized cross-over controlled trial. Intensive Care Med. 2017;43(11):1562-71.

 - Several bench studies and observational trials have shown that endotracheal tubes with new improved cuffs (shapes and material) reduce aspiration and VAP rates.
 - However, two recent RCTs failed to prove any benefit of ETTs with tapered cuffs and/or cuffs made of polyurethane over traditional ETTs with regards to aspiration or development of VAP. Hence, their use as of now is not supported by sound evidence.

19. **Ans. (a)**

 Klompas M, Branson R, Eichenwald E, et al. Strategies to Prevent Ventilator-Associated Pneumonia in Acute Care Hospitals: 2014 Update. Infect Control Hosp Epidemiol. 2014;35(8):915-36.

 - VAE is now the CDC's recommended surveillance metric for ventilated patients proposed to overcome the poor sensitivity and specificity of traditional VAP definitions.

- VAC is defined by greater than or equal to 2 days of stable or decreasing PEEP or FiO_2 followed by an increase in daily minimum PEEP greater than or equal to 3 cm of H_2O or daily minimum FiO_2 greater than or equal to 0.20 points sustained for greater than or equal to 2 calendar days.
- IVAC is considered when VAC is associated with infection indicators like fever, leukocytosis, and start of new antibiotics.
- Possible/probable VAP is present when IVAC is associated with purulent respiratory secretions and/or positive cultures from respiratory samples.

20. **Ans. (b)**
    - These novel tubes have drainage ports connected to an externalized lumen just above not below the ETT cuff. The rational for this technique is that secretions pool in the space between the laryngeal aperture and the ETT cuff.
    - Recent IDSA and SHAE guidelines recommend endotracheal tubes with subglottic secretion drainage ports for patients likely to require greater than 48 or 72 hours of intubation for prevention of VAP.
    - Reintubation of an already intubated patient with these tubes is not recommended as reintubation is associated with increase in risk of aspiration and VAP.

21. **Ans. (d)**
    - A surgical procedure can be classified as clean, clean-contaminated, contaminated, or dirty. SSI risk is definitely higher in contaminated and dirty procedures.
    - The aim of ASA (American Society of Anesthesiologists) score is to measure the intrinsic host susceptibility which is readily available at the time of surgery. ASA preoperative assessment score of 3, 4, or 5 increases the risk of SSI.
    - Duration of surgery is a marker of the complexity of the operative procedure as well as the skill of the operating team and increasing duration increases the risk of SSI.

22. **Ans. (d)**

    O'Grady NP, Alexander M, et al. Guidelines for the prevention of intravascular catheter-related infections. Clin Infect Dis. 2011;52(9):e162-93.
    - Exit site dressing should be replaced whenever it is damp, loosened, or soiled.
    - It should also be changed periodically after proper hand hygiene.
    - Replace gauze dressings every 2 days and transparent dressings every 7 days.
    - Gauze dressings are favored when exit site is bloody or moist.

23. **Ans. (a)**

    Berríos-Torres SI, Umscheid CA, Bratzler DW, et al. Centers for Disease Control and Prevention Guideline for the Prevention of Surgical Site Infection, 2017. JAMA Surg. 2017;152(8):784-91.
    - TKA is a clean surgical procedure. In clean and clean-contaminated procedures, an additional prophylactic antimicrobial agent dose after the surgical incision is closed in the operating room is not recommended, even in the presence of a drain.
    - Antimicrobial prophylaxis should be administered at a time so that its therapeutic concentration in serum is established at the time of incision.

Chapter 8 Infection Control

24. **Ans. (b)**
 Berríos-Torres SI, Umscheid CA, Bratzler DW, et al. Centers for Disease Control and Prevention Guideline for the Prevention of Surgical Site Infection, 2017. JAMA Surg. 2017;152(8):784-91.
 - A CLABSI is a laboratory-confirmed bloodstream infection (BSI) in a patient who had a central line within the 48 hour period before the development of the BSI, and that is not related to an infection at another site.
 - A CRBSI is a bloodstream infection attributed to an intravascular catheter by quantitative culture of the catheter tip or by differences in growth between catheter and peripheral venipuncture blood culture specimens. Differential time to positivity of more than 2 hours confirms that catheter is the source of BSI in this patient.

25. **Ans. (d)**
 Makris D, Luna C, Nseir S. Ten ineffective interventions to prevent ventilator-associated pneumonia. Intensive Care Medi. 2018;44(1):83-6.

26. **Ans. (d)**
 O'Grady NP, Alexander M, Burns LA, et al. Guidelines for the prevention of intravascular catheter-related infections. Clin Infect Dis. 2011;52(9):e162-93.
 - Guidewire exchanges are not recommended if the catheter is suspected to be infected.
 - Guidewire exchange can be used to replace a malfunctioning nontunneled catheter, if no evidence of infection is present.
 - Tubing used to administer blood, blood products, or fat emulsions must be replaced within 24 hours, however, tubing used to administer propofol infusions should be changed every 6 or 12 hours or when the vial is changed. Option D is true.

27. **Ans. (b)**
 Damani N. Manual of Infection Prevention and Control, 3rd edition. New York: Oxford University Press; 2012.
 Sequence in option B is correct order of donning of personal protective equipment (PPE). Correct sequence of removing PPE is: remove gloves first, remove apron/gown gently, wash your hands, remove eye protection, remove mask last, and finally decontaminate your hands.

28. **Ans. (d)**
 Damani N. Manual of Infection Prevention and Control, 3rd edition. New York: Oxford University Press; 2012.
 - High-risk body fluids and tissues include blood and body fluids contaminated with blood, amniotic fluid, vaginal secretions, semen, human breast milk, cerebrospinal fluid, peritoneal fluid, pleural fluid, pericardial fluid, synovial fluid and unfixed tissues, and organs.
 - Low-risk materials include urine, vomit, saliva (with the exception of dentistry), and feces, unless they are visibly stained with blood or originated from patients with suspected/confirmed infection.

CHAPTER 9

Infectious Diseases

Rajeev Soman, Neha Gupta

QUESTIONS

1. A 45-year-old lady admitted with dyspnea, fever, and chest pain. X-ray chest revealed 3 peripheral triangular-shaped opacities. Hemogram revealed WBC-25,000/cmm, procalcitonin >10. Treated with piperacillin-tazobactam. Worsening status and hence, changed to IV colistin next day. No improvement over 4 days. Chest physician suspected bronchiolitis obliterans organizing pneumonia (BOOP) and started steroids. Further worsening occurred. PET scan was done which revealed uptake in lung lesions, left side of neck and splenic lesions. Referred for ID opinion—on enquiry, had a left tooth abscess 15 days before and was treated with ciprofloxacin. Tenderness over the left side neck was found. What is most likely?
    a. Aspergillosis
    b. Actinomycosis
    c. Infective endocarditis (IE)
    d. Lemierre's syndrome

2. A 55-year-old lady with chronic kidney disease on hemodialysis with history of mitral valve replacement (MVR) for rheumatic heart disease (RHD) developed fever and dyspnea. TEE showed vegetation. Blood culture positive for *Burkholderia cepacia*. Which of the following is true?
    a. Colistin or aminoglycoside should be used
    b. TMP SMX or ceftazidime or carbapenems should be used
    c. Cefepime or FQN are the drugs of choice
    d. Tigecycline is a good option if allergy

3. A 22-year-old gentleman had waded through flood water and was presented with myalgia, high bilirubin, CPK, LDH, creatinine and low platelets, subconjunctival suffusion, and hemorrhage. Anti-Leptospira IgM negative. The patient was critically ill and required invasive ventilation. This patient should be treated with:
    a. Oseltamivir
    b. Levofloxacin
    c. Ribavirin
    d. None of the above

4. A 52-year-old lady with compensated HCV cirrhosis, who had received interferon 2 months ago, was admitted with history of pain in right foot and leg (a small utensil had fallen on the foot), marked prostration fever and breathlessness. There was a small patch of psoriasis on the leg and red lesions up to the inguinal region. The patient developed hypotension (70/40 mm Hg) in the next 4 hours. Laboratory abnormalities showed hepatic dysfunction, renal failure, and coagulopathy. TTE showed suspicious vegetation. Abdominal and pelvic USG were normal and three blood cultures were done. Piperacillin-tazobactam was started. There was minimal response to vasopressor over 2 days. What is the most likely diagnosis?
   a. Infective endocarditis (IE)
   b. Staphylococcal toxic shock syndrome
   c. Streptococcal toxic shock syndrome
   d. *Clostridium sordellii* toxic shock syndrome

5. A 65-year-old gentleman with DM and CKD on chronic HD elsewhere developed cough and increasing infiltrate over 20 days. It showed nodules with ground glass appearance within them. He received treatment with antibiotics but no improvement occurred. He was started on anti-TB drugs empirically for 15 days without improvement. Serum GM is negative. What should be done?
   a. Sputum cytology
   b. Blood culture
   c. PET scan
   d. CT-guided biopsy

6. A 14-year-old youth had a fall from a swing in a playground where there were many cats. He sustained a compound fracture in the upper limb. Four days later severe pain and toxicity developed. There was crepitus and gas in the tissues seen on X-ray of the upper limb. Two days later amputation is done. Smear from the surgical specimen shows gram-positive rods. Which is the likely organism?
   a. *Streptococcus*
   b. *Vibrio vulnificus*
   c. *Pasteurella multocida*
   d. None of the above

7. In addition to debridement and amputation, what has proven benefit for survival in the above patient (Question 6)?
   a. Penicillin
   b. Hyperbaric oxygen
   c. Specific antiserum
   d. All of the above

8. A 38-year-old gentleman with RTA was treated with an intramedullary nail following which he developed infection and discharging sinus. Debridement and repeated nailing were done. Finally sequestrectomy and nail removal were done. Pus culture grew *Enterobacter cloacae* (only sensitive to colistin). He was to be treated with colistin colistimethate sodium (CMS). What is true about CMS?

a. 1 mU = 80 mg = 30 mg colistin base activity (CBA)
b. Dose should be 1–2 mU 8 hourly for a 60 kg person with normal renal function
c. Loading dose is optional
d. Low doses are needed in a patient on CRRT

9. A 55-year-old gentleman was treated elsewhere for massive gastrointestinal bleed. Patient's comorbidities included ischemic heart disease (post-PTCA) on clopidogrel and ASA. Subclavian line was inserted, antiplatelets agents stopped. X-ray chest showed a doubtful opacity right base? Healthcare-associated pneumonia. He was given piperacillin-tazobactam and levofloxacin for 10 days.
Following this, bleeding duodenal ulcer was injected and antibiotics stopped. Two peripheral blood cultures were negative. Blood culture from central line was positive for MRSA. Central line was removed and the tip which was sent for culture showed no growth. Which is the most correct statement?
a. Should be treated with vancomycin for 5 days
b. Should be treated with vancomycin for 14 days
c. TEE is a must
d. Unresolved how this should be treated

10. In the treatment of patients with fulminant *Clostridium difficile*-associated diarrhea with no oral access, what is preferred?
a. IV metronidazole with vancomycin by nasogastric tube and retention enema
b. Rifaximin 200 mg tds × 10 days
c. IV vancomycin with metronidazole by nasogastric tube and retention enema
d. Nitazoxanide 500 mg bd × 5 days

11. A 47-year-old gentleman previously healthy, presented with fever, headache, crops of skin lesions, and fluid filled vesicles which turned cloudy, mental changes, and dyspnea. He was admitted and taken on invasive ventilation. Which is the likely organism?
a. Cytomegalovirus (CMV)
b. *Mycoplasma*
c. Varicella-zoster virus (VZV)
d. Hantavirus

12. A 60-year-old diabetic, paddy farmer from Konkan, was working bare footed in his field during the 1st heavy rain and stormy weather. Ten days later developed leg abscesses. He was treated elsewhere with co-amoxiclav and ceftazidime for 10 days and had improved. One month later he has pyogenic arthritis of knee and brain abscess. What among the following is most likely to benefit him?
a. Vancomycin
b. Meropenem with cotrimoxazole
c. Penicillin
d. Albendazole

13. A 41-year-old gentleman with CKD, with swap live unrelated kidney transplant had received daclizumab. He was on cyclosporine A, MMF, prednisolone, TMP-SMX, and INH. After 4 months, he presented with diarrhea, oral ulcers, weight loss of 9 kg, and reducing absolute lymphocyte count. Colonoscopic biopsy showed ulceration and CMV inclusions. CMV-DNA >100. He was treated with vGCV.
    He had persistent fever, was on empiric cefoperazone sulbactam, and was changed to colistin after a positive culture for *A. baumannii* What is false about *A. baumannii*?
    a. It resists desiccation for 30 days
    b. It resists disinfectants for only 30 seconds
    c. It is fastidious in its nutritional requirement
    d. It develops antimicrobial resistance during treatment

14. A 45-year-old obese, nondiabetic male was operated for appendicectomy. Postoperatively, the wound did not heal, patient had severe pain, toxicity developed. He was on cefoperazone sulbactam. He was shifted to ICU and underwent extensive debridement. Operative specimen showed *Mucor* along with *Klebsiella pneumoniae* susceptible to tigecycline, colistin, and amikacin. Amphotericin B 75 mg IV and 50 mg locally started. Which among the following is the correct step?
    a. No need to start antibiotics
    b. Start colistin
    c. Start amikacin
    d. Start tigecycline

15. A 67-year-old lady with interstitial nephritis with worsening renal function was put on steroids, azathioprine, calcium, vitamin D, pantoprazole, and amlodipine. His WBC count reduced after 2 months which increased a little after G-CSF.
    He presented 1 year later with dyspnea, nonproductive cough for 2 weeks. Oral candidiasis was present. HRCT showed bilateral haziness. BAL was negative for any organism CMV PP65 came positive. Azathioprine was withdrawn.
    Valganciclovir started but the patient continued to worsen over 15 days. What could be the most likely reason?
    a. Resistant CMV
    b. PCP
    c. Gram-negative sepsis
    d. None of the above

16. What should be used as treatment for PCP in the above described patient?
    a. TMP SMX
    b. Clindamycin primaquine, if G6PD is normal
    c. Inhaled pentamidine
    d. Any of the above

17. A 36-year-old gentleman with diabetes mellitus for 4 years on oral hypoglycemic agents met with a road traffic accident with a closed fracture of tibia. Screw and plate fixation was done. Two weeks later patient developed fever and purulent discharge

from site. He was treated with amikacin, ofloxacin, clindamycin, and amoxiclav; and screw/plate was removed. Culture from screw site revealed *Enterobacter* species (sensitivity to amikacin, carbapenems, colistin, and tigecycline) and *Klebsiella pneumoniae*. Which of the antibiotic combination should not be used?
   a. Cefepime – tazobactam + colistin
   b. Carbapenem + colistin
   c. Carbapenem + colistin + rifampin
   d. Ertapenem + doripenem

18. A 61-year-old gentleman was admitted with pain in abdomen, fever, and mild jaundice since 2 months. He was initially treated with ceftriaxone, amikacin co-amoxiclav, and ofloxacin. CT scan abdomen showed biliary air and sludge. ERCP showed perforated duodenal (D1) ulcer and choledochoduodenal fistula. Bile culture grew citrobacter diversus with susceptibility to cefoperazone-sulbactam, piperacillin-tazobactam, amikacin, and carbapenem.
   Which is the correct choice of treatment?
   a. Piperacillin-tazobactam or meropenem or fluoroquinolone
   b. Cefoperazone-sulbactam or imipenem or aminoglycosides
   c. Piperacillin-tazobactam or imipenem or cefoperazone-sulbactam
   d. Meropenem or aminoglycosides or fluoroquinolone

19. A 60-year-old gentleman with DM, HTN, and ESRD on HD with Permacath for 18 months developed intermittent high grade fever with chills. His WBC count was 16,000/cmm and USG abdomen was normal. He was treated with cefoperazone-sulbactam and vancomycin. Fever continued, but the patient remained hemodynamically stable. There are no metastatic foci of infection and the Permacath exit site did not show any signs of infection. Blood culture grew *Flavobacterium* species.
   What is the option for systemic treatment among the following?
   a. Tigecycline
   b. Carbapenem
   c. Linezolid
   d. Any of the above

20. A 32-year-old lady with subarachnoid hemorrhage due to aneurysm underwent VP shunt done. She developed infected neck wound and features of meningitis. Culture grew MRSA.
   In addition to shunt removal, what would be your choice?
   a. Teicoplanin
   b. Linezolid
   c. Vancomycin
   d. Any of the above

ANSWERS

1. **Ans. (d)**
   - Aspergillosis lung lesions have a similar appearance. They occur in immuno-compromised especially neutropenic patients and SOT recipients. Neck tenderness is not a feature.
   - Actinomycosis can follow dental infection, but produces a localized jaw infection which is indolent and woody hard.
   - IE involving the right side of the heart produces septic pulmonary emboli, but no neck tenderness accompanies.
   - Lemierre's syndrome is lateral parapharyngeal space infection with jugular vein suppurative thrombophlebitis. The most common pathogen is the anaerobe *Fusobacterium necrophorum*. The microbiologic diagnosis may be made based on culture of blood, and culture of purulent material expressed from the site if present. Empiric therapy is with BL-BLI.

2. **Ans. (b)**
   - Colistin or aminoglycoside or cefepime has no activity against *B. cepacia*.
   - Treatment is governed by *in vitro* susceptibility. Ceftazidime, doripenem, meropenem, and minocycline are preferred agents.
   - Chloramphenicol and minocycline have useful activity. FQN is not useful despite some *in vitro* susceptibility.
   - Tigecycline does not have any reliable activity. Besides, it is not useful for bacteremia or endocarditis.

3. **Ans. (d)**
   - An acute disease with myalgia, jaundice, conjunctival suffusion, hemorrhages, ARDS, and alveolar hemorrhage occurring in an appropriate setting is highly suspicious of leptospirosis.
   - Immediate starting of specific treatment is necessary without waiting for confirmation by microbiology tests.
   - The organism can be cultured, but the diagnosis is more frequently made by serologic testing like the microscopic agglutination test (MAT), indirect hemagglutination, and ELISA.
   - Since the MAT, is not readily available, anti-Leptospira IgM ELISA is performed in suspected cases of leptospirosis, the sensitivity is only 70% hence a negative test does not rule out the diagnosis and needs to be repeated.
   - PCR is highly sensitive and specific. It is not widely available but is a promising tool for quick and accurate diagnosis.

4. **Ans. (c)**
   - IE may be suspected because of the suspicious vegetation, but cannot explain the skin-related findings and ARDS.
   - The unrelenting hypotension, renal and hepatic dysfunction, and the skin-related findings suggest that a toxin may be involved in the pathogenesis of the illness in this patient.

Staphylococcal TSS	Streptococcal TSS
Mortality 5%	Mortality 50%
Hypotension, kidney, liver, blood, lung, CNS involvement, and desquamating rash	Similar involvement, generalized rash, and necrotic soft tissue lesions
Not isolated frequently from blood culture. Hence, other causes need to be excluded	Isolated more frequently from blood culture

- *Clostridium sordellii* TSS can be rapidly fatal, but there may be no fever or rash as in this patient. The predisposing features are vaginal pack, postpartum endometritis, episiotomy, or a degenerated cervical myoma. None of these were applicable in this patient.

5. **Ans. (d)**
   - Sputum cytology may help to diagnose a malignant process but the sensitivity and specificity is low.
   - Blood culture, the sensitivity is around 15% only.
   - PET scan may be able to distinguish an infective process from a malignant process; however, the pace of the illness is too rapid for a malignant process.
   - CT-guided biopsy—the pace of the illness and the pattern of progression of the chest shadows are highly atypical for a usual bacterial pneumonia as well as for a malignant process. This patient had end stage renal disease and hemodialysis which are emerging as risk factors for mucormycosis. Therefore, CT-guided biopsy has the highest chance of yielding the diagnosis of pulmonary mucormycosis.

6. **Ans. (d)**
   - *Streptococcus* can produce necrotizing fasciitis but not usually after soil contaminated injury. It occurs often without previous external injury.
   - *Vibrio vulnificus* occurs by exposure of wound to swimming in warm water or ingestion of raw oysters. Cirrhosis of liver is an important predisposing factor.
   - Pasteurella multocida occurs after cat bite or a cat or a dog licking an open wound or inhalation of contaminated dust. It is a bipolar staining organism.
   - This case is likely to be gas gangrene due to Clostridia. They are typically rods with spores and Gram-positive, but can be Gram variable in clinical specimens.

7. **Ans. (a)**
   - Along with surgical debridement, antibiotic therapy is the only intervention that has a survival benefit.
   - Pending definitive etiologic diagnosis of the necrotizing process, empiric antibiotic treatment should cover group A Streptococcus, clostridium species, mixed aerobes, and anaerobes.
   - It should consist of the combination of penicillin (3–4 million units every 4 hours IV) plus clindamycin (600–900 mg every 8 hours IV) or tetracycline (500 mg every 6 hours IV).
   - Antibiotic agents with excellent *in vitro* activity against *C. perfringens* include penicillin, clindamycin, tetracycline, chloramphenicol, metronidazole, and a number of cephalosporins.

8. Ans. (a)
- When CMS is administered about 70% of it is excreted unchanged in urine with a T1/2 of 2.3 h and a small proportion is converted to active colistin. Colistin is filtered and extensively reabsorbed by tubules resulting in a long T1/2 of 14.4 h. The complex activation and excretion pattern of CMS require a loading dose to achieve a steady state quickly. Otherwise 5 half-lives (T1/2) are the time needed to achieve a steady state.
- As renal function declines, more CMS is converted to colistin. Hence, post-HD 3 mu OD is recommended recently.
- Colistin is filtered and extensively reabsorbed by tubules. In CRRT, there is no mechanism to return the filtered colistin. CRRT increases clearance of colistin. Hence, average steady state plasma colistin concentration (Cssavg) × 192 mg colistin base activity (CBA) is the daily dose for a patient on CRRT.

9. Ans. (b)
- When the culture from central line is positive and peripheral culture is negative, it is possible that there is no invasion yet of the bloodstream or there is invasion but the number of CFU is less than the detectable limit.
- Since *Staphylococcus aureus* is more likely associated with CLBSI and is more likely to be associated with metastatic infection, it is advised to treat for 5–7 days even if only the tip culture is positive.
- If culture from central line is positive as in this patient, treatment should be given for 14 days, even if the peripheral culture is negative. In this situation, the central line needs to be removed.

10. Ans. (a)
- Guidelines issued in 2010, SHEA and the IDSA recommend oral vancomycin as first-line therapy for severe CDAD (CDI)
- The major pharmacologic advantage of vancomycin over metronidazole is that vancomycin is not absorbed, so maximal concentrations of the drug can act intracolonically at the site of infection.
- The major advantage of metronidazole over vancomycin is that the cost of metronidazole is substantially lower. With respect to *in vitro* activity, risk of relapse, and potential for emergence of vancomycin resistant enterococci, the drugs appear to be relatively similar.
- The standard duration of antibiotic therapy for *C. difficile* diarrhea is 10–14 days.
- Intravenous vancomycin has no effect on *C. difficile* colitis since vancomycin is not excreted into the colon.

11. Ans. (c)
- CMV may produce mononucleosis like syndrome with a maculopapular rash, LN enlargement, myalgia, and throat involvement in a healthy individual.
- The rash in this case is characteristic of VZV.

12. **Ans. (a)**
    - Meropenem with cotrimoxazole may be the empiric choice, if melioidosis is suspected. The epidemiological setting, initial involvement with subcutaneous abscesses, septic arthritis, and brain abscess later with a history of partial response to ceftazidime are all consistent with this diagnosis.
    - Penicillin may be useful for actinomycosis, which can result from working in fields, but the patients clinical features are entirely different from *actinomycosis,* where local woody induration and discharging sinuses occur.

13. **Ans. (c)**
    - It has the genes that give it environmental hardiness and allow prolonged survival even in dry environments.
    - *Acinetobacter* has minimal nutritional requirement, allowing it to survive in clean water.
    - *Acinetobacter* species are capable of accumulating multiple antibiotic resistance genes, leading to the development of multidrug-resistant or pan-resistant strains.
    - Hetero-resistance, characterized by resistant subpopulations within a single strain, has been described in *Acinetobacter* strains.

14. **Ans. (d)**
    - While *K. pneumoniae* has been obtained from superficial swabs and may be a colonizer, there is substantial necrotic tissue and an angioinvasive pathogen alongside. Hence, there is a risk of dissemination and treatment is probably indicated.
    - Start tigecycline since it is useful for complicated SSTI; however, it will not work against bloodstream invasion, if it has already occurred.

15. **Ans. (b)**
    - The clinical illness with CMV reactivation is often another opportunistic infection such as PCP. Features of dyspnea, nonproductive cough for 2 weeks, not being on TMP SMX prophylaxis, and the HRCT appearance are consistent with PCP.
    - The diagnostic yield of BAL is less in transplant recipients as compared to HIV-infected patients and so negative BAL does not rule out the diagnosis.
    - A resistant CMV is unlikely in this patient. It occurs with suboptimal drug exposure to valganciclovir (vGCV).

16. **Ans. (b)**
    - Clindamycin primaquine is to be used in this patient, if G6PD is normal. Although TMP-SMX is the drug of choice for PCP, there is likelihood of additive myelotoxicity with vGCV.
    - Inhaled pentamidine is the alternative for PCP, but has produced inferior results. It does not work for systemic dissemination of this pathogen and is not available in India.

17. **Ans. (d)**
    Bulik CC, Nicolau DP. Double-carbapenem therapy for carbapenemose-producing Klebsiella pneumoniae. Antimicrob Agents Chemother. 2011;55:3002-4.

- Ertapenem + Doripenem is a new strategy which may work for KPC, but perhaps not for NDM which is the most common mechanism of carbapenem resistance in India.
- KPC has a high affinity for ertapenem and gets consumed in the interaction with it. This is exploited by adding ertapenem, as a consumer of KPC, to a regimen of doripenem which is a powerful carbapenem. This strategy was found effective *in vitro* and *in vivo* models.

18. **Ans. (a)**
    - The factors to be considered are kinetics of penetration into bile, efficacy against the organism and its tendency to develop resistance by induction of Amp C.
    - The "SPICE" group of organisms as *Serratia* species, *Pseudomonas aeruginosa*, indole positive protease, *Citrobacter* species, and *Enterobacter* species, develop resistance during treatment with cephalosporins despite initial susceptibility.

Agent	Bile penetration (x serum conc.)
Piperacillin	30–60x
Cefoperazone	8–12x
Ciprofloxacin	4x
Ofloxacin	1x
Meropenem	0.4x
Imipenem	Minimal
Aminoglycosides	Minimal

19. **Ans. (c)**
    - Linezolid is a good option for outpatient oral therapy of bacteremia in this patient.
    - The other option is vancomycin which could be given after dialysis.
    - Tigecycline is bacteriostatic and not useful for bacteremia due to very low blood levels.
    - Although *Flavobacterium* is gram-negative, its susceptibility pattern is like that of a Gram-positive organism and carbapenems are not useful despite *in vitro* results.

20. **Ans. (c)**
    - Vancomycin penetration is just adequate in the presence of meningeal inflammation, but has the support of the largest experience for this indication.
    - Teicoplanin has poor CSF penetration—hence, not used for meningitis. Linezolid has good CSF penetration, but is bacteriostatic.

CHAPTER 10

Gastrointestinal System

AJITH KUMAR AK, NITHYA CA

QUESTIONS

1. A 42-year-old gentleman presents with sudden onset of retrosternal excruciating pain started following an episode of severe retching and vomiting in the morning. His pain was atypical of any cardiac cause. A bedside 12 lead ECG was within normal limits. Air entry was equal on both sides clinically. Closer evaluation revealed an area of crepitus on the left side of the chest. The patient is hemodynamically stable at present except for tachycardia and maintains a saturation of 95% on 6 L of oxygen via mask. What is the most probable diagnosis at this stage?
   a. Effort esophageal rupture (Boerhaave syndrome)
   b. Mallory–Weiss syndrome
   c. Acute coronary syndrome
   d. Primary spontaneous tension pneumothorax

2. What would be the best modality to adequately evaluate the above patient?
   a. ECHO heart
   b. Upper GI endoscopy
   c. CT thorax and upper abdomen complemented by CT esophagogram
   d. Troponins

3. An 80-year-old diabetic patient was admitted in the ICU with left lower limb cellulitis. He was initiated on treatment with IV clindamycin (600 mg thrice daily). On day 7 of this admission, he developed persistent watery diarrhea and low grade fever (37.9°C), leukocytosis (17,000 cells/cumm) and his creatinine was 1.9 mg% and the lactate was 3 mmols/L. Which of the following statement is incorrect?
   a. *Clostridium difficile*-associated diarrhea is the most important diagnostic consideration
   b. *Clostridium difficile* manifestations can range from asymptomatic carriage and profuse diarrhea, to fulminant colitis and toxic megacolon
   c. High index of suspicion is important for diagnosis. Enzyme immune assays for both A and B toxins as well as *C. difficile* glutamate dehydrogenase (GDH) antigen and real time PCR help in confirmation of diagnosis
   d. Lower GI endoscopy should be done in all cases of suspected *C. difficile* disease and the absence of pseudomembrane rules out the disease.

4. The same patient in question no. 3 was diagnosed to have *Clostridium difficile*-associated diarrhea (CDAD) on the basis of CD toxin positivity. Which of the following statements is incorrect?
   a. Metronidazole and vancomycin used to treat *Clostridium difficile* infection can also predispose to *clostridium difficile* colonization
   b. Age seems to promote frequency and severity of CDAD
   c. 2% chlorhexidine (alcohol-based hand rub) is more effective than hand hygiene with soap and water for prevention of spread of the infection
   d. Toxin B is approximately 10 times more potent than toxin A

5. A 50-year-old male is brought to the emergency department with history of sudden onset of severe periumbilical abdominal pain. He had multiple comorbidities including hypertension, diabetes, and ischemic cardiomyopathy with severe LV dysfunction (EF = 20–25%) and was also on treatment for nonvalvular atrial fibrillation (on rivaroxaban 20 mg per day), which he had stopped 3 weeks ago. Which of the following statements is incorrect regarding the diagnosis and further evaluation of this patient?
   a. Mesenteric ischemia is the key consideration of diagnosis in this patient, and CECT abdomen with CT angiogram is the best way to evaluate and diagnose the pathology
   b. Colonoscopy is the diagnostic procedure of choice for patients suspected to have acute colonic ischemia
   c. Early surgical exploration with embolectomy/revascularization is the traditional option
   d. Surgical exploration is contraindicated in patients with clinical, radiographical, or laboratory evidence of bowel infarction, perforation, and peritonitis

6. Which of the following is incorrect regarding abdominal compartment syndrome?
   a. Primary abdominal compartment syndrome is due to disease or injury in the abdominopelvic region. Secondary abdominal compartment syndrome refers to etiologies that do not originate in the abdominopelvic compartment.
   b. Risk factors for intra-abdominal hypertension and abdominal compartment syndrome include patients resuscitated in trauma, burns, and postoperative patients.
   c. Immediate medical measures after treating abdominal compartment syndrome include analgesia/sedation/paralysis/supine positioning/consideration for nasogastric or rectal tubes for drainage of gas and flatus in patients with bowel distention.
   d. Renal arterial compression with resultant ischemia is the main mechanism of renal failure in abdominal compartment syndrome.

7. A 68-year-old gentleman is admitted with history of bleeding per rectum. He was passing bright red blood in moderate quantity for the past few hours. His medical history includes ischemic heart disease (on low dose aspirin). Which of the following is incorrect?
   a. Diverticulosis is the most common cause of lower GI bleeding in most series.
   b. Arterial bleed occurs in angiodysplasia (more severe) whereas venous bleeding occurs in diverticulosis (less severe).

c. Radionuclide scans utilizing (99mTc) sulfur colloid or 99mTc pertechnetate-labeled RBCs (autologous) are the most sensitive radiographic tests for lower gastrointestinal bleeding (can detect when bleeding occurs at 0.1–0.5 mL per minute).
d. CT angiography using multidetector row helical device could detect bleeding happening at 0.3–0.5 mL per minute, can localize site of bleeding with more accuracy.

8. A 47-year-old male comes to the emergency department with history of hematemesis since morning. He was diagnosed to have HBV-related cirrhosis liver 3 years ago. Patient was conscious and alert patient who was hemodynamically stable except for tachycardia 143/minute and saturation was 96% on room air. The Hb at bedside was 6.1 g% and it was decided to proceed with an early upper GI endoscopy. Which of the statements about variceal bleeding is most appropriate?
    a. Hemorrhage occurs in one-third of cirrhotic patients with varices, and acute variceal hemorrhage accounts for approximately one-third of all cirrhosis-related mortality.
    b. Treatment failure of variceal management is: fresh hematemesis or more than 100 cc of coffee ground aspirate after 2 hours of endoscopic treatment or initiation of drugs, or hypovolemic shock, or drop in Hb more than 3 g% in 24 hours.
    c. 50% of the variceal bleeds stop spontaneously.
    d. All of the above are correct.

9. Which of the following is most appropriate regarding TIPS in variceal bleeding?
    a. Colapinto catheter is passed via the internal jugular vein and wedged into the hepatic vein. Then the extruded needle is advanced to portal vein followed by stenting between portal and hepatic veins
    b. Heart failure, sepsis, severe tricuspid regurgitation, and pulmonary hypertension are absolute contraindications
    c. Complications of tips include encephalopathy, TIPS stenosis, arrhythmias, and hepatic capsular injury
    d. All of the above are true

10. Which of the following statement is incorrect regarding pharmacotherapy in variceal bleeding?
    a. Vasoactive medications (e.g. octreotide, vasopressin, and terlipressin) are portal vasoconstrictors and have been known to achieve hemostasis and reduce mortality
    b. Terlipressin has got sustained hemodynamic effects and is the only individual agent known to reduce mortality by itself
    c. We should always wait for the endoscopic confirmation of source of bleeding before starting vasoactive drugs even though the patient is at risk of varices
    d. Current recommendation is to provide both vasoactive medication and endoscopic therapy for esophageal varices

11. Which of the following are true regarding risk of bleeding from esophageal varices?
    a. Site (varices at gastroesophageal junction are more likely to bleed)
    b. Size (e.g. large varices filling more than one-third of esophagus are more likely to bleed than others)

c. Clinical appearance including "red signs" (e.g. varices with red whale marks are more likely to bleed)
   d. All above are correct.
12. **Which of the following is incorrect regarding abdominal paracentesis in cirrhotic patients?**
   a. It is a standard of care to routinely administer blood products to reverse the coagulopathy before the procedure, to prevent intractable bleeding
   b. It is better to avoid paracentesis in patients with distended superficial bowel loops and ileus. Also better to avoid puncture at sites of surgical scars
   c. Large volume paracentesis is defined as removal of more than 5 L of ascitic fluid at one sitting
   d. IV albumin supplementation appears to have a role in prevention of postparacentesis circulatory dysfunction (PCD) which is a hypovolemic state associated with hemodynamic deterioration and high renin levels. PCD can result in renal failure
13. **Which of the following regarding portal hypertension is not true?**
   a. The most common causes for portal hypertension in the world are cirrhosis of liver and schistosomiasis
   b. Schistosomiasis and portal vein thrombosis are major causes in nonwestern world (noncirrhotic portal hypertension)
   c. Hepatic venous pressure gradient is the gradient between portal vein and inferior vena cava. Normal gradient is between 1 and 5 mm Hg
   d. Hepatic venous pressure gradient measurement is required in all cases (for diagnosis) even if the patient has clinical features and risk factors for portal hypertension
14. **Which of the following is correct regarding spontaneous bacterial peritonitis versus secondary bacterial peritonitis in cirrhotic patients with ascites?**
   a. Abdominal examination could be deceivably unremarkable in SBP as well as secondary bacterial peritonitis (in spite of perforation)
   b. Ascitic fluid should be tapped before starting broad-spectrum antibiotics. Broad-spectrum antibiotics need to be initiated when the PMN is >250 cells/cumm even before the culture report comes.
   c. Runyon criteria help to diagnose secondary peritonitis by analyzing protein, glucose, and LDH in ascitic fluid.
   d. All of the above are correct
15. **A 45-year-old male in question 2 was shifted to the intensive care unit and underwent an endoscopy which revealed a large peptic ulcer with a visible vessel not bleeding actively. Endoscopic hemoclipping was done. Which of the following statements is incorrect regarding upper GI bleed?**
   a. The above endoscopic criteria belong Forrest Ia and the risk of rebleeding with medical management alone is 90%
   b. Proton pump inhibitors have been shown to significantly and consistently decrease rebleed and need for surgery, in patients with bleeding ulcers with or without undergoing endoscopic management, when compared with placebo or H_2 receptor antagonist

c. Rockall, Glasgow–Blatchford, and AIMS 65 criteria predict the risk of rebleeding and mortality in upper gastrointestinal bleeding
d. Prophylactic antibiotics have been shown to reduce the risk of infection and probably mortality in cirrhotic patients with upper gastrointestinal bleeding

16. A 22-year-old-girl has been admitted at intensive care unit in a state of altered consciousness. The relatives give history of paracetamol ingestion (650 mg × 20 tablets) about 5 days before. Encephalopathy grade II was diagnosed. An ABG revealed a pH of 7.22. Liver function tests reveal AST 6,500 IU/L with the ALT being 12,800 IU/L. Bilirubin was 10 mg% (direct bilirubin 6 mg%). The prothrombin time was 108 seconds and creatinine was 3.5 mg%. Which of the following statements regarding paracetamol-induced acute liver failure is incorrect?
    a. Short-term transplant free survival is more than 50% in acute liver failure due to acute paracetamol overdosage.
    b. Both prothrombin time more than 100 seconds and creatinine more than 3.4 mg% is an indication liver transplantation (Kings College criteria).
    c. The only indication warranting orthotopic liver transplant referral in this patient is the pH below 7.30.
    d. Paracetamol-induced acute liver failure could be prevented in vast majority of cases if N-acetyl cysteine is administered within 8 hours of ingestion.

17. A 52-year-old patient comes to the emergency department with history of sudden onset epigastric pain for the past 1 day which has increased in severity for the past few hours. Examination revealed a toxic patient whose heart rate was 142/min with systolic blood pressure of 82 mm Hg. Ultrasound showed CBD diameter of 9.2 mm and visible gall stones were present. The liver function tests revealed a bilirubin of 5 mg% (direct 3.8 mg%), ALP was 132 IU/L, and both the ALT and AST were above 190 IU/L. The amylase was 1500 units/L and the lipase 4000 units/L. Which one of the following statement is incorrect?
    a. The clinical, radiological, and laboratory features are suggestive of gallstone pancreatitis with cholangitis
    b. Emergency ERCP is indicated in the above patient, which is expected to help source control for sepsis and reduce severity of pancreatitis
    c. ERCP is not indicated in acute gallstone pancreatitis without cholangitis, in absence of CBD dilatation
    d. High bilirubin (direct as well as indirect) level is the most useful parameter in the liver function tests, which helps in the diagnosis of gallstone pancreatitis.

18. A 45-year-old-male is admitted to the intensive care unit with polytrauma, involving the abdomen, and lower extremities. The patient had massive exsanguination and was in profound shock at admission at the emergency and was aggressively resuscitated with crystalloids and blood products. Subsequently, he underwent an emergency exploratory laparotomy. Next day patient had abdominal distension. A CECT abdomen was ordered showed no fresh changes. The patient subsequently started dropping the urine output and ABGs were getting progressively hypotensive, acidotic with the lactate

climbing up gradually. A progressive increase in the peak and plateau pressures were recorded at ventilator monitors. Which of the following statements is incorrect in this patient in this context?
a. The ideal next step is to measure intra-abdominal pressure to rule out abdominal compartment syndrome
b. Intra-abdominal pressure should always be measured when the patient is actively exhaling
c. Abdominal compartment syndrome is defined as a sustained intra-abdominal pressure more than 20 mm Hg (with or without an abdominal perfusion pressure <60 mm Hg) with a new onset organ dysfunction
d. An emergency decompressive laparotomy/laparostomy might be lifesaving in this patient whose measured intra-abdominal pressure was >25 mm Hg.

19. The patient diagnosed to have acute pancreatitis did not improve clinically after 72 hours of supportive measures and had developed progressive worsening of multiorgan failure. A contrast enhanced CT abdomen on the 4th day of ICU admission showed large areas of necrosis of body and tail of pancreas and severe peripancreatic fluid collection was present. Which of the following statements regarding further management of this patient is incorrect?
a. No treatment is usually required for peripancreatic fluid collections (usually develop before 4 weeks)
b. The necrosed areas can be acute necrotic collection (occurs within less than 4 weeks) or walled of necrosis (develops after more than 4 weeks)
c. Infected pancreatic necrosis should be considered in patients who are diagnosed to have pancreatic necrosis and subsequently deteriorate with signs and symptoms of ongoing sepsis or fail to improve after 7–10 days of hospital admission.
d. Urgent surgical necrosectomy is indicated in all cases of infected necrosis which is in fact lifesaving.

20. A 26-year-old lady with primigravida in her 32 weeks of gestation presents to MICU with right hypochondriac. Examination revealed a conscious and oriented lady and icterus was seen, blood pressure was 162/98 mm Hg and heart rate was 112 per minute. Urine evaluation was showing protein (++). Complete blood count showed a platelet count of 76,000/cumm. The liver function tests revealed a total bilirubin of 5.6 mg% with direct bilirubin being 2.2 mg%. The AST (SGOT) was 96 IU/L and ALT (SGPT) was 88 IU/L. The peripheral smear revealed helmet cells <1%. The LDH was 970. Some of the differential diagnoses to be considered in the above lady are:
a. HELLP syndrome or preeclampsia with severe features
b. Acute fatty liver of pregnancy (AFLP)
c. TTP/HUS
d. All of the above

ANSWERS

1. **Ans. (a)**
   Wilson RF. *Spontaneous perforation of the esophagus*. Ann Thorac Surg. 1971;12(3):291-6.

   The differential diagnoses are as mentioned. The classic history with evidence of local crepitus (subcutaneous emphysema) is in favor of Boerhaave's syndrome. Crepitus could be felt in pneumothoraces too.

2. **Ans. (c)**
   Tonolini M, Bianco R. *Spontaneous esophageal perforation (Boerhaave syndrome): Diagnosis with CT-esophagography*. J Emerg Trauma Shock. 2013;6(1):58-60.

   CT finding includes thickened esophageal wall with fluid collection around (with or without air). Mediastinal widening is also noticed. Air fluid levels could be seen in pleural cavity, retroperitoneum, and lesser sac. Contrast esophagogram is challenging in uncooperative and unstable patients. It can be false negative in 10% of cases. Utilizing both modalities could be complementary.

3. **Ans. (d)**
   Goodhand JR. *Systematic review: Clostridium difficile and inflammatory bowel disease*. Aliment Pharmacol Ther. 2011;33(4):428-41.

   Lower GI endoscopy is not indicated in patients with classic clinical background and features with a positive laboratory test, and/or good response to empirical treatment. Pseudomembranes would be absent in patients with mild or partially treated infection, recurrence of infection, or in patients with inflammatory bowel disease.

4. **Ans. (c)**
   Jabbar U. *Effectiveness of alcohol-based hand rubs for removal of Clostridium difficile spores from hands*. Infect Control Hosp Epidemiol. 2010;31(6):56-70.

   Alcohol-based hand rubs (e.g. 2% chlorhexidine) do not eradicate *C. difficile* spores and are hence inferior to soap and water hand washing in preventing spread of infection. Moreover, soap and water must be the choice when dealing with the diarrheal episodes (stool) and handling patients with *C. difficile*.

5. **Ans. (d)**
   Cudnik MT. *The diagnosis of acute mesenteric ischemia: A systematic review and meta-analysis*. Acad Emerg Med. 2013;20(11):1087-100.

   Abdominal pain which is "out of proportion to the physical examination" is characteristic of intestinal ischemia. Pain control, anticoagulation, and antibiotics are the initial management strategy. Surgical exploration followed embolectomy/revascularization is the traditional treatment option, though angiographic interventions are also done increasingly.

6. **Ans. (d)**
   Kim CY, Suhocki PV. *Provocative mesenteric angiography for lower gastrointestinal hemorrhage: results from a single-institution study*. J VascInterv Radiol. 2010;21(4):477-83.

The major cause for renal impairment is venous compression with resultant increase in resistance thereby impairing the drainage.

7. **Ans. (b)**

   Strate LL, Gralnek IM. ACG clinical guideline: Management of patients with acute lower gastrointestinal bleeding. Am J Gastroenterol. 2016;111(4):459-74.

   Venous bleeding occurs in angiodysplasia (less severe whereas arterial bleed occurs in diverticulosis (more severe).

8. **Ans. (d)**

9. **Ans. (d)**

10. **Ans. (c)**

    de Franchis R. Stratifying risk and individualizing care for portal hypertension. J Hepatol. 2015;63(3):743-52.

    We need to start vasoactive medications (before endoscopically confirming the source of bleeding) sooner in all patients with past history of variceal bleeding or who are risk of having a variceal bleed.

11. **Ans. (d)**

12. **Ans. (a)**

    Yeon JE, Kwon MJ, Hyung LJ, et al. Effect of fresh frozen plasma (FFP) transfusion on prothrombin time (PT) and bleeding control in patients with chronic liver disease. Hepatology. 2010;52:908A.

    Studies have shown that clinically significant bleeding is very unlikely to occur after abdominal paracentesis even when the INR is as high as 8.7 with platelets as low as 19,000 per cumm. Giving unnecessary blood products will delay the procedure, can increase the cost and cause transfusion-associated lung injury.

13. **Ans. (d)**

    Pinzani M, Rosselli M, Zuckermann M. Liver cirrhosis. Best Pract Res Clin Gastroenterol. 2011;25(2):281-90.

    Inpatients with known risk factors for developing portal hypertension (e.g. cirrhosis), there is no need to do routine portal hepatic venous pressure gradient (HVPG) for diagnosis. HVPG might also help in monitoring and managing patients on nonselective beta-blockers for portal hypertension.

14. **Ans. (d)**

    Runyon BA, Hoefs JC. Ascitic fluid analysis in the differentiation of spontaneous bacterial peritonitis from gastrointestinal tract perforation into ascitic fluid. Hepatology. 1984;4(3):447-50.

    Apart from the above Runyon's criteria, if the culture shows polymicrobial picture or Gram stain shows multiple different bacteria again suggests perforation of gut.

15. **Ans. (a)**
Forrest JA, Finlayson ND, Shearman DJ. Endoscopy in gastrointestinal bleeding. Lancet. 1974;2(7877):394-7.

Forrest classification helps to predict rebleeding risk in medically managed peptic/gastric ulcers, based on endoscopic picture. PPIs have shown superiority over placebo or H2 receptor blockers.

16. **Ans. (b)**
Ostapowicz G, Fontana RJ, Schiødt FV, et al. Acute Liver Failure Study Group. Results of a prospective study of acute liver failure at 17 tertiary care centers in the United States. Ann Intern Med. 2002;137(12):947.

Transplant free survival is more than 50% (3 weeks survival criteria) in paracetamol overdose, hepatitis A, ischemia, and pregnancy-related acute fulminant failure. Many such patients will not require liver transplant.

The encephalopathy is grade II in this patient, the high PT and creatinine values become King College criteria only when the encephalopathy is grade III or IV.

17. **Ans. (d)**
Tenner S, Dubner H, Steinberg W. Predicting gallstone pancreatitis with laboratory parameters: a meta-analysis. Am J Gastroenterol. 1994;89(10):1863-6.

Elevated ALT (SGPT) level is the most useful predictive parameter among liver function tests, helping in the diagnosis of gallstone pancreatitis. A more than threefold elevation of ALT levels had a positive predictive value of 95% in one meta-analysis. In our patient, the CBD is also definitely dilated and stones are visible too.

18. **Ans. (b)**
Malbrain ML, Cheatham ML, Kirkpatrick A, et al. Results from the International Conference of Experts on Intra-abdominal Hypertension and Abdominal Compartment Syndrome. I. Definitions. Intensive Care Med. 2006;32(11):1722-32.

Most patients with suspected intra-abdominal hypertension in ICU setting might be already intubated and on ventilator. Intra-abdominal pressure should be measured at mid-axillary line, end expiration, with the patient in supine position after ensuring absence of intra-abdominal muscle contraction.

19. **Ans. (d)**
Wysocki AP, McKay CJ, Carter CR. Infected pancreatic necrosis: minimizing the cut. ANZ J Surg. 2010;80(1-2):58-70.

Surgical necrosectomy in the early phase (first 2 weeks) is associated with high morbidity and mortality. Surgical debridement is considered only after 4 weeks (at least 3 weeks) in view of intense on going retroperitoneal inflammation resulting in undemarcated necrotic areas from viable tissue, making safe surgery extremely challenging in the early weeks.

20. **Ans. (d)**

Pourrat O, Coudroy R, Pierre F. Differentiation between severe HELLP syndrome and thrombotic microangiopathy, thrombotic thrombocytopenic purpura and other imitators. Eur J Obstet Gynecol Reprod Biol. 2015;189:68-72.

There is always an overlapping of clinical presentation between HELPP syndrome and severe preeclampsia. High blood pressure and proteinuria are seen in 85% of HELLP patients. High blood pressure, proteinuria, and transaminitis would be seen in preeclampsia with severe features. Elevated transaminase is seen both in HELLP and AFLP. Hypertension and proteinuria are absent in AFLP though they are noted in 85% of HELLP patients. Hypoglycemia, coagulopathy, and renal failure are common in AFLP than with HELLP. Very high levels of LDH are seen in TTP/HUS when compared with HELLP and AFLP. Low ADAMST13 activity is considered typical of TTP. Schistocytes are higher in TTP (2 to 5%) than with HELLP (1%).

CHAPTER 11

Nutrition

SUBHAL DIXIT, KHALID ISMAIL KHATIB

QUESTIONS

1. **Critically ill patients are at high risk of malnutrition, if their:**
   a. NUTRIC score is < = 5 or a nutritional risk score-2002 (NRS-2002) score is > 3
   b. NUTRIC score is > = 5 or a nutritional risk score-2002 (NRS-2002) score is < 3
   c. NUTRIC score is < = 5 or a nutritional risk score-2002 (NRS-2002) score is < 3
   d. NUTRIC score is > = 5 or a nutritional risk score-2002 (NRS-2002) score is > 3

2. **The various methods to calculate energy requirement in critically ill patients are:**
   a. Predictive equations (Harris-Benedict, Mifflin, Penn-State, St. Jeorii)
   b. Fixed prescription formulae
   c. Indirect calorimetry
   d. All of the above

3. **In patients with pulmonary failure, ASPEN 2016 guidelines recommend all of the following, *except*:**
   a. Specialty high-fat/low-carbohydrate formulations designed to manipulate the respiratory quotient and reduce CO_2 production should not be used in ICU patients with acute respiratory failure
   b. Fluid restricted energy-dense EN formulations may be considered for patients with acute respiratory failure (especially if in a state of volume overload)
   c. Serum phosphate concentrations should be monitored closely and phosphate replaced appropriately when needed
   d. Serum magnesium concentrations should be monitored closely and magnesium replaced appropriately when needed

4. **According to ASPEN 2016 guidelines, which of the following statements about patients with acute renal failure/AKI are correct?**
   a. Patients with acute renal failure or AKI should not be placed on a standard enteral formulation and that standard ICU recommendation for protein (1.2–2 g/kg actual body weight per day) and energy (25–30 kcal/kg/d) provision should not be followed
   b. If significant electrolyte abnormalities develop in patients with acute renal failure or AKI, a specialty formulation designed for renal failure (with appropriate electrolyte profile) may not be considered

c. Acute renal failure or AKI patients receiving frequent hemodialysis or CRRT should receive increased protein, up to a maximum of 2.5 g/kg/d
d. Protein should be restricted in patients with renal insufficiency as a means to avoid or delay initiating dialysis therapy

5. In critically-ill patients with liver cirrhosis and hepatic failure, ASPEN 2016 guidelines recommend all of the following, *except*:
   a. Dry weight or usual weight should be used instead of actual weight in predictive equations to determine the amount of energy and protein to be provided
   b. Nutrition regimens should avoid restricting protein in patients with liver failure, and instead use the same recommendations as for other critically ill patients
   c. Enteral nutrition should be used preferentially when providing nutrition therapy in these patients
   d. Parenteral nutrition should be used preferentially when providing nutrition therapy in these patients

6. In patients with acute pancreatitis all statements are false, *except*:
   a. Specialized nutrition therapy should be given to patients with mild acute pancreatitis, instead of an oral diet, as tolerated
   b. Patients with moderate to severe acute pancreatitis should have a naso-/oro enteric (gastric/jejunal) tube placed and EN started at a trophic rate, within 24–48 hours of admission
   c. Use immune-enhancing formulation rather than standard polymeric formula to initiate EN in the patient with severe acute pancreatitis
   d. PN should be used over EN in patients with severe acute pancreatitis who require nutrition therapy

7. According to ASPEN 2016, immune-modulating formulations containing arginine and fish oils may be considered in patients with:
   a. Severe trauma
   b. Pancreatitis
   c. Liver failure
   d. Severe sepsis

8. Obese ICU patient with a history of bariatric surgery should receive the following supplementation prior to initiating dextrose-containing IV fluids or nutrition therapy.
   a. Protein
   b. Thiamine
   c. Lipids
   d. Fish oil

9. Which of the following are false for the burns patients?
   a. Enteral nutrition should be provided to the burn patients whose gastrointestinal tracts are functional and for whom intake is inadequate to meet the estimated energy needs
   b. Parenteral nutrition should be reserved for those burn patients for whom EN is not feasible or not tolerated

c. Patients with burn injury should receive protein in the range of 1.5-2 g/kg/d
d. Enteral nutrition should not be initiated very early (within 4-6 hours of injury) in a patient with burn injury

10. All of the following are tools used to assess nutrition risk in the ICU, *except*:
    a. NUTRIC score
    b. Mini nutritional assessment (MNA)
    c. Malnutrition universal screening tool (MUST)
    d. Dual energy X-ray absorptiometry (DXA)

11. The gold standard for assessment of energy needs in critically ill patients is:
    a. Calculated ideal body weight
    b. Indirect calorimetry
    c. Actual body weight
    d. Predictive weight based equations (Harris–Benedict formula)

12. Enteral nutrition should not be used in the presence of all, *except*:
    a. Intestinal obstruction/perforation
    b. Severe hemodynamic instability
    c. Gastrointestinal bleed
    d. ARDS

13. All the following statements regarding monitoring of enteral feeds are true, *except*:
    a. Monitoring for tolerance of enteral feed should be done daily
    b. There should be minimal interruption of feeding regimen due to "Nil Per Os" status for procedures or diagnostic tests
    c Gastric residual volume (GRV) should be regularly measured prior to giving enteral feed
    d Enteral feeding need not be interrupted for diarrhea unless it is infectious or it is associated with worsening abdominal distension

14. Which of the statements regarding maximizing efficacy of parenteral nutrition are true?
    a. Protocols should be formulated and nutrition support teams should be formed
    a. In the initial week of starting PN, use hypocaloric PN (80% of estimated energy requirement with adequate protein dose) and stop PN once enteral intake is two-thirds of energy targets
    b. Routine monitoring of fluid status, electrolytes, LFTs, blood glucose, calcium, magnesium and phosphate levels, and lipid profile
    c. All of the above

15. The amino acid which becomes conditionally essential during stress is:
    a. Glutamine
    b. Thiamine
    c. Leucine
    d. Isoleucine

ANSWERS

1. **Ans. (d)**

   Kondrup J. Nutritional-risk scoring systems in the intensive care unit. Curr Opin Clin Nutr Metab Care. 2014;17(2):177-82.

   The NUTRIC score is designed to identify critically-ill patients at risk of malnutrition and who will benefit by nutritional interventions. The score is based on 6 variables with a maximum score of 10. Higher the score, higher is the risk of adverse outcomes. Patients with a score of >= 5 are at high risk of malnutrition. Similarly, patients with a nutritional risk score-2002 (NRS-2002) score of > 3 are at risk of malnutrition while those with a NRS 2002 score of >5 are at high risk.

2. **Ans. (d)**

   McClave SA, Taylor BE, Martindale RG, et al. Guidelines for the provision and assessment of nutrition support therapy in the adult critically ill patient: Society of Critical Care Medicine (SCCM) and American Society for Parenteral and Enteral Nutrition (A.S.P.E.N.). J Parenter Enteral Nutr. 2016;40(2):159–211.

   Clinicians should determine energy requirements to establish the goals of nutrition therapy. Energy requirements in critically-ill patients may be calculated through simplistic formulas (25-30 kcal/kg/d), published predictive equations, or indirect calorimetry. In the absence of facility to perform IC, the other methods may be used.

3. **Ans. (d)**

   McClave SA, Taylor BE, Martindale RG, et al. Guidelines for the provision and assessment of nutrition support therapy in the adult critically ill patient: Society of Critical Care Medicine (SCCM) and American Society for Parenteral and Enteral Nutrition (A.S.P.E.N.). J Parenter Enteral Nutr. 2016;40(2):159–211.

   A small trial comprising of 20 patients lead to the use of high-fat/low-carbohydrate formulations designed to manipulate the respiratory quotient and reduce CO_2 production. But, a later and larger RCT failed to reproduce the results of the earlier trial. Patients with respiratory failure and volume over-expansion, pulmonary edema, and acute renal failure/AKI have poorer outcomes as compared to patients without these complications. Fluid-restricted and energy-dense nutrient formulation (1.5-2 kcal/mL) should be considered for these patients. Hypophosphatemia may be present in about one-third of critically-ill patients and in mechanically ventilated patients, it may be a cause of difficult weaning and its supplementation leads to better weaning outcomes.

4. **Ans. (c)**

   McClave SA, Taylor BE, Martindale RG, et al. Guidelines for the provision and assessment of nutrition support therapy in the adult critically ill patient: Society of Critical Care Medicine (SCCM) and American Society for Parenteral and Enteral Nutrition (A.S.P.E.N.). J Parenter Enteral Nutr. 2016;40(2):159–211.

   Energy and protein requirements are as for other critically-ill patients and are calculated using either IC or published predictive equations or simplistic body weight based formulae. These patients may benefit from the use of feeding preparations with lesser potassium and phosphate content. Patients on HD or CRRT lose protein due to amino acid loss during CRRT and also due to catabolism. These patients require more protein supplementation (up to 2.5 g/kg/d). Restricting protein intake in patients with renal insufficiency does not delay initiation of HD.

5. **Ans. (d)**
   McClave SA, Taylor BE, Martindale RG, et al. Guidelines for the provision and assessment of nutrition support therapy in the adult critically ill patient: Society of Critical Care Medicine (SCCM) and American Society for Parenteral and Enteral Nutrition (A.S.P.E.N.). J Parenter Enteral Nutr. 2016;40(2):159–211.

   There is a high risk of malnutrition in seriously ill patients with liver cirrhosis and liver failure, which is proportional to the degree of liver dysfunction. Ascites and edema lead to increased water content and increased weight, rendering weight-based equations extremely unreliable. Protein restriction (for encephalopathy prevention) leads to further malnutrition and decreased lean body mass. Enteral nutrition leads to increased muscle mass and better nutrition status in critically ill patients with hepatic failure and also reduces infectious and other complications in post-transplant period.

6. **Ans. (b)**
   Sun JK, Li WQ, Ke L, et al. Early enteral nutrition prevents intra-abdominal hypertension and reduces the severity of severe acute pancreatitis compared with delayed enteral nutrition: a prospective pilot study. World J Surg. 2013;37(9):2053-60.

   Wereszczynska-Siemiatkowska U, Swidnicka-Siergiejko A, Siemiatkowski A, et al. Early enteral nutrition is superior to delayed enteral nutrition for the prevention of infected necrosis and mortality in acute pancreatitis. Pancreas. 2013;42(4):640-6.

   Patients with mild pancreatitis do not require specialized nutrition therapy as rate of complications and mortality is very low and oral diet is usually tolerated. Studies in patients with moderate to severe pancreatitis have demonstrated reduced mortality and reduced infectious complications, organ failure, and ICU length of stay in patients started on early enteral nutrition (by either gastric/jejuna route). Though, small studies have shown benefit of immunonutrition in these patients. Probiotics are generally considered as safe and have been demonstrated to reduce complications in patients with severe pancreatitis.

7. **Ans. (a)**
   Immune modulating formulations have failed to show benefit with regards to clinical outcomes (mortality, infectious complications, and hospital length of stay). Even then ASPEN 2016 guidelines have recommended the use of immune modulating formulations in severe trauma and traumatic brain injury. Immune modulating formulations have been shown to have outcome benefits in the postoperative SICU patient.
   McClave SA, Taylor BE, Martindale RG, et al. Guidelines for the provision and assessment of nutrition support therapy in the adult critically ill patient: Society of Critical Care Medicine (SCCM) and American Society for Parenteral and Enteral Nutrition (A.S.P.E.N.). J Parenter Enteral Nutr. 2016;40(2):159–211.

8. Ans. (b)

Fujioka K, DiBaise JK, Martindale RG. Nutrition and metabolic complications after bariatric surgery and their treatment. JPEN J Parenter Enteral Nutr. 2011;35(5):52S-9S.

Patients who have undergone bariatric surgery in the form of sleeve gastrectomy or Roux-en-Y gastric bypass procedures are at increased risk of malabsorption and micronutrient deficiency. Hence, thiamine should be supplemented prior to IV dextrose to prevent the precipitation of Wernicke's encephalopathy and Korsakoff's psychosis. These patients also need supplementation of iron, vitamin B12, calcium, and vitamin D.

9. Ans. (TTTF)

Rousseau AF, Losser MR, Ichai C, et al. ESPEN endorsed recommendations: nutritional therapy in major burns. Clin Nutr. 2013;32(4):497-502.

As for any other critically-ill patient, even the burns patient should be provided early enteral nutrition (starting within 4–6 hours of the injury). Enteral nutrition leads to lesser calorie delivery but better outcomes in terms of mortality and infections as compared to parenteral nutrition. Energy needs should be assessed by indirect calorimetry and it should be repeated weekly. ASPEN 2016, ESPEN 2013, and 2001 American burns association guidelines suggest a protein intake of 1.5–2 g/kg/d.

10. Ans. (d)

McClave SA, Taylor BE, Martindale RG, et al. Guidelines for the provision and assessment of nutrition support therapy in the adult critically ill patient: Society of Critical Care Medicine (SCCM) and American Society for Parenteral and Enteral Nutrition (A.S.P.E.N.). J Parenter Enteral Nutr. 2016;40(2):159–211.

MNA, MUST, SNAQ, Malnutrition Screening Tool, NUTRIC score, and Nutritional risk score-2002 (NRS-2002) are some of the screening and assessment tools used to assess nutrition risk in the ICU. The NUTRIC score and NRS-2002 assess both nutrition risk and disease severity. Muscle ultrasound and skeletal muscles CT scan are also emerging as tools for this purpose.

Serum albumin, serum transthyretin, serum transferring, and serum retinol binding protein are protein markers whose levels may change in acutely ill patients due to increased vascular permeability, altered hepatic synthesis due to acute or premorbid conditions. Hence these must not be used to judge the nutrition status and the risk of malnutrition in these patients.

11. Ans. (b)

Haugen HA, Chan LN, Li F. Indirect Calorimetry: A Practical Guide for Clinicians Nutr Clin Pract. 2007; 22:377

Indirect calorimetry measures total energy expenditure by measuring the respiratory gases (oxygen utilized and CO_2 produced) in a particular (resting) state. It accurately predicts nutritional needs if variables affecting it are understood and avoided or minimized as far as possible. Predictive weight-based equations (Harris–Benedict formula or other formulae), though used widely for this purpose, are often inaccurate due to injuries and acute illnesses.

12. Ans. (d)

McClave SA, Chang WK. Feeding the hypotensive patient: does enteral feeding precipitate or protect against ischemic bowel? Nutr Clin Pract. 2003;18(4):279-84.

Enteral nutrition should be used in all patients with an intact and functional gastrointestinal tract. In the presence of intestinal obstruction/perforation, in severe hemodynamic instability (due to gut ischemia) and in the presence of active gastrointestinal bleed, enteral nutrition should not be started.

13. Ans. (c)

Passier RH, Davies AR, Ridley E, et al. Periprocedural cessation of nutrition in the intensive care unit: opportunities for improvement. Intensive Care Med. 2013;39(7):1221-6.

Montejo JC, Minambres E, Bordeje L, et al. Gastric residual volume during enteral nutrition in ICU patients: the REGANE study. Intensive Care Med. 2010;36(8):1386-93.

Critically-ill patients being given enteral feeding may develop intolerance to the feeds which will be manifested as abdominal pain or distension, vomiting, high gastric aspirate, diarrhea, reduced stool output, or abnormal X-rays of the abdomen. NPO orders for diagnostic or therapeutic procedures lead to feeding interruption. Intolerance and inappropriate length of NPO orders lead to failure to achieve target energy goals. Gastric residual volumes do not correlate with complications (aspiration pneumonia) and should not be routinely used to monitor enteral feeding. Enteral feeds should be interrupted only if GRV >500 mL.

14. Ans. (d)

Mousavi M, Hayatshahi A, Sarayani A, et al. Impact of clinical pharmacist-based parenteral nutrition service for bone marrow transplantation patients: a randomized clinical trial. Support Care Cancer. 2013;21(12):3441-8.

Jeejeebhoy KN. Permissive underfeeding of the critically ill patient. Nutr Clin Pract. 2004;19(5):477-80.

Critically-ill patients initiated on parenteral nutrition are at-risk of complications and protocols and nutrition support teams decrease these. Monitoring electrolytes and other parameters and hypocaloric feeding reduce complications and refeeding syndrome. Parenteral nutrition should be stopped as early as feasible once enteral feeding supplies majority of the calories.

15. Ans. (a)

Oudemans-van Straaten HM, Bosman RJ, Treskes M, et al. Plasma glutamine depletion and patient outcome in acute ICU admissions. Intensive Care Med. 2001;27(1):84–90.

Glutamine is required by rapidly dividing cells and its level is depleted in patients with critical illness. Its concentration on ICU admission is an independent predictor of ICU mortality. During stress, it is said to become a conditionally essential amino acid.

CHAPTER 12

Endocrine and Metabolic System

Anand Tiwari

QUESTIONS

1. A 58-year-old female patient admitted to intensive care unit with dyspnea on exertion, she was afebrile, heart rate on monitor was 120 beats/min and blood pressure was 100/70 mm of Hg, and pulse oximeter showed a saturation of 94% on high flow oxygen 10 L/min on O_2 mask. Laboratory reports showed WBC—88 × 10^3, Hgb—9 gm%, Hct—25, platelet—75 × 10^3, ABG report sent to laboratory got delayed results showed pH—7.29, pCO_2—34.2, pO_2—21 mm of Hg, HCO_3—16.6. Very low pO_2 in above ABG is in line with following possibility.

   a. Severe acute respiratory distress syndrome (ARDS)
   b. Laboratory error
   c. Leukocyte larceny.
   d. Sampling error (mixed sample).

2. A 56-year-old male presented to emergency room (ER) with history of fatigue, generalized weakness, and weight loss of 3 kg since last 6 months. Last 4 days he is complained of abdominal pain, anorexia, nausea, and vomiting. On examination, the patient is thin cachectic lethargic, afebrile heart rate 118 beats/min, blood pressure 85/65 mm of Hg in supine and 70 systolic on sitting up, respiratory rate 24 breaths/min, chest is clear, cardiac sound normal, per abdominal examination soft diffuse mild tender, bowel sounds sluggish, neurologically no focal deficit.

   Laboratory finding: WBC—12,500, 10% eosinophils, hemoglobin—8.7 gm%, Hct—29.2%, serum sodium—129 mEq/L, potassium—5.0 mEq/L, blood urea nitrogen (BUN) 65, Serum creatinine—1.7 mg%, arterial blood gas (ABG)—pH—7.42, pCO_2—34, pO_2—80 mm of Hg, HCO_3—22, BSL—58 mg%.

   Hypotension persisted despite administration of 2 liters of normal saline.

   Clinical history in above case leads to the probable diagnosis of:

   a. Septic shock
   b. Pulmonary embolism
   c. Adrenocortical insufficiency
   d. Cardiogenic shock.

3. Correct action while managing above patient with hypotension not responding to optimum fluid therapy and vasopressor would be:
   a. Begun on hydrocortisone 100 mg intravenously every 8 hourly
   b. Perform ACTH stimulation test
   c. Use injection dexamethasone as it does not interfere with cortisol test
   d. Perform serum cortisol test.

4. A 65-year-old elderly female brought to emergency room with history of cough since 4 days, progressive altered mentation. On examination she is drowsy, winces to pain delayed tendon reflexes, pupils equal reacting to light hypothermic (temperature 35.4°C), Pulse—58 beats/min, blood pressure 110/70 mm Hg, on general appearance she had dry coarse skin, scaly elbows and knees, yellowness in skin without scleral icterus, coarse hair, macroglossia and hoarseness. She had history of taking tablet thyroxine 25 mcg daily since last 4 years. TFT studies are sent, and BSL—98 mg%. Present evaluation suggests following working diagnosis:
   a. Meningitis
   b. Hypoglycemia
   c. Atypical pneumonia
   d. Myxedema coma

5. Plan of care in above patient will include all of the following *except*:
   a. Rapid thyroid hormone replacement
   b. Steroids until evidence of intact adrenal function secured by cortisol measurement on blood sample obtained on admission
   c. Active rewarming
   d. Early intubation and mechanical ventilation.

6. Elderly male patient was transferred to ICU from wards for altered sensorium. His pulse rate was 128 beats/min, blood pressure was 100/55 mm of Hg, his parameters on day 1 of admission to wards were, pulse rate: 82 beats/min, blood pressure: 128/84 mm of Hg and poor appetite. Following were the laboratory parameters.

Blood reports	Day 1	Day 3
Hemoglobin	16.4 g/dL	18.4 g/dL
Blood urea nitrogen	18 mg/dL	56 mg/dL
Glucose	100 mg/dL	89 mg/dL
Sodium	135 mEq/L	151 mEq/L
Creatinine	1.1 mg/dL	1.2 mg/dL

Most likely diagnosis in above patient is:
   a. AKI (acute kidney injury)
   b. SIADH (syndrome of inappropriate antidiuretic hormone)
   c. Dehydration
   d. Occult gastrointestinal hemorrhage.

7. What is the calculated osmolarity in:

Sodium	139 mEq/L
Potassium	3.5 mEq/L
Chloride	112 mEq/L
Bicarbonate	18 mEq/L
BUN and creatinine	28 mg/dL and 1.5 mg/dL
Glucose	180 mg/dL

   a. 157 mOsm/L
   b. 274 mOsm/L
   c. 298 mOsm/L
   d. 310 mOsm/L.

8. A 50-year-old female patient admitted to neuro-ICU with severe headache diagnosed to have SAH underwent DSA and found to have aneurysmal bleed (ACOM). She underwent successful clipping of ACOM aneurysm and while recovering on day 10 develops altered mental status and lethargy. Scan shows no evidence of cerebral vasospasm or infarct no evidence of hydrocephalus.

   Laboratory parameters:

   Na—119 mEq/L

   CVP: 2 cm of H_2O, hematocrit—38 (was increased above baseline) BUN—50 mg%

   Urine spot sodium—65

   Most likely explanation of hyponatremia is due to:
   a. SIADH (Syndrome of inappropriate antidiuretic hormone)
   b. Diabetes insipidus
   c. Renal failure
   d. CSW (Cerebral salt wasting)

9. A 24-year-old male after admission to ICU for diabetic ketoacidosis is much improved. His vital signs are pulse rate 84 beats/min, blood pressure 120/70 mm of Hg, respiratory rate 18 breaths/min, and spO_2 95% on room air. His blood sugar level was 200 mg%, and urine ketone was still moderate. Patient was tolerating clear liquids and asked for food, resident doctor on duty after assessing above state discontinued IV fluids and ordered diabetic diet 25 kcal/kg and subcutaneous insulin dosage. However, sister on duty withholds dose of subcutaneous insulin as his diet tray is delayed from cafeteria for an hour.

   Which of the following action regarding insulin is justified in this patient?
   a. Insulin infusion should be stopped as it risks hypoglycemia
   b. Switched to subcutaneous insulin dose after receipt of meals
   c. Insulin infusion to be continued during transition period of switching to subcutaneous insulin for an hour
   d. Infusion of 5% dextrose and 45% saline to be continued with insulin infusion.

10. All of the following are common laboratory pitfall in diabetic ketoacidosis *except*:
    a. Patient in diabetic ketoacidosis may present with leukocytosis in absence of infection.
    b. Normal or low concentration of potassium early in ketoacidosis reflect a severe potassium deficit.
    c. Abnormally low sodium concentration due to osmotic effect of glucose drawing fluids from intracellular to extracellular space, produces a fall of 1.6 mEq/L of sodium for every increase in 100 mg/dL in blood glucose concentration more than 100 mg/dL
    d. Nitroprusside reaction provides a semi-quantitative estimation of beta-hydroxybutyrate (BOHB) which is a main ketoacid in diabetic ketoacidosis.

11. A 30-year-old young female whose BMI is 35, suffering from depressive illness, she is brought into ER with hyperpyrexia, agitation, found to have tachycardia and warm peripheries, accompanying friends also brought an empty bottle of tablet thyroxine found near the patient and further asking informed that she has been taking this tablet often on as measure of reducing weight. All of the following is justified in management of this patient *except*:
    a. Gastric lavage and emesis induction
    b. Beta blockers
    c. High dose corticosteroids
    d. Propylthiouracil (PTU) and iodide.

12. A 45-year-old female is shifted to ICU for postoperative observation after undergoing subtotal thyroidectomy. She complains of difficulty in breathing, decrease in $SpO_2 \leq 92\%$ and stridor. She was started on high flow oxygen. Which of the following actions to be taken immediately *except*:
    a. Remove all bandages and examine neck for swelling.
    b. Immediate tracheostomy
    c. Fiberoptic laryngoscopy may be warranted in patient with airway issues without apparent wound hematoma to assess vocal cord function.
    d. If neck hematoma is compromising patient airway open surgical incision at bedside to release collection of blood and immediately transfer patient to operating room.

13. A 25-year-old female patient admitted to intensive care unit (ICU) with acute onset breathlessness, accompanying brother gives history of no premorbid conditions. He gives history of domestic conflict a day prior. On examination, she appears anxious, complaining of perioral numbness, tingling sensation in limbs, respiratory rate of 28 breaths/min, chest is clear, and SpO_2 is 98%, heart rate 110 beats/min, blood pressure 130/70 mm of Hg while checking blood pressure sister noticed appearance of carpopedal spasm.

    In the given context, working diagnosis is:
    a. Acute asthmatic attack
    b. Hyperventilation syndrome
    c. Pheochromocytoma
    d. Pulmonary embolism.

14. A patient of severe traumatic brain injury with no signs of brainstem reflexes, pupils nonreacting, apnea test positive is identified as brain death. Family is counseled and he is identified as potential organ donor. Which of the following medication will be considered for improving function of impaired heart prior to transplant?
    a. Levosimendan
    b. Thyroxine
    c. Digoxin
    d. Corticosteroids.

15. A 48-year-old female patient, postoperative case of total thyroidectomy is being monitored in ICU. She complains of tingling sensation, Chvostek sign is positive. ECG shows mild prolongation of QT interval.

    Possible cause in above clinical context is:
    a. Hypercarbia
    b. Hypoxia
    c. Hypocalcemia
    d. Hypercalcemia.

16. A 45-year-old adult female patient of post-trans-sphenoid pituitary surgery was admitted in intensive care unit with altered mentation, lethargy, weakness and irritability, she had one episode of seizure, her laboratory parameters were: Na—160 mEq/L, K—3.5 mEq/L; Blood glucose 105 mg%, blood urea 45 mg% creatinine 1.2 mg%, serum osmolality 336 and urine osmolarity—180 mOsm/kg, considering her weight to be 70 kg total water deficit in the patient is:
    a. 3.5 liters
    b. 4.5 liters
    c. 5 liters
    d. 5.5 liters

17. In above clinical context (question 16) if correction is planned for serum sodium from 160–140 mEq/L at correction rate of 0.5 mEq/L. considering insensible loss of water 30 mL/hour what should be the rate replacement of free water with (IV 5% dextrose, 0.45 saline or plain water by the tube)?
    a. 125 mL/hour
    b. 155 mL/hour
    c. 165 mL/hour
    d. 175 mL/hour

18. A 58-year-old male, chronic alcoholic, with decreased appetite and food intake since last few months, complains of white patches in mouth and gingivitis on off resulting in poor intake, his BMI was 18.3 kg/m². His laboratory test on day 1:

    Na—(126 mEq/L) (K⁺3.7 mEq/L), (Calcium 2 mmol/L, Magnesium 0.5 mmol/L), Cl⁻ 101 mEq/L, (pO$_4^{3-}$ 0.9 mmol/L).

    He was started on parenteral nutrition with 25 kcal/kg/day.

Altered mentation, confusion and lethargy was detected, there was marked fluid retention within 72 hours.

Laboratory	Day 1	Day 3
Sodium (mEq/L)	128	127
Potassium (mEq/L)	3.7	3.0
Calcium (mmol/L)	2.3	2.0
Magnesium (mmol/L)	0.5	0.45
Phosphate (mmol/L)	0.9	0.5

In above clinical situation most likely cause of clinical deterioration is due to:
a. Alcohol withdrawal
b. Refeeding syndrome
c. Hypomagnesemia
d. Hypokalemia.

19. A 56-year-old female with history of metastatic breast cancer presents with altered sensorium, she is afebrile, no focal neurological deficit, had weight loss and dehydration, serum calcium was 15 mg%. All of the following actions are justified *except*:
a. Calcitonin (4 IU/kg)
b. IV saline infusion
c. IV furosemide injection
d. Glucocorticoid administration.

ANSWERS

1. **Ans. (c)**
   Pardesi O, Bittner EA. Leukocyte larceny: a cause of pseudohypoxemia. Can J Anaesth. 2016;63:1374-5. Fox MJ, Brody JS, Weintrab LR. Leukocyte larceny: cause of spurious hypoxemia. Am J Med. 1979;67(5):742-6.

   Leukocyte larceny (aka pseudohypoxemia) is a phenomenon of artificially low pO_2 on ABG due to markedly increased oxygen consumption by increased malignant leukocytes. The degree of pO_2 decay is increased by delay in processing the sample and can be blunted sending sample in ice box and shortening the processing time. In such instances pulse-oximetry is often a better measure of oxygenation.

2. **Ans. (c)**
   Angelis M, Yu M, Takanishi D, et al. Eosinophilia as a marker of adrenal insufficiency in the surgical intensive care unit. J Am coll Surg. 1996;183(6):589-96.

   This is a classic presentation of patient with chronic compensated adrenocortical insufficiency. Usually most likely explanation for such patient hypotension is septic shock which may also respond poorly to the fluids however history of chronic illness and laboratory data showing eosinophilia and hypoglycemia provides strong evidence for adrenocortical insufficiency.

3. **Ans. (c)**
   Asare K. Diagnosis and treatment of adrenal insufficiency in critically ill patient. Pharmacotherapy. 2007;27(11):1512-28.

   Ideally hydrocortisone 200–300 mg/day administrated in divided doses or as continuous infusion is the preferred corticosteroid in patient with septic shock. Given the severity of illness simply sending a random sample for cortisol determination is inappropriate. Rapid ACTH stimulation should be performed to confirm clinic suspicion; however presumptive treatment with dexamethasone 4 mg should begin immediately since unlike hydrocortisone it does not interfere with serum cortisol estimation.

4. **Ans. (d)**
   Wall CR. Myxedema coma: diagnosis and treatment. Am Fam Phys. 2000;62(11): 2485-90.

   Myxedema coma is an extreme complication of hypothyroidism and occurs when compensatory responses to hypothyroidism are overwhelmed by precipitating factor such as infection. High index of suspicion should be kept as myxedema coma is misnomer because most patients exhibit neither nonpitting edema known as myxedema, nor coma instead cardinal manifestation is deterioration of patient mental status. 80% of myxedema coma occurs in female and almost exclusively in patient 60 years and above. Patients with myxedema coma usually have long-standing hypothyroidism and clinical features of fatigue, constipation, weight gain, cold intolerance, deep voice, coarse hair, and dry pale cool skin. Common precipitating factors include infection particularly pneumonia, urosepsis and certain medication.

5. **Ans. (c)**

   Goldberg PA, Inzucchi SE. Critical issues in endocrinology. Clin Chest Med. 2003;24(4):583-606, vi.

   Patient suspected of myxedema coma should be treated presumptively with thyroid hormone, admitted to intensive care unit, mechanical ventilation may be necessary, because of possibility of secondary hypothyroidism and associated hypopituitarism hydrocortisone should be administered until adrenal insufficiency has been ruled out. patient with hypothermia should be covered with regular blanket, active rewarming or use of warming blanket should be avoided as it increases risk of peripheral vasodilation, and may lead to hypotension and cardiovascular collapse.

6. **Ans. (c)**

   https://www.mayoclinic.org/diseases-conditions/dehydration/symptoms-causes/syc-20354086 [Accessed June, 2019,11.45 pm IST]

   Total body water is 60% of weight in males and 50% of ideal body weight in female. It decreases with increasing age. Dehydration in elderly is a major health concern, severe dehydration in elderly may lead to confusion, irritability, low blood pressure, change in sodium level, blood urea, hemoconcentration and can precipitate seizures and renal failure.

7. **Ans. (c)**

   https://www.ncbi.nlm.nih.gov/books/NBK448090/figure/article-22866.image.f1/ [Accessed June, 2019,11.48 pm IST]

   Serum osmolarity is calculated as (2X Na + glucose mg%/18+BUN/2.8 +ETOH/3.7)

8. **Ans. (d)**

   Momi J, Tang CM, Abcar AC, et al. Hyponatremia—What is cerebral salt wasting? Perm J. 2010;14(2):62-5.

   Hyponatremia in the setting of central nervous system event is a diagnostic challenge both SIADH (syndrome of inappropriate ADH) and CSW (cerebral salt-wasting syndrome) are likely etiology. SIADH is a euvolemic to mildly hypervolemic state where as CSW is a volume depleted state. A correct and timely diagnosis is important in order to obtain a good outcome, because two conditions are treated differently.

9. **Ans. (c)**

   Avanzini F, Marelli G, Donzelli W, et al. Transition from intravenous to subcutaneous insulin, diabetes care. Am Diab Assoc. 2011;34(7):1445-50.

   In critically ill patients with diabetes or hyperglycemia who are admitted to intensive care unit, intravenous insulin is recommended. Treatment of patients in postacute phase when patient starts tolerating oral feeds switching is recommended to subcutaneous insulin. Complexity of transition process demands nursing and medical speciality choosing best time to stop intravenous insulin and plan correct subcutaneous dose calibrated to meet patients' needs to prevent relapse hyperglycemia or hypoglycemia. Insulin therapy must be continuous in DKA as half-life of intravenous dose of insulin just minutes till subcutaneous insulin is given and its action starts. So they have to be bridged over time.

CHAPTER 12 Endocrine and Metabolic System

10. **Ans. (d)**

    Laffel L. Ketone bodies: a review of physiology, pathophysiology and application of monitoring to diabetes. Diabetes Metab Res Rev. 1999;15(6):412-26.

    Ketone bodies produced in ketoacidosis are acetoacetate, beta-hydroxybutyrate (BHB) and acetone. Beta-hydroxybutyrate is most common and acetone is least abundant. The frequently employed nitroprusside test only detects acetoacetate in blood and urine, the test is inconvenient, does not assess best indicator of ketosis (3BHB), provides only semiquantitative assessment of ketone levels and is associated with false positive results.

11. **Ans. (d)**

    Shilo L, Kovatz S, Hadavi R, et al. Massive thyroid hormone overdose, kinetics, clinical manifestations and management. Isr Med Assoc J. 2002;4(4):298-9.

    Thyroxin overdose may be accidental or unintentionally ingested, most commonly by children and adolescents. It may occur in young and older adults in attempt to loose weight, with suicidal intentions or undeclared purposes. Therapy for overdose includes gastric lavage, beta-blockers, and steroids. Beta-blocker ameliorates the metabolic effects of hormone on cardiac system controlling tachycardia and prevents arrhythmias. Glucocorticoids (dexamethasone) decreases conversion of LT4 to T3 the active hormone. PTU (Propylthiouracil)/Iodide therapy are not effective if thyroid storm is due to excessive ingestion of thyroxin; as PTU (Propylthiouracil) mainly affects synthesis of the endogenous hormone while Iodide mainly affects release of the same. Neither of the two drugs have effect on peripheral activity of thyroid hormone.

12. **Ans. (b)**

    Naik SM, Ranishankara S, Bhat S, et al. Post-thyroidectomy hematoma: a rare but potentially fatal complications. Otolarngol Online J. 2015;5(3):1-8.

    Post-thyroidectomy airway distress can be due to vocal cord paralysis, hypocalcemia or postthyroidectomy hematoma. Hematoma is usually due to major vessel ligature slippage or reopening of cauterized veins common in surgery done for large thyroid and deadspace postoperatively. Patient presents with respiratory distress, pain or pressure sensation in neck, progressive neck swelling, and suture-line bleeding. Postoperative case includes attention to drain, careful monitoring in recovery room and appreciation of subtle signs of respiratory distress and immediate shift to OT with 100% oxygen. Vocal cord paralysis is a possibility if no hematoma should be checked as damage to recurrent laryngeal nerve is possibility.

13. **Ans. (b)**

    Parasa M, Saheb SM, Vemuri NN. Cramps and tingling: A diagnostic conundrum. Anesth Essays Res. 2014;8(2):247-9.

    Hyperventilation is a condition in which breathing in excess of metabolic requirement results in hypocapnia secondary to various medical conditions like asthma, chronic bronchitis, emphysema, Copd, pulmonary embolism, and encephalitis and brain tumor. Hyperventilation can also occur in reponse to extreme stress, fear and anxiety.

Hyperventilation secondary to anxiety can result in tetany. Tetany is a syndrome of sharp flexion of wrist and ankle joint (carpopedal spasm), muscle twitching, cramps and convulsions, sometimes with attack of stridor is due to hyperexcitability of nerves and muscles caused by extracellular ionized calcium.

14. Ans. (b)

Cooper LB, Milano CA, Williams M, et al. Thyroid hormone use during cardiac transplant organ procurement. Clin Transplant. 2016;30(12):1578-83.

Acute hypothyroidism after brain death results in hemodynamic impairment that limits availability of donor hearts. Thyroid hormone infusions can halt that process and lead to increased utilization of donor organs.

15. Ans. (c)

Tredici P, Grosso E, Gibelli B, et al. Identification of patients at high risk of hypocalcaemia after total thyoidectomy. Acta Otorhinolaryngol Ital. 2011;31(3):144-8.

Hypocalcemia remains a major postoperative complication of total thyroidectomy. Primary cause of hypocalcemia is secondary to hypothyroidism following damage or devascularization of one or more parathyroid gland during surgery. Hypocalcemia can be asymptomatic, particularly if calcium levels are only mildly reduced or symptomatic with typical manifestation such as Chvostek and Trousseau sign, muscle spasm and paresthesia.

16. Ans. (c)

Kim SW. Hypernatremia: successful treatment. Electrolyte Blood Press. 2006;4(2);66-71.

Hypernatremia is defined as sodium concentration in excess of 145 mmol/L. Correction of hypernatremia must occur slowly to prevent rapid fluid movement into brain and cerebral edema changes that can lead to seizures and coma. The total body water is 60 and 50% of lean body weight in young men and women respectively. When calculating the amount of free water to be given insensible losses and some part of urine and GI losses must be added to the calculations. Maximun safe rate at which plasma sodium concentration should be corrected lowered is 0.5 mEq/L/hour and no more than by 12 mEq/L per 24 hour.

17. Ans. (b)

Kim SW. Hypernatremia: successful treatment. Electrolyte Blood Press. 2006;4(2);66-71.

Rate of replacement 0.5mEq/hour. Insensible losses and some part of urine and gastrointestinal losses must be added to the calculation. Water deficit = 0.6 × body weight (1 − 140/Na), 0.5 × body weight for female.

18. Ans. (b)

Mehanna HM, Moledina J, Travis J. Refeeding syndrome: What it is, and how to prevent and treat it. BMJ. 2008;336(7659):1495-8.

Refeeding syndrome is a well-described but often forgotten condition. It can be defined as the potentially fatal shifts in fluid and electrolytes that may occur in malnourished patient receiving artificial feeds either (enterally or parenteraly).

These shift results from hormonal and metabolic changes and may cause serious clinical complications. The hallmark biochemical feature of refeeding syndrome is hypophosphatemia; however, the syndrome is complex and may also feature abnormal sodium and fluid balance changes in glucose, protein, and fat metabolism, thiamine deficiency, hypokalemia, and hypomagnesemia.

19. **Ans. (c)**

    Lumachi F, Brunello A, Roma A, et al. Cancer-induced hypercalcemia: Anticancer Res. 2009;29(5):1551-5.

    The mainstay of cancer-related hypercalcemia is hydration with normal saline and intravenous bisphosphonates. Loop diuretics are no longer recommended except if there is a evidence of fluid overload. Steroids might still play role for those rare lymphomas that secrete active vitamin D, calcitonin can be used initially with bisphosphonates in case of severe symptoms and very high calcium levels to incur rapid response and allow time for bisphonates to work.

CHAPTER 13

Neurocritical Care

Sunil Karanth, Gaurav Kakkar

QUESTIONS

1. Which is the correct sequence of the blood vessels revealing decreasing order of incidence of intracranial aneurysms?
   a. Anterior communicating, internal carotid, middle cerebral artery, and posterior circulation
   b. Anterior communicating, middle cerebral artery, internal carotid, posterior circulation
   c. Anterior communicating, posterior circulation, middle cerebral artery, internal carotid
   d. Anterior communicating, posterior circulation, internal carotid, middle cerebral artery

2. Pathogenetically brain damage can occur with SAH during the early brain injury (EBI) and delayed cerebral ischemia (DCI). The difference between the two pathogenetic mechanisms is:
   a. Both mechanisms are similar and mere continuation of the spectrum of pathogenetic mechanisms
   b. EBI is not described in spontaneous SAH and is only seen in traumatic SAH
   c. EBI is seen early and is a global process, while DCI is a more focal process occurring after 72 hours
   d. DCI is never seen in traumatic SAH

3. In the prevention of DCI which of the following statements is most true:
   a. Triple H therapy is recommended for preventing DCI
   b. Currently there is no way to treat DCI effectively
   c. Induced hypertension has shown to be beneficial in an RCT
   d. Maintaining euvolemia with the help of transpulmonary thermodilution technique is found to be more efficacious than CVP or fluid responsive based therapy in the prevention of DCI

4. Which one of the following is false regarding sodium balance in SAH?
   a. Both hypernatremia and hyponatremia are described in the course of the illness as a part of natural history
   b. Hypernatremia is associated with a higher mortality in SAH
   c. The nadir of hyponatremia is seen between days 6 and 12
   d. Hyponatremia can develop due to any of the central causes like SIADH, cerebral salt wasting glucocorticoid deficiency, hypovolemia, etc.

5. Amongst the various ECG changes in SAH, the most likely feature which is associated with higher mortality is:
   a. Sinus tachycardia
   b. ST-T changes
   c. QTc prolongation
   d. Peaked T wave inversion

6. A 60-year-old gentleman presented to ER with sudden onset of headache and confusion. At evaluation he was noted to have a GCS of E2M5V3. There were no lateralizing signs or cranial nerve involvement. Mild neck rigidity was noted. He was hemodynamically stable, but had a heart rate of 130/minute. ECG changes were as below:

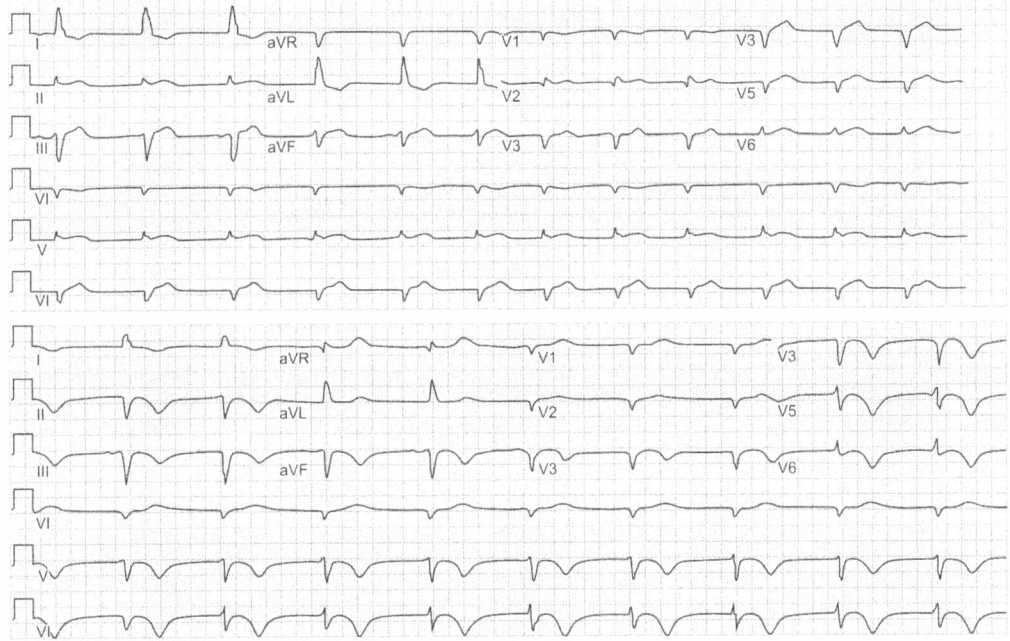

A screening echo was done which revealed EF of 40% with global LV dysfunction and apical ballooning. Troponin I was elevated. Cardiology opinion was sought. What will be your next course of action?
   a. Shift the patient for an urgent coronary angiogram
   b. Shift the patient for a CT brain
   c. Load the patient with antiplatelets
   d. Consider thrombolysis

7. A 50-year-old male presents with Grade 4 SAH due to a ruptured ACOM aneurysm. The family consent for a definitive procedure for repair of the ruptured aneurysm. Which of the following statements regarding the 2 modalities of therapy is false?
   a. Clipping has a greater incidence of rebleeding in comparison to endovascular repair

b. Patients with endovascular stenting had a better overall functional outcome than clipping
c. In patients with a poor clinical condition there is no proof to suggest that any of the modality is better
d. Morbidity is higher in surgical clipping due to want of a surgery to obtain control

8. Which of the following trials assessing magnesium as a therapeutic intervention does not test the efficacy of this drug for SAH patients?
   a. MASH
   b. IMASH
   c. MAGPIE
   d. FASTMAG

9. The following is true about measurement of flow velocities using transcranial Doppler (TCD):
   a. TCD can be measured in all patients with vasospasm
   b. Lindegaards index is the ratio of velocity of intracranial middle cerebral artery and extracranial external carotid artery
   c. Lindegaard index of more than 3 is highly specific to indicate vasospasm
   d. TCD uses a velocity of 3 MHz for its doppler signals

10. A 45-year-old male presented with Fischer Grade 4 SAH. He underwent endovascular coiling of the ruptured ACOM aneurysm day 3 of admission he developed sudden worsening of the GCS. What could be the most likely cause of his worsening?
    a. Hydrocephalus
    b. Seizures
    c. Early vasospasm
    d. All of the above

11. Which of the following statements is false regarding hydrocephalus as a consequence to SAH?
    a. Hydrocephalus can occur acutely or as a delayed complication
    b. Acute hydrocephalus can be managed acutely with temporary measures, while delayed hydrocephalus may need a more permanent diversion procedure
    c. Hydrocephalus is a very rare complication of SAH
    d. Sudden deterioration of GCS in the course of the illness, hydrocephalus could be one of the differentials

12. A 54-year-old gentleman, hypertensive, presented to ER at 11 am with a history of left-sided weakness of the upper and lower limbs. He was last noted to be normal the night before, after dinner. He woke up at 6 am with the left-sided hemiparesis. Initially taken to a nearby clinician dealing with alternative medicine, he was then referred to your hospital. CT brain showed a dense MCA sign on the right side. What is going to be your next course of action after stabilizing his airway breathing and circulation?
    a. Consider him for thrombolysis
    b. Commence on antiplatelets and other supportive measures

c. Perform a 4-vessel cerebral angiography and consider intervention if there is large vessel occlusion
d. Perform a diffusion-weighted MR and NIHSS score, if a mismatch exists in the presence of a large vessel occlusion consider him for mechanical thrombectomy

13. A 60-year-old gentleman developed sudden onset of slurring of speech and left-sided hemiparesis at 9 am. He was brought to the hospital emergency department by 1 pm. The delay happened as he was brought in his private vehicle and was held up in traffic. On evaluation in the ER, he was found to be having a dense left hemiplegia with a slurring of speech. A CT brain was done which revealed subtle hypodensities on the right side in the MCA territory in the frontoparietal region. An MRI was done with diffusion and flair was done which revealed a large infarct involving nearly half the hemisphere. The calculated NIHSS score was 25.
The medical facility did not have access to an interventional facility and the nearest facility was at least 6 hours away. What will be your next course of action?
a. Consider thrombolysis as he has arrived within the window period of 4.5 hours
b. Commence on antiplatelets and other supportive measures
c. No intervention and repeat an imaging of the brain after 24 hours
d. None of the above

14. A 40-year-old lady developed sudden onset of aphasia with right-sided hemiplegia. Within 1 hour, she presented to the ER of a nearby hospital. At presentation a stroke code was initiated. On examination she was found to be having a dense right hemiplegia with aphasia. She was found to be having a BP of 200/110 mm Hg. CT brain was performed which was normal. What action will you perform as the head of ER?
a. Immediate control of hypertension to target a BP of <185/100 mm Hg
b. Thrombolysis
c. Perform a digital substraction angiography and prepare for mechanical thrombectomy
d. None of the above

15. A 50-year-old gentleman, who is diabetic, presented to the ER from a peripheral town 8 hours following development of aphasia and right hemiplegia. Due to lack of facilities he was referred to a higher center in the metropolitan city. On admission in the ER, he was evaluated in the ER and found to be having a GCS of E1M5V1. He was also noted to be hypoxic due to pooling of secretions and was electively intubated for airway protection. Following stabilization he was taken up for a CT brain which showed a large left MCA infarction with a midline shift of 0.5 cm. The family has financial constraints and was keen to continue all measures only if he had a reasonable chance to survive with a reasonable quality of life. What will you tell the family regarding further direction of care?
a. Agree to their concerns and allow them to palliate the gentleman
b. Convince them and proceed with decompressive craniectomy
c. Continue all nonsurgical methods of therapy and intervention
d. Wait for 6 hours and repeat the CT after 6 hours

16. A 70-year-old gentleman presented with right hemiparesis. His presentation to the hospital was 8 hours after the onset of hemiparesis. He is a known case of coronary artery disease, hypertensive, and diabetic. His BP at presentation was 160/100 mm Hg. An MRI at admission revealed a small left basal ganglia infarct. MRA revealed a 90% occlusion of the left internal carotid artery. Antiplatelets were commenced. What is your next course of action?
    a. Discharge the patient on antiplatelets
    b. Plan for a carotid revascularization procedure at the earliest
    c. Control of hypertension
    d. None of the above

17. What is the next step in the management of this patient?

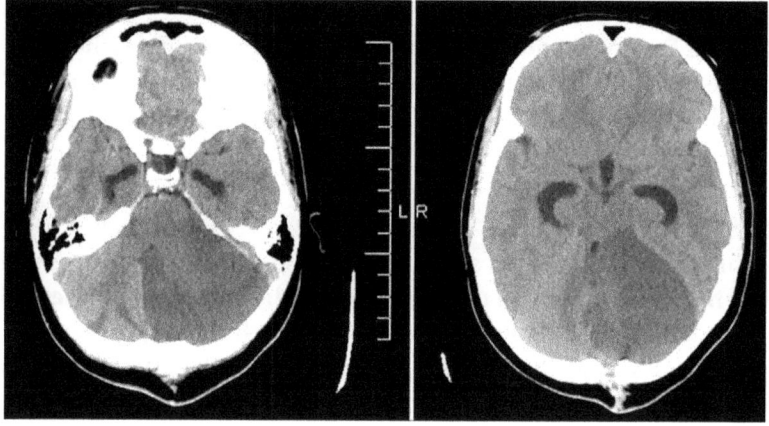

    a. Ventriculostomy
    b. Ventriculostomy with suboccipital craniectomy
    c. Ventriculostomy with suboccipital craniectomy only if no improvement happens in the sensorium, or further worsening happens
    d. None of the above

18. A 28-year-old lady on oral contraceptives presented to ER with left-sided headache and right hemiparesis. A CT scan performed showed an infarct in the high parieto-occipital infarct. A possibility of cerebral venous thrombosis was suspected and a CT venogram was done which confirmed the diagnosis revealing a thrombus in the posterior part of the superior sagittal sinus. Anticoagulation in the form of therapeutic dose of enoxaparin was commenced after relevant work up was sent. 48 hours later, patient has worsening of her weakness with a drop in the GCS to E3M6V3. An urgent CT is done reveals a slight increase in the size of the infarct with significant mass effect secondary to a hemorrhagic conversion. What will be your next step?
    a. Stop the anticoagulation
    b. Reduce the dose of anticoagulation
    c. Continue anticoagulation despite the hemorrhagic conversion
    d. Repeat a CT venogram

19. A 65-year-old patient presented to ER with a left-sided hypertensive gangliocapsular bleed. At presentation his BP is 220/140 mm Hg. What will be the systolic BP targets you would accept for this patient based on the current available literature?
    a. <130 mm Hg
    b. 140–160 mm Hg
    c. 160–180 mm Hg
    d. >180 mm Hg

20. A 29-year-woman had presented with a confused state after a sudden collapse at work in the last 6 hours. Her CT head noncontrast and DSA images were as above. She is transferred to the neurointensive care with a GCS of E3V4M6 (13/15). Consider the correct option out of the following:

    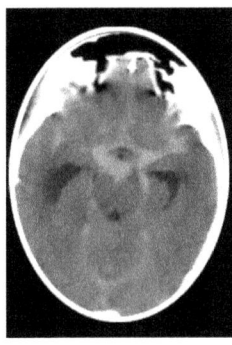 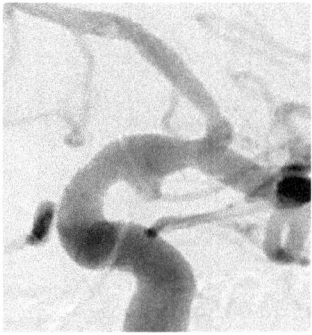

    a. The CT head is suggestive of an intracranial bleed
    b. Tranexamic acid is useful in prevention of rebleeding in early presenting cases
    c. Preferred definitive treatment is surgical clipping of the aneurysm than endovascular treatment
    d. Nimodipine 60 mg every 4 hours per oral route must be started immediately
    e. She could get delayed cerebral vasospasm until further 07 days

21. A 58-year-old male presented to emergency with right-sided weakness, headache, and history of collapse. In the ED he was conscious, oriented with right hemiparesis.

    Blood pressure was elevated to 188/95 mm Hg whilst other parameters were normal. CT head noncontrast and CT angiography shown as above. Consider the correct option out of the following in this patient's further treatment:

    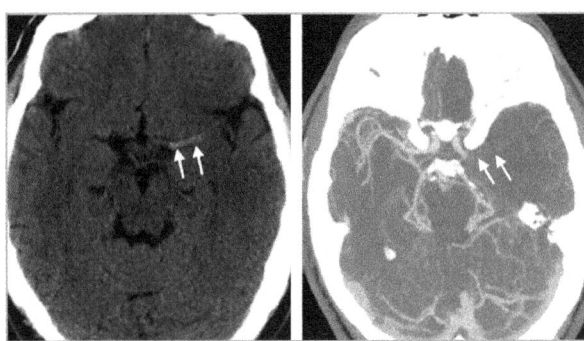

a. IV thrombolysis is contraindicated due to intracerebral bleed seen on the CT
b. Mechanical thrombectomy with bridging thrombolysis is most suited
c. Scan shows a hypodense MCA sign due to clot in the left MCA
d. The above scan and finding is associate with poor outcome
e. It would be prudent to lower the presenting blood pressure

22. A 64-year-old is ventilated in neuro-ICU for 6 days post intracerebral hematoma. He has suffered two seizure episodes for which he is on appropriate anticonvulsants. His serum sodium is 118 mmol/L. Which one of following is likely toward the diagnosis of SIADH?

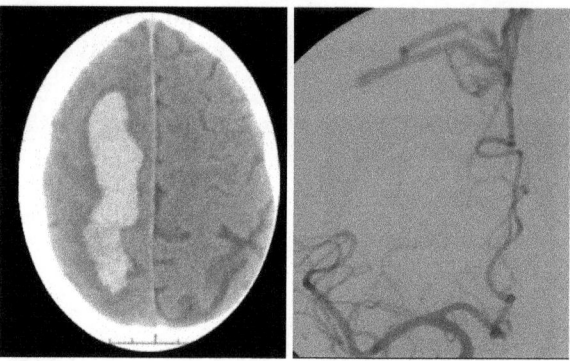

a. Urinary Na less than 18 mmol/L
b. Treatment by water restriction
c. Plasma osmolarity greater than urinary osmolarity
d. Pitting edema
e. Hypovolemia is likely in this case

23. A 63-year-old female is 4 days post admission in the neurocritical care unit after presenting with a right-sided stroke, which was outside the window period. She is currently ventilated and the noncontrast CT Head is as above. Choose the best option:

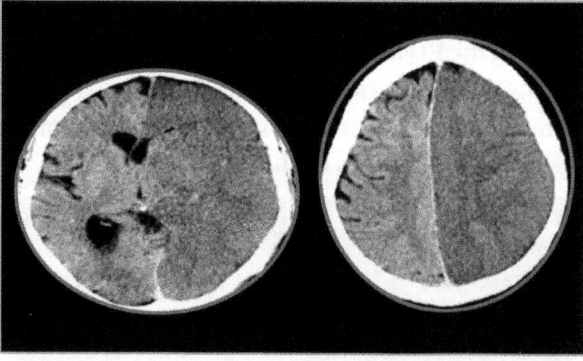

a. CT shows a complete right internal carotid artery infarction
b. There are signs of raised ICP on the right side
c. An urgent decompressive craniectomy should be considered on the left side
d. Decompressive craniectomy is likely to improve outcome
e. Medical management with hypertonic saline is a better treatment option

24. A 51-year-old male with known atrial fibrillation, diabetes mellitus, and hypertension presents with inability to balance, slurred speech and ataxia of 4 hours duration. The most appropriate treatment option for clinical suspicion of acute thrombotic stroke of a major intracranial vessel is:
    a. Immediate thrombolysis by paramedics or in triage
    b. Only thrombolysis once CT head confirms thrombotic stroke
    c. Bridging thrombolysis and thrombectomy after CT head confirms thrombotic stroke
    d. Only mechanical thrombectomy once CT head confirms thrombotic stroke
    e. Blood alcohol levels, IV fluids, and monitoring in HDU

25. A 54-year-old male recovered from a decompressive craniectomy which was performed for severe intracranial edema and raised ICP after his admission for ischemic stroke. At his 12 months follow-up visit, he is independent for his daily activities within the house, but is not fully recovered to join back work. Which of the following best describes his Glasgow Outcome Scale (GOS)?
    a. GOS 1
    b. GOS 2
    c. GOS 3
    d. GOS 4
    e. GOS 5

26. An 18-year-old presents with a history of recurrent TIAs over the preceding 9 months. The blood investigations and all cardiac investigations were normal. The MRI and DSA images show the following abnormalities. What is the most likely diagnosis from the MRA and DSA image given below?

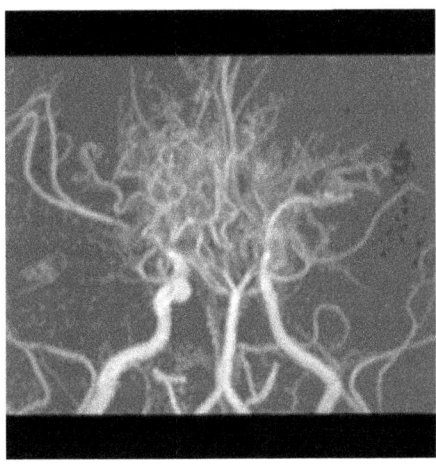
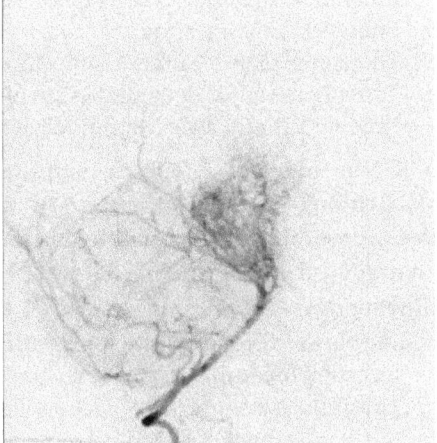

    a. Moya-Moya disease
    b. Intracranial aneurysm
    c. TB vasculitis
    d. Meningitis
    e. None of the above

27. A 46-year-old male was brought to ED after he collapsed at work complaining of sudden onset severe headache. On arrival to the ED the GCS was E1V1M2 with bilaterally reacting pupils. The CT head and angiography (as below) images revealed extensive Fischer Grade-4 subarachnoid hemorrhage with intraventricular extension. There was a basilar tip aneurysm along with other multiple intracranial aneurysm. The most realistic treatment strategy for this patient is:

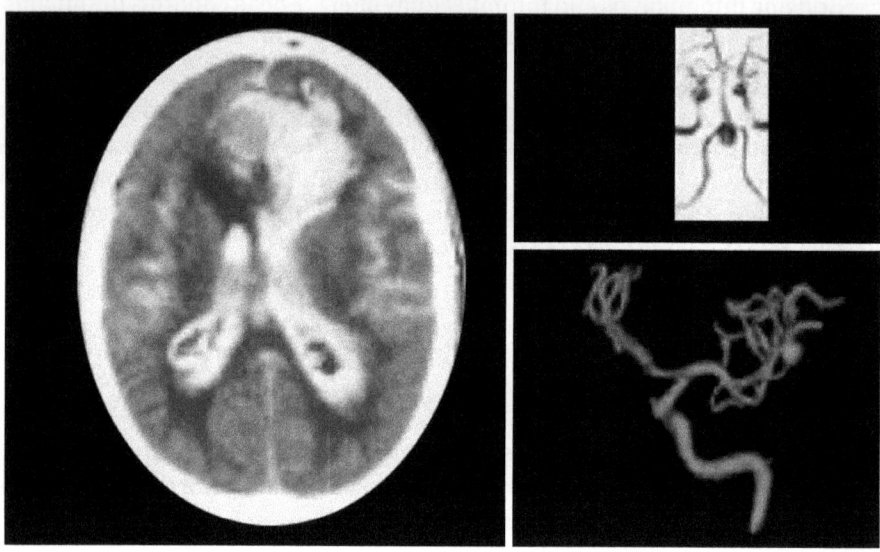

   a. Immediate decompressive craniectomy
   b. Brainstem death testing
   c. Transfer to DSA for urgent multiple coilings
   d. Transfer to OT for decompression and multiple clippings
   e. Urgent EVD and await neurological assessment for further definitive treatment

28. A 37-year-old school teacher is in the neurological ward on her day 11 post a left MCA coiling. She was admitted with an SAH following aneurysmal rupture earlier. She recovered well and had been transferred to the ward 2 days ago without any neurological deficit. She started complaining of weakness of her right upper limb and slurring of speech. A noncontrast CT head did not show any changes from the post coiling earlier CT scans. The most rational treatment plan would be:
   a. Insertion of lumbar drain for suspected hydrocephalus
   b. Thrombolysis for possible Ischemic stroke
   c. Induced hypertension and urgent cerebral angiography for possible cerebral vasospasm
   d. Urgent decompressive craniectomy for likely raised ICP
   e. Neurorehabilitation and speech therapy referral for assessment and treatment

29. The above patient has both TCD and DSA done on an urgent basics. According to the following images of TCD and DSA, pick the correct statement:

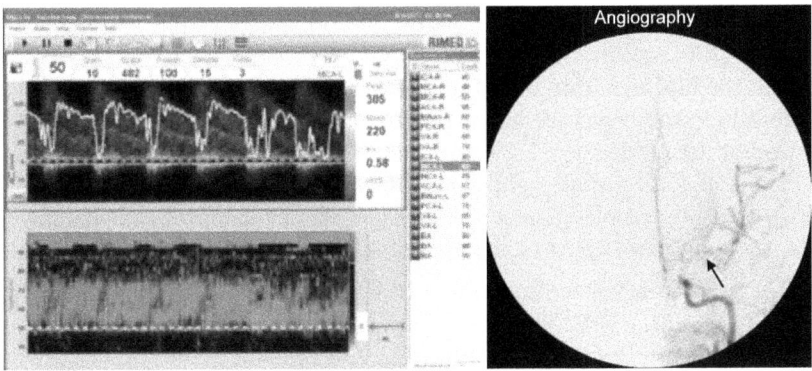

a. Image of DSA and TCD indicate MCA spasm
b. Milrinone is the recommended drug to be used for cerebral vasodilatation
c. Patient is likely to have left sided weakness
d. Nimodipine 60 mg every 6 hours is indicated
e. The above images do not explain the symptoms of the patient

30. An 18-year-old male is on his day 10 in the neuro-ICU after sustaining a diffuse axonal injury following a road traffic collision which resulted in an isolated head injury. He is on an appropriate type and dose of NG feed which is being well absorbed. He is being ventilated on a weaning strategy via a tracheostomy. The plan for stress ulcer prophylaxis for the given clinical scenario would be:
    a. Stress ulcer prophylaxis is indicated due to admission in neuro-ICU
    b. Ventilation is a risk factor for GI bleed and indicates stress ulcer prophylaxis
    c. Incidence of upper GI bleeding in neuro-ICU is declining, so none required
    d. Stress ulcer prophylaxis should be stopped as enteral feed is fully established
    e. TPN is indicated as a long-term measure for nutritional support

31. A patient admitted with WFNS Grade 2 SAH develops hydrocephalus over the 48 hours of admission to the hospital. The neurosurgical team decides to insert an external ventricular drain (EVD). Regarding EVD in neuro-ICU, pick the correct statement:
    a. Does not accurately monitor ICP
    b. Zero mark should be at the level of the external auditory meatus
    c. Should never be clamped
    d. Is an uncommon cause of CNS infection
    e. Inserted in operating rooms has better outcomes than ICU insertion

32. A 68-year-old man is admitted with right-sided weakness. CT head confirms a left MCA thrombotic stroke and he is started on a bridging thrombolysis with tPA and also being taken up for mechanical thrombectomy. His NIHSS score is 19 and he is uncooperative on the DSA table. Pick the correct statement regarding the anesthetic management of the patient:
    a. GA is contraindicated
    b. Sedation has better outcome
    c. Invasive monitoring is usually required intraoperatively
    d. Postoperative ventilation is a predictor of poor outcome
    e. Postoperative monitoring with tanscranial Doppler improves outcome

33. The treatment of aneurysmal SAH was revolutionized following the ISAT (International Subarachnoid Treatment) study in 2003 and 2005 worldwide. Pick the correct option based on the findings from the ISAT study:
    a. Landmark study revolutionizing the treatment of traumatic SAH
    b. Absolute risk reduction of 7.4% at 1 year mortality favoring Coiled vs. Clipped aneurysms
    c. Intraprocedural rupture greater in coiling than with clipping
    d. Post procedure rebleeding at first year greater with clipping than coiling
    e. Long-term follow-up was a strength of this trial

34. A neurology resident wishes to calculate the NIHSS score on a recently admitted patient of stroke. Regarding NIHSS Score please pick the correct statement:
    a. Tool to quantify the impairment caused by a Brain SOL
    b. 11 items carrying a score of 0–4 for each
    c. Maximum possible score is 44
    d. Score of 0 indicates abnormal function or death
    e. It is not a validated tool for predicting patient outcome

35. Nimodipine is commonly used in the treatment of patients with SAH. Pick the most appropriate statement regarding the drug and its relevant use in SAH:
    a. Poor evidence for treating post aneurysmal SAH vasospasm
    b. Best administered IV for vasospasm treatment
    c. Binds specifically to L type voltage-gated calcium channels
    d. Beneficial effects cease after 7 days post ictus
    e. Should be administered after definitive treatment of the aneurysm

36. A phenytoin loading dose was erroneously given as a bolus to a patient rather than an infusion. Which statement is most appropriate?
    a. Acute sodium channel blockade causes wide QRS complexes
    b. Patient is prone to ventricular dysrhythmias
    c. Sodium bicarbonate is indicated
    d. Cerebellar features are seen in phenytoin toxicity
    e. All of the above

37. A patient admitted post 2nd day clipping of intracranial aneurysm is in the ICU. Poor neurological recovery prompts an EEG which is shown as below. Pick the most appropriate diagnosis from the EEG:

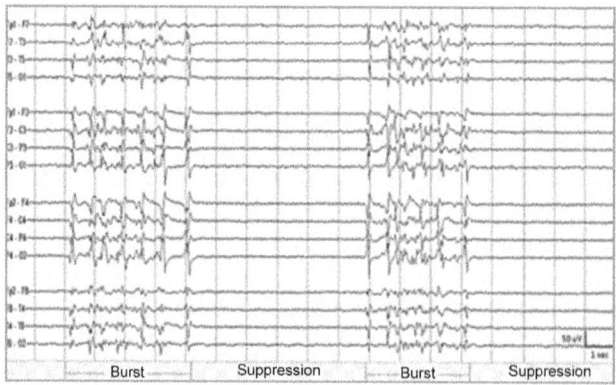

State the diagnosis from the EEG Strip:
a. Status epilepticus
b. Brain dead
c. Burst suppression
d. Normal brain
e. None of the above

38. The following are the CT image and the microdialysis graph of a patient admitted with SAH in the neuro-ICU. Pick the incorrect statement regarding microdialysis in this patient:

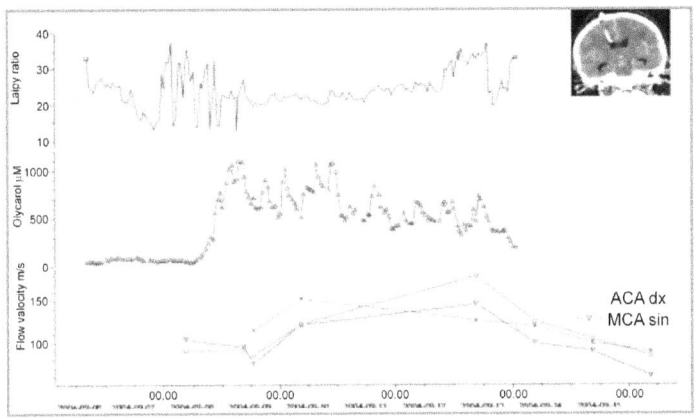

Microdialysis Graph: Lactate/pyruvate ratio; Glycerol and TCD Flow Velocity
a. Indicates normal brain activity
b. Indicates ischemia as seen by the suddenly rising lactate/pyruvate ratio above normal levels from initial downward trend
c. Dramatic increase in glycerol indicates brain damage
d. TCD flow velocity shows spasm much later than the biomarkers
e. Tip of the EVD is seen in the ventricles in the CT

39. Which is the most appropriate statement for the following graph with cerebral blood flow in mL/100 g/min on the y axis:

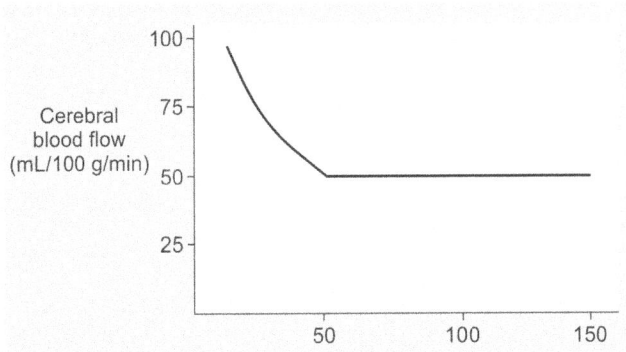

a. Depicts relation between cerebral blood flow arterial paCO$_2$
b. Depicts relation between intracranial pressure and cerebral volume
c. Depicts relation between cerebral blood flow and arterial pO$_2$
d. Depicts autoregulation of cerebral blood flow and MAP

40. **The presence of "Plateau Wave" on the ICP trace suggests:**
    a. Sudden surges in ICP to 50–80 mm Hg lasting 5–20 minutes
    b. Smaller surges in ICP to 20 mm Hg for 1–2 minutes
    c. Failing compliance of the brain to ICP and risk for ischemia
    d. Interference artefact
    e. None of the above

41. **All of the following are risk factors for a poor outcome in post aneurysmal subarachnoid hemorrhage (SAH), *except*:**
    a. Male sex
    b. Presence of comorbid conditions
    c. Posterior circulation aneurysm
    d. World Federation of Neurosurgeons (WFNS) grade IV
    e. Multiple aneurysms

42. **Proven therapies in the management of vasospasm for SAH include all of the following, *except*:**
    a. Triple H therapy
    b. Oral nimodipine
    c. Antifibrinolytics
    d. Balloon angioplasty
    e. IV milrinone with intra-arterial vasodilatation

43. **For overall management of SAH patients, pick the most appropriate statement:**
    a. The ISAT study demonstrated a better outcome for Clipped vs. Coiled aneurysms
    b. The overall case mortality for SAH is 10%
    c. Intraoperative hypothermia improves neurological outcome
    d. CT is 100% sensitive in detecting aneurysms
    e. Best results are at tertiary centers

44. **Regarding hyperacute thrombotic stroke service, pick the most appropriate statement:**
    a. IV thrombolysis has better results than mechanical thrombectomy (MT)
    b. Combined IV thrombolysis and mechanical thrombectomy has best results
    c. MT has a higher procedural mortality than thrombolysis
    d. MT is only useful for distal clots
    e. IV thrombolysis is better for large vessel clots

ANSWERS

1. **Ans. (a)**

   Gasparotti R, Liserre R. Intracranial aneurysms. Eur Radiol. 2005;15:441-7

   Eighty-five percent of saccular aneurysms arise from the arteries of the circle of Willis. The most frequent location is the anterior communicating artery (35%), followed by the internal carotid artery (30%—including the carotid artery itself, the posterior communicating artery, and the ophthalmic artery), the middle cerebral artery (22%), and finally, the posterior circulation sites, most commonly the basilar artery tip. Multiple aneurysms are found in approximately 30% of patients.

2. **Ans. (b)**

   Geraghty JR, Testai FD. Delayed cerebral ischemia after subarachnoid hemorrhage: beyond vasospasm and towards a multifactorial pathophysiology. Curr Atheroscler Rep. 2017;19:50.

   Kusaka G, Ishikawa M, Nanda A, et al. Signaling pathways for early brain injury after subarachnoid hemorrhage. J Cereb Blood Flow Metab. 2004;24:916-25.

   A concept of early brain injury (EBI) for the immediate brain injury during the first 72 hours after the hemorrhage has been proposed. EBI is another factor that affects neurological outcome. Aneurysmal rupture leads to transient global ischemia, which is caused by increasing intracranial pressure, decreasing cerebral perfusion pressure, and decreasing cerebral blood flow, and toxic activity of the subarachnoid hemorrhage. These mechanisms induce multifactorial derangement, such as microcirculatory constriction, endothelial cell apoptosis, blood–brain barrier disruption, brain edema, and thromboinflammatory cascade.

   Although a clear picture of DCI remains unknown, several pathophysiological mechanisms contribute to development of DCI. These mechanisms are cerebral vascular dysregulation, including cerebral vasospasm and microcirculatory dysfunction, microthrombosis, cortical spreading depolarization, and neuroinflammation.

3. **Ans. (b)**

   Meyer R, Deem S, Yanez ND, et al. Current practices of triple-H prophylaxis and therapy in patients with subarachnoid hemorrhage. Neurocrit Care. 2011;14:24-36.

   Steiner T, Juvela S, Unterberg A, et al. European Stroke Organization guidelines for the management of intracranial aneurysms and subarachnoid haemorrhage. Cerebrovasc Dis. 2013;35:93-112.

   Gathier CS, van den Bergh WM, van der Jagt M, et al. Induced hypertension for delayed cerebral ischemia after aneurysmal subarachnoid hemorrhage: a randomized clinical trial. Stroke. 2018;49:76-83.

   Monnet X, Teboul JL. Transpulmonary thermodilution: advantages and limits. Crit Care. 2017;21:147.

   Tagami T, Kuwamoto K, Watanabe A, et al. Effect of triple-H prophylaxis on global end-diastolic volume and clinical outcomes in patients with aneurysmal subarachnoid hemorrhage. Neurocrit Care. 2014;21:462-9.

Mutoh T, Kazumata K, Terasaka S, et al. Early intensive versus minimally invasive approach to postoperative hemodynamic management after subarachnoid hemorrhage. Stroke. 2014;45:1280-4.

Current evidence does not support use of triple H therapy. Based on several case series, induced hypertension was a highly anticipated intervention for patients with DCI. An RCT was designed to evaluate the effectiveness of induced hypertension which was terminated prematurely because of its ineffectiveness for cerebral perfusion and slow recruitment. Currently, there is no way to treat DCI definitively. Appropriate interventions, including induced hypertension and endovascular treatment, are recommended based on the needs of individual patients. It is difficult to accurately evaluate volume status and maintain normovolemia. Several studies have reported the utility of transpulmonary thermodilution (TPTD) in SAH management. An RCT was performed to assess the efficacy of TPTD-based management compared with fluid balance or central venous pressure-guided management. However, TPTD-based management neither decreased DCI nor improved functional outcomes.

4. **Ans. (b)**
Okazaki T, Hifumi T, Kawakita K, et al. Target serum sodium levels during intensive care unit management of aneurysmal subarachnoid hemorrhage. Shock. 2017;48:558-63.

Uozumi Y, Mizobe T, Miyamoto H, et al. Decreased serum sodium levels predict symptomatic vasospasm in patients with subarachnoid hemorrhage. J Clin Neurosci. 2017;46:118-23.

Hyponatremia is associated with a greater mortality in SAH while hypernatremia has no bearing on mortality. The threshold of hyponatremia associated with poor neurological outcomes was addressed in a retrospective observational study involving 131 patients. In this study, multiple regression analysis showed that minimum sodium levels in the ICU were associated with unfavorable neurological outcomes at hospital discharge, and receiver operating characteristics curve analysis derived a cutoff value of 132 mmol/L.

5. **Ans. (c)**
Zhang L, Qi S. Electrocardiographic abnormalities predict adverse clinical outcomes in patients with subarachnoid hemorrhage. J Stroke Cerebrovasc Dis. 2016;25:2653-9.
Prolongation of QTc was associated with neurologic pulmonary edema and delayed cerebral ischemia (DCI), ST depression with hospital death, nonspecific ST-T changes with neurologic pulmonary edema, delayed cerebral ischemia, and death.

6. **Ans. (b)**
Abd TT, Hayek S, Cheng JW, et al. Incidence and clinical characteristics of takotsubo cardiomyopathy post-aneurysmal subarachnoid hemorrhage. Int J Cardiol. 2014;176:1362-4.
Tsuchihashi K, Ueshima K, Uchida T, et al. Transient left ventricular apical ballooning without coronary artery stenosis: a novel heart syndrome mimicking acute myocardial infarction. Angina Pectoris-Myocardial Infarction Investigations in Japan. J Am Coll Cardiol. 2001;38:11-8.

Since the patient has presented with altered sensorium and unexplained drop in GCS, a CT brain will be warranted Takotsubo cardiomyopathy, also known as stress-induced cardiomyopathy, broken heart syndrome or apical ballooning syndrome was reported in about 0.8-4.5% of patients with SAH. It is defined as reversible LVD, electrocardiographic changes and myocardial enzymes release mimicking myocardial infarction (MI) in the absence of obstructive coronary artery disease. Takotsubo cardiomyopathy is caused by high catecholamine release following acute emotional or physical stresse. The characteristics of these SAH patients are different from those of other patients with Takotsubo cardiomyopathy in other contexts: they are younger and always present with signs of heart failure and no chest pain. Thus, it is defined as neurogenic stress cardiomyopathy (NSC) or stunned myocardium. The mortality of these patients is about 25% higher than 1% of patients with Takotsubo cardiomyopathy, and it could be explained by the impact of severe associated neurological comorbidities first. ECG changes are seen in over 60% of patients with SAH.

7. **Ans. (a)**
   Lindgren A, Vergouwen MD, van der Schaaf I, et al. Cochrane Database of Systematic Reviews Endovascular coiling versus neurosurgical clipping for people with aneurysmal subarachnoid haemorrhage (Review). Endovascular coiling versus neurosurgical clipping for people with aneurysmal subarachnoid haemorrhage. Cochrane Database Syst Rev. 2018;8:CD003085.
   Coiling is known to have a better outcome in terms of functional recovery in comparison to clipping when done in patients presenting with a more stable clinical condition. The risk of rebleeding is higher in endovascular therapy, as compared to coiling. However, in patients presenting with a poor outcome both have similar outcomes.

8. **Ans. (c)**
   MAGPIE tests magnesium as a therapeutic intervention for preeclampsia.

9. **Ans. (b)**
   Transcranial Doppler is possible in only 75% of patients. Lindegaard specificity l is better with higher values. A cut off of more than 6 is highly specific to suggest vasospasm. TCD uses a low frequency probe of 2 MHz.

10. **Ans. (d)**

11. **Ans. (c)**
    Hydrocephalus is fairly common seen with an incidence of 15-80%. It can happen acutely or as a delayed complication with the needing a more permanent procedure.

12. **Ans. (d)**
    Nogueira RG, Jadhav AP, Haussen DC, et al. DAWN Trial Investigators. Thrombectomy 6 to 24 hours after stroke with a mismatch between deficit and infarct [published online ahead of print November 11, 2017]. N Engl J MedM. doi: 10.1056/NEJMoa1706442.
    Albers GW, Marks MP, Kemp S, et al. DEFUSE 3 Investigators. Thrombectomy for stroke with perfusion imaging selection at 6-16 hours. N Engl J Med.2018;378:708-18.

The DAWN trial used clinical imaging mismatch (a combination of NIHSS score and imaging findings on CTP or DW-MRI) as eligibility criteria to select patients with large anterior circulation vessel occlusion for treatment with mechanical thrombectomy between 6 hours and 24 hours from last known normal. This trial demonstrated an overall benefit in function outcome at 90 days in the treatment group (mRS score 0-2, 49% versus 13%; adjusted difference, 33%; 95% CI, 21-44; posterior probability of superiority >0.999).

The DEFUSE 3 trial used perfusion-core mismatch and maximum core size as imaging criteria to select patients with large anterior circulation occlusion 6-16 hours from last seen well for mechanical thrombectomy. This trial showed a benefit in functional outcome at 90 days in the treated group (mRS score 0-2, 44.6% versus 16.7%; RR, 2.67; 95% CI, 1.60-4.48; P<0.0001).109. DAWN and DEFUSE 3 are the only RCTs showing benefit of mechanical thrombectomy >6 hours from onset. Therefore, as of now, only the eligibility criteria from these trials should be used for patient selection.

13. **Ans. (b)**

    Hacke W, Donnan G, Fieschi C, et al. ATLANTIS Trials Investigators; ECASS Trials Investigators; NINDS rt-PA Study Group Investigators. Association of outcome with early stroke treatment: pooled analysis of ATLANTIS, ECASS, and NINDS rt-PA stroke trials. Lancet. 2004;363:768-74.

    Though, the patient has presented within the extended window period of 3-4.5 hours, it is a large stroke with a very NIHSS score. So he is not an ideal candidate for thrombolysis. If he was in a center with expertise available for endovascular intervention, he could have been considered as a candidate for mechanical thrombectomy.

14. **Ans. (a)**

    Patient eligible for thrombolysis or mechanical thrombectomy need to have the BP immediately reduced to a systolic BP <185 mm Hg and diastolic BP <110 mm Hg. This can be achieved emergently through a combination of IV or oral agents and the BP targets should be maintained so over the next 24 hours to prevent risk of hemorrhage.

15. **Ans. (b)**

    Vahedi K, Hofmeijer J, Juettler E, et al. DECIMAL, DESTINY, and HAMLET Investigators. Early decompressive surgery in malignant infarction of the middle cerebral artery: a pooled analysis of three randomised controlled trials. Lancet Neurol. 2007;6:215-22.

    The pooled results of RCTs demonstrated significant reduction in mortality when decompressive craniectomy was performed within 48 hours of malignant MCA infarction in patients <60 years of age, with an absolute risk reduction in mortality of 50% (95% CI, 34-66) at 12 months. These findings were noted despite differences in the clinical trials in terms of inclusion and exclusion criteria, percent of MCA territory involved, and surgical timing. At 12 months, moderate disability (ability to walk) or better (mRS score 2 or 3) was achieved in 43% (22 of 51) of the total surgical group and 55% (22 of 40) of survivors compared with 21% (9 of 42; P = 0.045) of the total nonsurgical group and 75% (9 of 12; P = 0.318) of the nonsurgical survivors. At 12 months, independence (mRS score 2) was achieved in 14% (7 of 51) of the total surgical group and 18% (7 of 40) of survivors compared with 2% (1 of 42) of the total nonsurgical group and 8% (1 of 12) of the nonsurgical survivors.

16. Ans. (b)

    Ois A, Cuadrado-Godia E, Rodríguez-Campello A, et al. High risk of early neurological recurrence in symptomatic carotid stenosis. Stroke. 2009;40:2727-31.

    De Rango P, Brown MM, Chaturvedi S, et al. Summary of evidence on early carotid intervention for recently symptomatic stenosis based on meta-analysis of current risks. Stroke. 2015;46:3423-36.

    Johansson EP, Arnerlöv C, Wester P. Risk of recurrent stroke before carotid endarterectomy: the ANSYSCAP study. Int J Stroke. 2013;8:220-7.

    Past data have indicated that the risk of recurrent stroke caused by symptomatic carotid stenosis is highest early after the initial event. Although there is evidence that early or emergency revascularization via either CEA or carotid angioplasty and stenting may be safe in selected cases, there are no high-quality prospective data supporting early versus late carotid revascularization in all cases. Revascularization between 48 hours and 7 days after initial stroke is supported by the data in cases of nondisabling stroke (mRS score 0-2). Imaging within 24 hours of admission is feasible and recommended to facilitate CEA/carotid angioplasty and stenting in eligible patients in the 48- to 72-hour window.

17. Ans. (c)

    Raco A, Caroli E, Isidori A, et al. Management of acute cerebellar infarction: one institution's experience. Neurosurgery. 2003;53:1061-605.

    Ventriculostomy is a well-recognized effective treatment for the management of acute obstructive hydrocephalus and is often effective in isolation in relieving symptoms, even among patients with acute ischemic cerebellar stroke. Thus, in patients who develop symptoms of obstructive hydrocephalus from a cerebellar stroke, emergency ventriculostomy is a reasonable first step in the surgical management paradigm. If cerebrospinal diversion by ventriculostomy fails to improve neurological function, decompressive suboccipital craniectomy should be performed. Although a risk of upward herniation exists with ventriculostomy alone, it can be minimized with conservative cerebrospinal fluid drainage or subsequent decompression if the cerebellar infarct causes significant edema or mass effect.

18. Ans. (c)

    Despite the hemorrhagic conversion, anticoagulation is not stopped in this setting of a venous infarct as the mechanism of hemorrhage is different related to increased venous back pressure.

19. Ans. (b)

    Anderson CS, Heeley E, Huang Y, et al.; INTERACT2 Investigators. Rapid blood-pressure lowering in patients with acute intracerebral hemorrhage. N Engl J Med. 2013;368: 2355-65.

Qureshi AI, Palesch YY, Barsan WG, et al.; ATACH-2 Trial Investigators and the Neurological Emergency Treatment Trials Network. Intensive blood- pressure lowering in patients with acute cerebral hemorrhage. N Engl J Med. 2016;375:1033-43.

Aggressive control of BP was recommended by INTERACT 2. But subsequently a subgroup analysis of INTERACT 2 and ATACH 2 showed that a very aggressive BP control resulted in increased risk of acute kidney injury. Hence optimal BP of 140–160 mm Hg in patients with hypertensive intracranial bleeds.

20. **Ans. (d)**

Connolly ES, Rabinstein AA, Carhuapoma JR, et al. Guidelines for the management of aneurysmal subarachnoid hemorrhage stroke. 2012;43(6):1711-37.

The risk factors for poor outcome in SAH include female sex, WFNS grade 4, multiple aneurysms, posterior circulation aneurysms, low presenting GCS, delayed presentation, and presence of major comorbidities. SAH is a neurological condition with high morbidity and mortality and usually half of the patients do not reach hospital alive. Of the remaining at least 20% end up with complications especially from delayed cerebral vasospasm which can happen up to 2 weeks post ictus. Tranexamic acid has shown some benefit in prevention of rebleeding in aneurysms that are presenting late. The ones that present early after rupture, tranexamic has no role in preventing rebleeding.

Triple therapy and oral nimodipine are proven therapies for SAH management and are recommended in the 2012 ASA/AHA guidelines. Angioplasty and IV milrinone are performed for vasospasm treatment in some centers of the world but its benefit is not consistent and is currently not a universally recommended and acceptable treatment as per the international guidelines.

21. **Ans. (b)**

Palaniswami M, Yan B. Mechanical thrombectomy is now the gold standard for acute ischemic stroke: implications for routine clinical practice. Interv Neurol. 2015;4(1-2):18-29.

The images show the classical left MCA "Dot Sign" due to the presence of a thrombus in the left MCA. The sign is hyperdense not hypodense.

Mechanical thrombectomy and bridging thrombolysis are the most effective treatment nowadays for acute ischemic stroke done as part of hyperacute stroke service. The clinical outcomes are getting better with good mRS scores of at least 40% in the best reported studies. The blood pressure should not be lowered to allow collaterals to flow until the offending vessel is restored.

22. **Ans. (b)**

Bersten AD, Soni N. Oh's Intensive Care Manual, 5th edition. Burlington, MA: Butterworth Heinemann; 2003.

In SIADH, there is serum hyponatremia with fluid retention and increased urinary sodium excretion. The serum osmolarity is normal to low while the urine osmolarity is raised. It is a volume-loaded state and the treatment is fluid restriction. The only way to differentiate from cerebral salt wasting is clinically judging the volume status in each, as the latter is a volume-depleted state.

23. **Ans. (c)**
    Bansal H, Chaudhary A, Singh A, et al. Decompressive craniectomy in malignant middle cerebral artery infarct: an institutional experience. Asian J Neurosurg. 2015;10(3);203-6.

    Computed tomography shows malignant left ICA infarction and edema of the left side with midline shift. Malignant ischemic strokes presenting outside the window period may result in severe cerebral edema of the affected side. Hypertonic saline is increasingly being preferred over mannitol to reduce the pressure effects. However, in this case time has passed for any medical management due to signs of raised ICP. Decompressive craniectomy is required for the cerebral edema to resolve. It however has shown increased survival without increasing functional outcome in some of the latest reported studies.

24. **Ans. (c)**
    Muralidharan R. External ventricular drains: management and complications. Surgical Neurology International. 2015;6(Suppl 6):S271-S274.

    Bridging thrombolysis and thrombectomy after CT head confirms thrombotic stroke.

    Once a hemorrhage is ruled out by the CT head and a thrombotic major vessel stroke identified with a CTA, bridging thrombolysis is started immediately and the patient is shifted to the intervention laboratory for a mechanical thrombectomy. If the thrombotic stroke is a small vessel distal stroke, then thrombolysis is still given and patient is reviewed for resolution of symptoms and considered for thrombectomy. Recent trials have confirmed that the best outcome after thrombotic stroke is via both a bridging thrombolysis and mechanical thrombectomy for major vessel strokes, rather than the two options practiced individually in isolation.

25. **Ans. (e)**
    Weir J, Steyerberg EW, Butcher I, et al. Does the extended Glasgow Outcome Scale add value to the conventional Glasgow Outcome Scale? J Neurotrauma. 2012;29(1):53-8.

    Glasgow Outcome Scale of 5 indicates full independence for in-house daily activities but not returned to work.

    Glasgow Outcome Scale is a clinical tool used to categorize the outcome of patients after traumatic head injury as follows:
    1. Death
    2. Persistent vegetative state with minimal response
    3. Severe disability
    4. Moderate disability
    5. Good recovery.

26. **Ans. (a)**
    Tarasów E, Kułakowska A, Łukasiewicz A, et al. Moya-moya disease: diagnostic imaging. Polish Journal of Radiology. 2011;76(1):73-9.

    Moya-Moya Disease. "Puff of Smoke appearance" on DSA and MRA images.

    Moya-Moya is a rare CNS disease in which the CNS arteries are blocked at the base of the brain. This results in clusters of tiny vessels trying to compensate for the blockage giving ITA typical "puff of smoke appearance" which mean Moya-Moya in Japanese. The patient presents with recurrent TIAs and strokes. Whilst it cannot be cured, endovascular treatment or surgery provides good results, by providing alternate blood flow.

27. **Ans. (e)**

   Connolly ES, Rabinstein AA, Carhuapoma JR, et al. Guidelines for the management of aneurysmal subarachnoid hemorrhage: a guideline for healthcare professionals from the American Heart Association/American Stroke Association. Stroke. 2012;43(6):1711-37.

   There is a basilar tip aneurysm on the DSA image and also seen are multiple aneurysms. The Fischer grade on the CT head is Grade 4 because there is extensive intraventricular blood from the SAH. The WFNS classification also has it as Grade 4 SAH as the patient is likely to be in a comatosed state. Most urgent rational treatment is to insert an EVD to drain CSF and monitor ICP. The prognosis is extremely poor and most centers await some neurological recovery before performing any definitive procedure.

28. **Ans. (c)**

29. **Ans. (a)**

   Connolly ES, Rabinstein AA, Carhuapoma JR, et al. Guidelines for the Management of Aneurysmal Subarachnoid Hemorrhage Stroke. 2012;43(6):1711-37.

   (For Q. 28 and Q. 29) The image is of DSA and TCD indicating MCA spasm. In the TCD there is increased peak velocity in the MCA segment whilst the MCA shows severe spasm on the actual DSA run. Milrinone is likely to be used for cerebral vasodilatation although there is no level-1 evidence for its use. It is a common practice in some Canadian and North American centers. The patient is likely to have right-sided weakness. Nimodipine 60 mg every 4 hours is indicated and has level-1 evidence for its use, from as soon as the patient is admitted.

30. **Ans.(d)**

   Cook DJ, Griffith LE, Walter SD, et al. The attributable mortality and length of intensive care unit stay of clinically important gastrointestinal bleeding in critically ill patients. Critical Care. 2001;5(6):368-75.

   All patients admitted to neurocritical care do not require stress ulcer prophylaxis. Only patients at risk require gastric protection and they are patients on ventilation, renal support or the ones who are coagulopathic or with previous history of gastric ulcers. The incidence of upper GI bleeding in neuro-ICU patients is declining over the years due to better ICU care and better treatment of *Helicobacter pylori*. Stress ulcer prophylaxis should be stopped as soon as enteral feed is established. The H2 receptor antagonists can cause encephalopathy in rare cases.

31. **Ans. (b)**

   Muralidharan R. External ventricular drains: management and complications. Surgical Neurology International. 2015;6(Suppl 6):S271-S274.

   External ventricular drain insertion in neuro-ICU is one of the most important interventions. It is also one of the most important measures to monitor ICP and reduce elevated ICP by CSF drainage. The EVD catheter should be zeroed and placed at the level of the "Foramen of Monroe" which should be at the level of the external auditory meatus in supine position and in-between the eyebrows in the lateral position.

The EVD should always be clamped during transfer or patient movement to avoid over or underdrainage of CSF which can cause catastrophic consequences. Infection is a common complication of EVD catheters and poses a continual challenge. The outcome of EVD insertion in ICU and OR is not known to be different, however complete sterility is a must irrespective of the place of the procedure.

32. **Ans. (d)**
Palaniswami M, Yan B. Mechanical thrombectomy is now the gold standard for acute ischemic stroke: implications for routine clinical practice. Interv Neurol. 2015;4(1-2):18-29.

In hyperacute thrombotic stroke the recommended treatment is bridging thrombolysis and clot evacuation by mechanical thrombectomy if presentation is within window period. Thrombolysis alone is only useful in small vessels and is unable to dissolve large vessel clots. MT is useful for large vessel clots and is unable for clot evacuation of very small distal vessels. Complications of MT are lesser with significantly better outcomes.

During MT, no one anesthetic (GA or Sedation) is superior to another. Options need to be tailored for individual scenario. GA is recommended for posterior circulation strokes due to the risk of clot migration and brainstem stroke. TCD and invasive monitoring are usually not required as time is of the essence to minimize "door to needle" time. Postoperative ventilation is a predictor of poor outcome.

33. **Ans. (b)**
Darsaut TE, Jack AS, Kerr RS, et al. International subarachnoid aneurysm trial – ISAT Part II: Study protocol for a randomized controlled trial. Trials. 2013;14:156.

International Subarachnoid Treatment was a landmark study revolutionizing the treatment of aneurysmal SAH and no traumatic SAH. It demonstrated a 7.4 absolute risk reduction in death for Coiling vs. Clipping. Intraprocedural rupture was less with coilings whilst postoperative rebleeding rates were more with coilings. Its critique was that long-term follow-up in years was missing.

34. **Ans. (b)**
Sartor EA, Albright K, Boehme AK, et al. The NIHSS Score and its Components can Predict Cortical Stroke. J Neurol Disord Stroke. 2013;2(1):1026.

The NIHSS score is a validated tool to quantify the degree of impairment caused by stroke. It has 11 items carrying a score of 0–4 for each. The maximum possible score is 42. A score of 0 indicates normal function. It is also a validated tool for predicting patient outcome.

35. **Ans. (c)**
Connolly ES, Rabinstein AA, Carhuapoma JR, et al. Guidelines for the management of aneurysmal subarachnoid hemorrhage. Stroke. 2012;43(6):1711-37.

Nimodipine treatment should start as soon as the diagnosis of SAH is made with an oral dose of 60 mg every 4 hours. It has level I evidence and should be continued for at least 21 days post the day of the bleeding. It blocks L-type voltage-gated calcium channels and is best given orally or via a nasogastric tube.

36. **Ans. (e)**
    Robertson K, von Stempel CB, Arnold I. When less is more: a case of phenytoin toxicity. BMJ Case Reports. 2013;2013:bcr2012008023.

    Phenytoin toxicity causes acute sodium channel blockade leading to wide QRS complexes. The patient gets prone to ventricular dysrhythmias and sodium bicarbonate is used in the treatment. Cerebellar features like ataxia are seen in phenytoin toxicity. There should be regular phenytoin levels on patients who are on the drug and repeat levels should be done in case of systemic illnesses where volume of distribution or polypharmacy is likely to affect the drug levels.

37. **Ans. (c)**
    The EEG is typical of burst suppression with periods of high voltage activity alternating with periods of no activity in the brain. It might be seen in deep anesthesia, comatosed states or hypothermia. It is sometimes deliberately achieved in states like refractory status or brain surgery where brain is at risk of hypoperfusion.

38. **Ans. (a)**
    Darvesh AS, Carroll RT, Geldenhuys WJ, et al. In vivo brain microdialysis: advances in neuropsychopharmacology and drug discovery. Expert Opinion on Drug Discovery. 2011;6(2):109-127.

    The image depicting microdialysis and TCD is not that of a normal brain. The L/P ratio curve indicates ischemia as seen by the suddenly rising lactate/pyruvate ratio above normal levels from the initial downward trend. The dramatic increase in glycerol indicates brain damage whilst the TCD flow velocity shows spasm much later than the actual rise in biomarkers. The tip of the EVD is also seen in the ventricles in the CT head image.

39. **Ans. (c)**
    Graph depicts relationship between cerebral blood flow (CBF) and arterial partial pressure of oxygen (paO_2). In the normoxemic range there is no effect on CBF. When there is reduction of paO_2 below 50 mm Hg, cerebral blood flow increases significantly thereby increasing the ICP if not corrected.

40. **Ans. (a)**
    Plateau wave in ICP = Sudden surges in ICP to 50–80 mm Hg lasting 5–20 minutes B wave in ICP = Smaller surges in ICP to 20 mm Hg for 1–2 minutes A waves in ICU = Failing compliance of the brain to ICP and risk for ischemia.

41. **Ans. (a)**
    Connolly ES, Rabinstein AA, Carhuapoma JR, et al. Guidelines for the management of aneurysmal subarachnoid hemorrhage. Stroke. 2012;43(6):1711-37.

    The risk factors for poor outcome in SAH include female sex, WFNS grade 4, multiple aneurysms, posterior circulation aneurysms, low presenting GCS, delayed presentation, and presence of major comorbidities. SAH is a neurological condition with high morbidity and mortality and usually half of the patients do not reach hospital alive. Of the remaining at least 20% end up with complications especially from delayed cerebral vasospasm.

42. **Ans. (b)**
    Connolly ES, Rabinstein AA, Carhuapoma JR, et al. Guidelines for the management of aneurysmal subarachnoid hemorrhage. Stroke. 2012;43(6):1711-37.

    Triple therapy and oral nimodipine are proven therapies for SAH management and are recommended in the 2012 ASA/AHA guidelines. Triple H however has weakened over the last decade but avoidance of hypovolemia is key in SAH management. Angioplasty and IV milrinone are performed for vasospasm treatment in some centers of the world but its benefit is not consistent and is currently not a universally recommended and acceptable treatment as per the international guidelines.

43. **Ans. (e)**
    Connolly ES, Rabinstein AA, Carhuapoma JR, et al. Guidelines for the management of aneurysmal subarachnoid hemorrhage. Stroke. 2012;43(6):1711-37.

    The ISAT study was a landmark study which recommended coiling over clipping for aneurysmal SAH treatment. CT scan is not 100% sensitive and digital subtraction angiography should be done to rule out an aneurysm. It is a condition with high mortality nearing about 50%. The proven therapies to improve outcome are oral nimodipine and HHH. Hypothermia has no benefit in treating SAH patients. Outcomes are better if these complex patients are managed at tertiary care centers.

44. **Ans. (b)**
    Palaniswami M, Yan B. Mechanical thrombectomy is now the gold standard for acute ischemic stroke: implications for routine clinical practice. Interv Neurol. 2015;4(1-2):18-29.

    In hyperacute thrombotic stroke the recommended treatment is bridging thrombolysis and clot evacuation by mechanical thrombectomy if presentation is within window period. Thrombolysis alone is only useful in small vessels and is unable to dissolve large vessel clots. MT is useful for large vessel clots and is unable for clot evacuation of very small distal vessels. Complications of MT are lesser with significantly better outcomes.

    During MT, no one anesthetic (GA or Sedation) is superior to another. Options need to be tailored for individual scenario. GA is recommended for posterior circulation strokes due to the risk of clot migration and brainstem stroke. TCD and invasive monitoring are usually not required as time is of the essence to minimize "door to needle" time. Postoperative ventilation is a predictor of poor outcome.

CHAPTER 14

Trauma

SUSHIL KUMAR YADAV

QUESTIONS

1. A 40-year-old female met with an accident. On examination in casualty, she was having breathing difficulty and hypotension (blood pressure 66/46 mmHg), and cyanotic. She had an open femur fracture with exposed bone. On auscultation decreased air entry on right side of the chest. The initial line of treatment priority should be:
   a. Central line insertion and beginning of emergency type O blood transfusion
   b. Control of hemorrhage with external compression
   c. Thoracostomy tube insertion in the right hemithorax
   d. Endotracheal intubation with manual in line cervical stabilization

2. According to ATLS guidelines, primary survey in a trauma patient includes all *except*?
   a. Circulation with hemorrhage control
   b. Breathing and ventilation
   c. Assessment of neurological status
   d. Ample history

3. Which of the following is not an important physiologic change/adaptation of pregnancy which can affect the response to injury?
   a. Increased cardiac output
   b. Increased plasma volume
   c. Decreased coagulation factors
   d. Compression of inferior vena cava

4. In a traumatic brain injury patient with signs of raised intracranial pressure (ICP), which of the following has no role in reducing ICP?
   a. Decompression craniotomy
   b. Hyperosmolar therapy
   c. Steroids
   d. Cerebrospinal fluid drainage

5. A trauma patient is brought to casualty room with suspected pelvic injury, which one of the following is true about pelvic trauma?
   a. Early stabilization can be achieved with a sheet or belt encircling the pelvis at the level of the iliac crests
   b. Unstable pelvic fracture and shock have a mortality of up to 30%
   c. Springing of the pelvis should be done to assess stability
   d. The weakest point of the pelvic ring is pubic rami

6. In a severe traumatic brain injury which one is not a useful prognostic variable?
   a. Glasgow coma scale
   b. Pupillary reaction to light
   c. Sensory neurological deficit
   d. Injury occurred in a low-middle income country

7. A 36-year-old female patient came to emergency department with comminuted fracture of tibia-associated tense swollen leg following road traffic accident with suspicion of acute compartment syndrome, all are correct *except*?
   a. Passive stretching exacerbates pain
   b. Palpable distal pulses rules out the diagnosis
   c. The anterior compartment is most likely affected
   d. Coagulopathy increases the risk of compartment syndrome

8. A 20-year-old male patient had a road traffic accident and sustained fractured of his tibia. He is having open reduction and internal fixation. During the operation there is sudden loss of end tidal carbon dioxide. This was followed by fall in blood pressure. What is the most likely diagnosis?
   a. Hemorrhage
   b. Fat embolism
   c. Hyponatremia
   d. Myocardial ischemia

9. Which of the following statement is incorrect in high cervical spinal injury in a trauma patient?
   a. Bradycardia and hypotension are most likely to be due to developing spinal shock
   b. Hemorrhage should be sought and excluded in the hypotensive patient
   c. Maintain mean arterial pressure of 90 mmHg for adequate cord perfusion
   d. Abdominal breathing is a sign of impending respiratory deterioration

10. A 23-year-old woman is admitted to the emergency department after major trauma. She has suffered a crush injury to her chest and back with widespread chest wall contusions and bilateral open femur fractures. Her vital signs before prehospital intubation and resuscitation were as follows: respiratory rate 32, heart rate 130 bpm, blood pressure 82/36. Most likely to cause hypotension in her could be?
    a. Tension pneumothorax
    b. Cardiac tamponade
    c. Hypovolemia
    d. Aortic dissection

11. A 26-year-old female at 30 weeks estimated gestational age, presented with history of trauma after a motor vehicle crash. The patient is hypotensive on arrival and after 2 liters of crystalloids, she remains hypotensive. What could be appropriate next line of management in this patient?
    a. Transfuse 2 units of packed red blood cells
    b. Elevation of the backboard to 30° to the left

c. Administer colloids
d. Start norepinephrine 0.1 mcg/kg/hr

12. A patient arrives at emergency department being involved in motor vehicle accident. The patient is conscious, hypotensive, and complains of abdominal pain. What is the most appropriate modality to detect free intra-abdominal fluid?
   a. Emergent abdominal CT scan
   b. Abdominal ultrasonography
   c. Diagnostic peritoneal lavage
   d. Flat and upright abdominal radiographs

13. Which is not a part of Beck's triad seen with cardiac tamponade?
   a. Pulmonary hypertension
   b. Decreased heart sounds
   c. Jugular venous distension
   d. Hypotension

14. Which of the following is not an advantage that sonography has in trauma over computed tomography (CT)?
   a. Ultrasound evaluation can be done within seconds to minutes
   b. Ultrasound can be done at bedside
   c. Ultrasound can be done in the hemodynamically unstable patient
   d. Ultrasound has a higher sensitivity than CT for free intra-abdominal fluid

15. A 33-year-old male driving a four wheeler at high speed without wearing seat belt, leaves the road and crashes with a full frontal impact into a pole. Which of the following injury patterns may occur from this type of impact?
   a. Injuries involving the knee, femur or hips
   b. Shear injuries such as laceration to liver, kidney or solid abdominal viscera
   c. Acute neck flexion, hyperextension or both resulting in a cervical spinal cord injury
   d. All of above

16. In patient with a pneumothorax following stab wound, the chest tube is best inserted at which level?
   a. Just below clavicle
   b. Between 8th and 9th intercostal space
   c. Between 2nd and 3rd intercostal space, in anterior axillary line
   d. Between 4th and 5th intercostal space, just anterior to mid-axillary line

17. An 18-year-old male had motor vehicle accident, he complains of deep aching pain and burning sensation in his left leg. A firmness of the anterior left leg is noted on deep palpation and there is decreased two point discrimination. What is definitive treatment for this patient?
   a. Angioplasty
   b. Leg elevation
   c. Fasciotomy
   d. Analgesia

18. Which one is not an indication for cesarean section during laparotomy for abdominal trauma during pregnancy?
    a. Maternal shock after 28 weeks period of gestation
    b. Unstable thoracolumbar spinal cord injury
    c. Mechanical limitation for maternal repair
    d. Threat to maternal life from exsanguination

19. What is the pathophysiological mechanism of trauma-induced coagulopathy?
    a. Hypothermia and acidosis
    b. Shock and endothelial dysfunction
    c. Loss of coagulation factors and platelets or dilution of coagulation factors
    d. All

20. Which of the following is correct regarding pediatric trauma?
    a. Fractures of bones are more common in pediatric patient
    b. >80% of injuries are penetrating
    c. The most common cause of head injury in the first year of life is accidental injury
    d. Apnea, hypoxia occurs five times more than hypotension and hypovolemia in pediatric age group

21. A 30-year-old female was involved in a head-on collision with another vehicle. She was an unrestrained passenger and is brought to the hospital with Glasgow coma scale of 6. A quick survey does not reveal any frank bleeding, but the patient remains hypotensive. Which of the following is least likely to account for the patient's low blood pressure?
    a. Hemothorax
    b. Spleen rupture
    c. Retroperitoneal bleeding
    d. Subdural hematoma

22. A 20-year-old female while driving two wheeler met with an accident, comes to casualty. She is groaning and speaking in a low voice and has multiple abrasions over chest, with blood pressure of 80/50 mmHg and has a respiratory rate of 22. She is cold to touch and there is extensive subcutaneous emphysema on the right upper chest and neck. What is the next step of management?
    a. CT thorax
    b. Arterial blood gas
    c. C tube thoracostomy
    d. Blood transfusion

23. Following a road traffic accident, an adult patient presents to casualty. On arrival he was alert and fully oriented even though he was unconscious at the scene. After some time he suddenly loses consciousness with left side dilated pupil. What is the most likely diagnosis?
    a. Fat emboli in retina
    b. Acute subdural hematoma

c. Ruptured aneurysm
d. Epidural hematoma

24. What is the ideal method to open airway in an unconscious patient that will not require cervical spine in line stabilization precautions?
   a. Lift the tongue laterally
   b. Tilt head and lift chin
   c. Lift the neck from behind
   d. Jaw thrust with chin lift

25. Which of the following is true regarding the Advanced Trauma Life Support (ATLS) classification system of hemorrhagic shock?
   a. Class I shock is equivalent to voluntary blood donation
   b. In Class II, shock is associated with change in vital signs including tachycardia, tachypnea, and a significant decrease in systolic blood pressure
   c. Class III hemorrhage can usually be managed by simple administration of crystalloids
   d. Class IV hemorrhage involves loss of over 20% of blood volume loss and can be considered as life-threatening

26. Which one is not an extracranial cause of secondary brain injury in trauma patient?
   a. Hypotension
   b. Hypercarbia
   c. Hypoxemia
   d. Uncontrolled fits

27. On the basis of American College of Surgeons Committee on Trauma recommendations, all of the following patients should be transported to a trauma center *except*?
   a. A 40-year-old male who fell 8 feet from a stair case, with isolated hip fracture and normal vital signs
   b. A 17-year-old with Glasgow Coma Scale score of 12 following head injury
   c. Penetrating injury to head, neck and torso
   d. Two or more proximal long bone fractures

ANSWERS

1. **Ans. (d)**

    American College of Surgeons. ATLS Advanced Trauma Life Support, 10th edition. Chicago: ACS.

    Control of airway remains the utmost priority in trauma patients with multiple injuries. The best given option for control of the airway is endotracheal intubation with restriction of cervical spine motion, which requires at least two persons to maintain neutral position of head and one to insert the endotracheal tube. Assessment of adequacy of ventilation, treating obvious hemorrhage, and assessment of patient's neurologic status can occur simultaneously, but priority is given to secure an adequate airway.

2. **Ans. (d)**

    American College of Surgeons. ATLS Advanced Trauma Life Support, 10th edition. Chicago: ACS

    According to ATLS guidelines, assessment and management is based on extent and mechanism of injuries, vital parameters. Preference of sequential management depends on initial assessment of the patient. It includes rapid primary survey with simultaneous resuscitation of vital parameters, and detailed secondary survey followed by definitive care. The primary survey consists of ABCDEs of trauma care and identifies immediate life-threatening conditions by following respective sequence:
    - Airway maintenance with manual in line stabilization
    - Breathing and ventilation
    - Circulation with control of hemorrhage
    - Disability (neurological status assessment)
    - Exposure/Environmental control

    Primary survey can be supported by adjuvants:
    - ECG
    - Pulse oximetry
    - Ventilator rate
    - ABG and capnography
    - Urinary and gastric catheter
    - Imaging X-rays

3. **Ans. (c)**

    Irwin RS. Irwin and Rippe's Intensive Care Medicine, 8th edition. Philadelphia: Wolters Kluwer Health; 2017.

    Physiologic: Maternal Adaptation to Pregnancy
    System Alternations:
    - *Cardiovascular:*
        - Cardiac output increased 20–30%
        - Blood pressure decreased
        - Peripheral vascular resistance decreased

- *Pulmonary system:*
  - Tidal volume increased
  - Respiratory rate increased
  - Functional residual capacity reduced
- *Renal system:*
  - Renal artery perfusion increased
  - Glomerular filtration rate
  - Increased creatinine clearance
  - Increased BUN, serum creatinine
  - Serum uric acid decreased
  - Urinary stasis increased
  - Dilated renal pelvis and ureters
- *Hematologic system:*
  - Plasma volume increased more than RBC volume
  - Increased leukocytosis
  - Increased liver-produced clotting factors
  - Increased fibrinogen, hypercoagulable state

4. **Ans. (c)**

   Carney N, Totten AM, O'Reilly C, et al. Guidelines for the Management of Severe Traumatic Brain Injury, Fourth Edition. Neurosurgery. 2017;80(1):6-15.

   Decompressive craniectomy has been done to decrease intracranial pressure with improvement in outcome of traumatic brain injury (TBI) patients. However, there is lack of sufficient evidence to support it as a Level I recommendation. Hyperosmolar therapy (mannitol and hypertonic saline) helps to decrease intracranial pressure by reducing blood viscosity, leading to improved microcirculatory flow of blood constituents and resultant constriction of pial arterioles, leading to decreased cerebral blood volume and intracranial pressure.

   There is no role of steroids to decrease intracranial pressure and improve outcome. In patients with TBI, high dose methylprednisolone is associated with increased mortality.

   Cerebrospinal fluid (CSF) drainage by extraventricular drainage (EVD) system in TBI is a topic of debate. An EVD can help in intracranial pressure monitoring as well as CSF drainage. There was lack of evidence for Level I or II recommendation. Other methods to decrease intracranial pressure are: prophylactic hypothermia, ventilation therapy, anesthetic, and sedative.

5. **Ans. (d)**

   Waldmann C, Soni N, Rhodes A. A Oxford Desk Reference Critical Care. Oxford: Oxford University Press; 2008.

   The mortality from pelvic trauma may approach 50% in patients with an unstable pelvic fracture and shock. The pubic rami is the weakest point of the pelvic ring. Springing of the pelvis can exacerbate bleeding and thus should not be part of routine practice in patients with acute pelvic trauma. Early stabilization can be achieved with a sheet or belt.

This should encircle the hips at the level of the greater trochanters. Not all patients with pelvic fractures must have a thoracoabdominal pelvic contrast CT prior to surgical intervention. Some patients will be too unstable for CT to be performed.

6. **Ans. (c)**
   Perel P, Arango M, Clayton T, et al. MRC CRASH Trial Collaborators. Predicting outcome after traumatic brain injury: practical prognostic models based on large cohort of international patients. BMJ. 2008;336(7641):425-9.

   The MRC CRASH trial was performed in which the model includes age, Glasgow coma scale, pupillary reaction to light, injury occurred in a low-middle income country, extra cranial injury, and CT scan findings. There is no role of sensory deficit.

7. **Ans. (b)**
   Newton EJ, Love J, et al. Acute complications of extremity trauma. Emerg Med Clin North Am. 2007;25(3):751-61.
   Farrow C, Bodenham A, Troxler M. Acute limb compartment syndromes. Contin Educ Anaesth Crit Care Pain. 2011;11(1):24-8.

   Acute compartment syndrome results from increased pressure within a fascia-bound muscular compartment, resulting in compression of structures enclosed in the compartment including neurovascular structures. Most commonly affected are volar compartment of forearm and anterior compartment of leg. Passive stretching of affected limb increases pain. Highest incidence is noted in fractures (75%), most commonly in tibial fracture. Patients with coagulopathy are at increased risk of compartment syndrome due to bleeding within compartment. Affected limb can still have palpable distal pulses and normal capillary refill time, complete loss of pulses is usually a late sign. Tissue pressure should be measured in suspicious case of compartment syndrome.

8. **Ans. (b)**
   Gupta A, Reilly CS. Fat embolism. Contin Educ Anaesth Crit Care Pain. 2007;7(5):148-51.

   Fat embolism may occur by entry of depot fat globules from disrupted bone marrow into the bloodstream in areas of trauma (mechanical) and by production of toxic intermediaries of fat present in the plasma (biochemical). The tibia is a long bone and fracture that requires the intramedullary nail. During the process of inserting the intramedullary nail there is increased pressure, which may lead to fat embolism. Fat embolism syndrome has a classic triad of respiratory signs (dyspnea, tachypnea, and hypoxemia), neurological abnormalities, and petechial rash. During fat embolism there can be hypoxia, pulmonary edema, coagulation disorder, and loss of carbon dioxide due to sudden increase in the dead space. Management of fat embolism syndrome includes prevention, timely diagnosis, and supportive treatment.

9. **Ans. (a)**
   Cadogan M. Trauma! Spinal Injury. [online] Available from http://www.lifeinthefastlane.com/trauma-tribulation-016. [Last accessed June, 2019].
   Casha S, Christie S. A systematic review of intensive cardiopulmonary management after spinal cord injury. J Neurotrauma. 2011;28(8):1479-95.

Traumatic spinal cord injury (SCI) can be primary injury or secondary cord damage due to hypotension/hypoxia. High cervical cord lesions lead to interruption of sympathetic outflow with resultant bradycardia and hypotension (neurogenic shock). Spinal shock, reflecting absence of reflexes below the level of the lesion due to transient "concussion" of the cord should be excluded. To prevent secondary injury, a MAP of 90 mmHg is currently recommended to optimize perfusion and to decrease ischemic penumbra. Abdominal breathing indicates failure of the thoracic musculature, sign of impending respiratory failure.

10. **Ans. (c)**
   American College of Surgeons. ATLS Advanced Trauma Life Support, 10th edition. Chicago: ACS.

   Most common cause of hypotension following major trauma is hypovolemic, hemorrhagic shock. In all multiply-injured patients, a significant element of hypovolemia should be considered and should be treated early. Spinal shock doesn't usually cause hypotension, but neurogenic shock may do. The other causes may be an alternative or contributory factor to hypotension, but are less common than hypovolemia.

11. **Ans. (b)**
   American College of Surgeons. ATLS Advanced Trauma Life Support, 10th edition. Chicago: ACS.

   The most likely etiology is supine hypotensive syndrome. Internal bleeding should be entertained, however the next step is to address the decreased venous return from periphery. During third trimester, the gravid uterus compresses and may completely occlude the inferior vena cava when lying in supine position. This results in a significant decrease in venous return to the heart. To relieve compression on the IVC, the patient should be tilted to the left on the background to 30°. Following advanced trauma life support guidelines, after 2 liters of crystalloids, additional ethology should be sought. Supine hypotension syndrome and etiologies should be sought including hemorrhage.

12. **Ans. (b)**
   American College of Surgeons. ATLS Advanced Trauma Life Support, 10th edition. Chicago: ACS.

   Focused assessment with sonography for trauma (FAST) is the study of choice in unstable patient with abdominal trauma. It has almost replaced diagnostic peritoneal lavage, which has higher false negative results. CT is the most sensitive test for intra-abdominal free fluid. However, it is recommended only for the hemodynamically stable patient. Abdominal radiographs can detect abdominal free air. They cannot detect free intra-abdominal fluid.

13. **Ans. (a)**
   American College of Surgeons. ATLS Advanced Trauma Life Support, 10th edition. Chicago: ACS.

   The Beck's triad of symptoms includes jugular venous distension (JVD), hypotension, and muffled heart sounds in the presence of cardiac tamponade. A widening pulse pressure may be found. In younger children or patients in hypovolemic shock, JVD may not be noticeable.

14. **Ans. (d)**

    American College of Surgeons. ATLS Advanced Trauma Life Support, 10th edition. Chicago: ACS.

    CT has a higher sensitivity than ultrasound for detection free intra-abdominal fluid. Approximately 200 cc of free intra-abdominal fluid is necessary to have a positive FAST exam. CT requires transportation of the trauma patient to a radiology suite, whereas ultrasound can be done at the bedside and CT is advised for hemodynamically stable trauma patient.

15. **Ans. (d)**

    American College of Surgeons. ATLS Advanced Trauma Life Support, 10th edition. Chicago: ACS.

    There could be any of the two predictable pathways in this kind of an impact—down and under the dashboard, where knees hit the dashboard and energy gets transferred to the upper legs leading to dislocated knees or femur fracture or dislocated hips. After the knees impact, the upper body flexes forward and up and over the steering wheel. The chest or abdomen impacts the steering wheel and the head impacts the wind shield. Second predictable injury, the up-and-over component include: (1) anterior flail chest; (2) compression injuries to hollow or solid abdominal viscera; (3) shear injuries like lacerations to the aorta or liver or other solid viscera; (4) injury to the brain following compression injury with scalp lacerations, skull fractures or cerebral contusions or from deceleration or shear forces; (5) acute flexion of neck, hyperextension or both resulting in cervical spinal cord injury.

16. **Ans. (d)**

    American College of Surgeons. ATLS Advanced Trauma Life Support, 10th edition. Chicago: ACS.

    Pneumothorax can be treated with insertion of a chest tube between the fourth and fifth intercostal spaces, just anterior to mid axillary line. Placement of tube too high can lead to damage to subclavian vessels. Too low can result in damage to the liver and spleen. Chest tube with trocars should be avoided due to the risk of injuring the heart and lung. In pregnant patient, the chest tube should be placed one or two levels higher as the diaphragm is higher in pregnancy.

17. **Ans. (c)**

    American College of Surgeons. ATLS Advanced Trauma Life Support, 10th edition. Chicago: ACS.

    Compartment syndrome is an acute emergency. If compartment syndrome is suspected, fasciotomy should be performed within 4-6 hours of symptom onset. The goal of treatment is to reduce the intracompartmental pressure and prevent further tissue ischemia and necrosis. The viability of compartment should be assessed during fasciotomy and nonviable muscle must be derided to minimize the risk of infection.

18. **Ans. (a)**

    Jain V, Chari R, Maslovitz S. Edmonton A-Guidelines for the Management of a Pregnant Trauma Patient. J Obstet Gynaecol Can. 2015;37(6):553-74.

Cesarean section should not be added in an abdominal trauma pregnant patients, unless required, owing to prolongation of operative time and increased blood loss (of around 1 liter). Vaginal delivery is encouraged even in the postoperative period. During laparotomy for trauma, indications for cesarean section are:
- Maternal shock, with pregnancy nearing term
- Threat to maternal life from exsanguination
- Mechanical limitation for maternal repair
- Increased risk of fetal distress exceeding risk of prematurity
- Unstable thoracolumbar spinal cord injury

The outcome of postmortem cesarean section (C-section) depends on the duration of the gestation and the time interval between maternal death and fetus delivery. Postmortem C-section is justified if the estimated age is about 26–28 weeks. If the time interval between maternal death and delivery is less than 5 minutes, the fetal prognosis is considered excellent. If the time interval since maternal death is prolonged to around 20 minutes, fetal prognosis is poor.

19. **Ans. (d)**

    Schöchl H, Maegele M, Solomon C, et al. Early and individualized goal directed therapy for trauma induced coagulopathy. Scand J Trauma Resusc. Emerg Med. 2012–20:15.

    Trauma-induced coagulopathy (TIC) describes the impairment of physiological clot formation and stability in trauma patients.

    Trauma-induced coagulopathy can result from several pathophysiological mechanisms:
    - (Local and systemic) hyperfibrinolysis
    - Loss of coagulation factors and platelets or dilution of coagulation factors
    - Hypothermia and acidosis
    - Shock and associated endothelial dysfunction

    The combination of hypothermia, metabolic acidosis, and coagulation abnormality has been termed as "lethal triad of trauma".

20. **Ans. (d)**

    American College of Surgeons. ATLS Advanced Trauma Life Support, 10th edition. Chicago: ACS.

    Most common pediatric trauma is blunt trauma which involves the brain, resulting in apnea, hypoventilation, hypoxia which occurs five times more than hypovolemia with hypotension.

    Due to incompletely calcified, more pliable bone skeleton in pediatric age group, bone fractures are less likely to occur in children as compared to adults. Nonaccidental injury is the most common cause of head injury in the first year of life.

21. **Ans. (d)**

    American College of Surgeons. ATLS Advanced Trauma Life Support, 10th edition. Chicago: ACS.

    Hypotension in a trauma patient is almost never due to brain injury. If there is no frank source of bleeding and the patient remains hypotensive, one should suspect a peripheral

Chapter 14 Trauma

cause, unless it is case of an infant or small child. The most common sources of bleeding in trauma patients are the chest, abdomen, and pelvis. The liver and spleen are two organs that often can bleed significantly. In the chest, a massive hemothorax can cause significant blood loss and should be suspected if there is an opacification on the chest X-ray. Another very common cause of hemorrhage is a pelvic or femur fracture. In rare cases, neurogenic shock may cause hypotension.

22. Ans. (c)

American College of Surgeons. ATLS Advanced Trauma Life Support, 10th edition. Chicago: ACS.

Airway should always be the first priority. One should always be suspicious of a reversible cause of respiratory distress. Subcutaneous emphysema with respiratory distress is a pneumothorax until proven otherwise. In the field needle compression can be done, in emergency department tube thoracostomy is preferred.

23. Ans. (d)

American College of Surgeons. ATLS Advanced Trauma Life Support, 10th edition. Chicago: ACS.

Epidural hematomas are typically caused by a tear of the middle meningeal artery from a temporal skull fracture. It appears as a hyperdense biconvex mass between skull and dura. Clinical presentation is highly variable. The classic scenario is a lucid interval following a period of altered consciousness from which the patient deteriorates, developing a dilating pupil and hemiparesis on the contralateral side.

24. Ans. (b)

American College of Surgeons. ATLS Advanced Trauma Life Support, 10th edition. Chicago: ACS.

The simplest way to ensure an open airway in an unconscious patient is to do a head tilt and chin lift maneuver which lifts the tongue from back of the throat.

25. Ans. (a)

American College of Surgeons. ATLS Advanced Trauma Life Support, 10th edition. Chicago: ACS.

The classification of hemorrhagic shock defined by the ATLS classification system of the American College of Surgeons includes Class 1 hemorrhage, which is up to 15% of total blood volume and is equivalent to 1 unit of voluntary blood donation. There is not much change in heart rate or respiratory rate, blood pressure or pulse pressure. Class II hemorrhage involves loss of 15–30% of total blood volume with clinical signs including tachycardia and tachypnea with slightly decreased systolic blood pressure and can generally be resuscitated with crystalloid solutions but may require blood transfusions. In Class III hemorrhage, 30–40% of total body volume is lost. Patients with obviously inadequate perfusion; marked tachycardia and tachypnea, cool, clammy extremities; hypotension; and significant changes in mental status. The resuscitation of these patients requires blood transfusion in addition to crystalloid administration. Class IV hemorrhage involves loss of greater than 40% of blood volume and represents life-threatening hemorrhage, requiring immediate transfusion for resuscitation and frequently require immediate surgical intervention.

26. **Ans. (d)**

    McHugh GS, Engel DC, Butcher I, et al. Prognostic value of secondary insults in traumatic brain injury: results from the IMPACT study. J Neurotrauma. 2007;24(2):287-93.

    Secondary brain injury can have extra or intracranial causes. Extracranial causes include hypotension, hypoxemia, hypercarbia, disturbance of blood coagulation, and infection. At macroscopic level intracranial causes include intracranial hematoma, brain swelling, cerebral edema, uncontrolled fits.

    At cellular level, a cascade of events contributing to secondary injury may result in cerebral cell ischemia and cell death. Secondary insults are more commonly associated with the cardiorespiratory disturbance and are independent predictors of poor outcome.

27. **Ans. (a)**

    American College of Surgeons. ATLS Advanced Trauma Life Support, 10th edition. Chicago: ACS.

    The American College of Surgeons Committee on Trauma has developed a field triage decision scheme to identify trauma victims with a significant risk of dying on basis of: (1) abnormal physiological signs, (2) anatomical area of injury, (3) mode of injury, and (4) concurrent or comorbid state. Major physiologic abnormalities include Glasgow Coma Scale less than or equal to 13, SBP <90 mmHg, respiratory rate <10 or >29 per minute and <20 respiratory rate in infant. Significant anatomical considerations include penetrating injuries to the torso, head and neck, and proximal extremities, chest wall instability, crush injuries, combination of trauma with burns to greater than 10% of body surface area, paralysis, two or more proximal long bone fractures, pelvic fractures, open or depressed skull fractures or traumatic amputation above the wrist or ankle. Significant mechanisms of injury include a death in the same passenger compartment or ejection from the automobile, high-impact (greater than 5 miles per hour) auto-pedestrian injuries, or a pedestrian thrown or run over. The comorbid factors include pediatric or elderly (<5 or >55) patients or known history of insulin-dependent diabetes or cardiac, respiratory, or psychotic disorders. These criteria should serve as guidelines for medical control and the prehospital care providers.

CHAPTER 15

Cardiovascular System

DIVYESH PATEL

QUESTIONS

1. A 60-year-old male presents with history of chest pain since last 30 minutes. ECG done was suggestive of ST elevation in lead II, III and aVF. Patient has HR of 90/min and BP 150/90 mm Hg. What is the best definitive step in management of this patient?
    a. Aspirin
    b. Aspirin with clopidogrel
    c. Aspirin with prasugrel
    d. IV thrombolysis

2. A 30-year-old male was attended by 108 ambulance at a rave party for complaints of sudden onset acute severe chest pain since last 1 hour. Friends give history of consumption of illicit drug. Patient is conscious and alert but distressed with pain. On examination HR 130/min and BP 170/90 mm Hg and cold extremities. ECG done is suggestive of ST elevation in V1-V4 leads. Patient is loaded with antiplatelets and statins and shifted to tertiary care hospital. On arrival to ER, patient is agitated and distressed with chest pain. On examination HR 140/min and BP 150/90 mm Hg and extremities cold and maintaining SpO_2 of 97% on room air. What is the next best step in management of this patient?
    a. IV benzodiazepine
    b. IV thrombolysis
    c. Primary PCI
    d. IV beta blockers

3. A 65-year-old male, a known case of HTN and IHD with reduced EF (30%), presents with history of breathlessness since last 2 days. On examination HR 120/min, BP 180/100 mm Hg and extremities cold. On chest examination patient has RR of 26/min and SpO_2 92% on room air and bilateral basal crepts present on auscultation. ECG is not suggestive of any new changes. Patient was diagnosed to have acute heart failure. What is the best choice of therapy in this patient?
    a. IV vasodilators
    b. IV diuretics
    c. IV dobutamine
    d. IV diuretics with IV vasodilators

4. A 55-year-old male (no comorbids) is admitted in surgical ICU for treatment of fracture shaft femur left. Patient underwent surgery on admission day and was shifted to ward. On postoperative day 4, patient had sudden episode of breathlessness, fever and hypotension and hence was shifted back to ICU. On arrival, patient was conscious but confused. On examination HR 120/min and BP 80/40 mm Hg and neck veins engorged and lactates 5.4 mmol/dL, RR 34/min and SpO_2 90% with oxygen at 4L/min through face mask and chest clear. What is the immediate best investigation to approach to diagnosis?
   a. Chest X-ray
   b. CT pulmonary angiography
   c. Bedside echocardiography
   d. HRCT thorax

5. A 55-year-old male (no comorbids) is admitted in surgical ICU for treatment of fracture shaft femur left. Patient underwent surgery on admission day and was shifted to ward. On postoperative day 4, patient had sudden episode of breathlessness and hypotension and hence was shifted back to ICU. On arrival to ICU, HR 120/min and BP 80/40 mm Hg and neck veins engorged and lactates 5.4 mmol/dL. RR 34/min and SpO_2 90% with oxygen at 4L/min through face mask and chest clear. ECG is suggestive of sinus tachycardia. What is the next best step in management of this patient?
   a. IV heparin
   b. SC enoxaparin
   c. IV thrombolysis
   d. IV antibiotics

6. A 55-year-old male (no comorbids) is admitted in surgical ICU for treatment of fracture shaft femur left. Patient underwent surgery on admission day and was shifted to ward. On postoperative day 4, patient had sudden episode of breathlessness and hypotension and hence was shifted back to ICU. On arrival to ICU, HR 120/min and BP 70/40 mm Hg and neck veins engorged and lactates 5.4 mmol/dL. RR 34/min and SpO_2 90% with oxygen at 4L/min through face mask and chest clear. ECG is suggestive of sinus tachycardia. Bedside echocardiography is suggestive of dilated RA and RV with pulmonary hypertension. A presumptive diagnosis of pulmonary embolism is made. What is the anticoagulant of choice?
   a. SC enoxaparin
   b. SC fondaparinux
   c. IV heparin
   d. Oral rivaroxaban

7. A 55-year-old female (no comorbids) is admitted in surgical ICU for treatment of fracture shaft femur left. Patient underwent surgery on admission day and was shifted to ward. On postoperative day 4, patient had sudden episode of breathlessness and hypotension and hence was shifted back to ICU. On arrival to ICU, HR 120/min and BP 70/40 mm Hg and neck veins engorged and lactates 5.4 mmol/dL. RR 34/min

and SpO$_2$ 90% with oxygen at 4L/min through face mask and chest clear. ECG is suggestive of sinus tachycardia. Bedside echocardiography is suggestive of dilated RA and RV with pulmonary hypertension. A presumptive diagnosis of pulmonary embolism is made. The following are absolute contraindications of IV thrombolysis *except*:
a. History of intracranial hemorrhage
b. History of spine surgery 1 month back
c. Intracranial malignancy
d. Menstruation

8. A 34 week pregnant female was admitted with sudden onset left lower limb pain and breathlessness. On examination left calf is swollen and tender. On examination HR 120/min and BP 90/50 mm Hg and SpO$_2$ of 94 % with 4L oxygen through face mask. Emergent lower limb Doppler done was suggestive of DVT and bedside echocardiography was suggestive of dilated RA and RV with normal LV function. What is the anticoagulant of choice in this patient?
a. Heparin
b. Warfarin
c. Rivaroxaban
d. Apixaban

9. A 32-year-old IT engineer, morbidly obese is admitted with history of recent air travel 1 week back. Since travel patient has complaints of swelling and redness of right leg with complaints of breathlessness. ECG done was suggestive of sinus tachycardia and echocardiography report was normal. Which one of the following statements is true?
a. Negative d-dimer value rules out pulmonary embolism
b. Positive or increased d-dimer value establishes diagnosis of pulmonary embolism
c. V/Q scan is the best investigation of choice
d. Normal echocardiography rules out pulmonary embolism

10. A 32-year-old IT engineer, morbidly obese is admitted with history of recent air travel 1 week back. Since travel, patient has complaints of swelling and redness of right leg with complaints of breathlessness. On arrival to ER patient is noticed to be in shock and echocardiography screening is suggestive of dilated RA and RV. A presumptive diagnosis of pulmonary embolism is made and patient is started on IV thrombolysis. 10 minutes on thrombolysis patient suddenly becomes unresponsive. Monitor show a HR of 54/min. What is the next best response in management of this patient?
a. Stop thrombolysis and urgent CT of the brain
b. Check for pulse
c. Immediately intubate the patient
d. IV atropine

11. A 32-year-old IT engineer, morbidly obese is admitted with history of recent air travel 1 week back. Since travel patient has complaints of swelling and redness of right leg with complaints of breathlessness. On arrival to ER, patient is noticed to be in shock and echocardiography screening is suggestive of dilated RA and RV. A presumptive

diagnosis of pulmonary embolism is made and patient is started on IV thrombolysis. 10 minutes on thrombolysis patient suddenly becomes unresponsive. Monitor show a HR of 54/min. However on assessment pulse is absent. What is the next best step in management of this patient?
   a. Start chest compression
   b. IV adrenaline
   c. DC shock
   d. Call for help

12. A 54-year-old male, chronic smoker, DM and hypertensive, presents with history of severe substernal chest pain since last 30 minutes. On examination HR is 76/min and BP 150/90 mm Hg. ECG done is normal and troponin T done is negative and echocardiography does not suggest any RWMA. Which of the following is next best course of action?
    a. Discharge patient
    b. Repeat troponin T after 6 hours
    c. Plan upper GI endoscopy
    d. Plan for exercise stress test

13. A 54-year-old male, chronic smoker, DM and hypertensive presents with history of severe substernal chest pain since last 30 minutes. On examination HR is 76/min and BP 150/90 mm Hg. Patient has SpO_2 of 98% on room air and chest is clear. ECG is suggestive of acute anterior wall myocardial infarction. What is the next best step in management of this patient?
    a. Oxygen
    b. IV Morphine
    c. Sublingual nitrates
    d. Primary PCI

14. A 54-year-old male, chronic smoker, DM and hypertensive presents with history of severe substernal chest pain since last 30 minutes to secondary care hospital at 11:00 pm. On examination HR is 76/min and BP 150/90 mm Hg. Patient has SpO_2 of 98% on room air and chest is clear. ECG is suggestive of acute anterior wall myocardial infarction. However hospital cardiologist is not available for the night and no other hospital in town has a cardiology department and nearest higher cardiology center is 6 hours away. What is the next best step in management of patient?
    a. Wait till morning till cardiologist arrives
    b. Refer the patient to higher center
    c. Initiate IV thrombolysis and then refer the patient to higher center
    d. Give IV heparin and the refer the patient to higher center

15. A 54-year-old male, chronic smoker, DM and hypertensive presents with history of severe substernal chest pain since last 8 hours. On examination HR is 120/min and BP 80/50 mm Hg. Patient has SpO_2 of 98% on room air and chest is clear. ECG is suggestive of acute anterior wall myocardial infarction. The best management plan is:

a. IABP insertion
   b. IV thrombolysis
   c. Primary PCI
   d. Start IV noradrenaline

16. A 54-year-old male, chronic smoker, DM and hypertensive presents with history of severe substernal chest pain since last 30 minutes to secondary care hospital at 11:00 pm. On examination HR is 76/min and BP 150/90 mm Hg. Patient has SpO_2 of 98% on room air and chest is clear. ECG is suggestive of acute anterior wall myocardial infarction. 10 minutes after arrival in ICU patient has pulseless VT. What is the best step in management?
   a. DC shock
   b. IV cordarone
   c. IV lignocaine
   d. Chest compression

17. A 54-year-old male, chronic smoker, DM and hypertensive presents with history of severe substernal chest pain since last 30 minutes. On examination HR is 120/min and BP 80/50 mm Hg. Patient has SpO_2 of 98% on room air and chest is clear. ECG is suggestive of acute anterior wall myocardial infarction. Echocardiography done is suggestive of LV ejection fraction of 40%. Patient is loaded with antiplatelets, statin and anticoagulants and is being taken for primary PCI. The vasopressor of choice for the patient is:
   a. Dopamine
   b. Dobutamine with dopamine
   c. Noradrenaline
   d. Adrenaline

18. A 54-year-old male, chronic smoker, DM and hypertensive presents with history of severe substernal chest pain since last 30 minutes. On examination HR is 120/min and BP 80/50 mm Hg. Patient has SpO_2 of 98% on room air and chest is clear. ECG is suggestive of acute anterior wall myocardial infarction. Echocardiography done is suggestive of LV ejection fraction of 40%. Patient is loaded with antiplatelets, statin and anticoagulants and is being taken for primary PCI. For optimization of hemodynamic status, parameters for assessment of preload/fluid responsiveness are used. Which of the following statement is true?
   a. Pulse pressure variation >13% is sensitive and specific indicator of preload responsiveness in mechanically ventilated patients without inspiratory movement and arrhythmia
   b. PAOP >15 indicates patient is not fluid responsive
   c. Pulse pressure variation is a useful test of preload responsiveness during weaning from ventilation.
   d. CVP 10 mm Hg indicates patient is fluid responsive.

19. A 54-year-old male, chronic smoker, DM and hypertensive presents with history of severe substernal chest pain since last 30 minutes. On examination HR is 120/min and BP 80/50 mm Hg. Patient has SpO_2 of 98% on room air and chest is clear. ECG is suggestive of acute anterior wall myocardial infarction. Echocardiography done is suggestive of LV ejection fraction of 40%. Patient is loaded with antiplatelets, statin and anticoagulants and is being taken for primary PCI. Patient is planned for IABP insertion by cardiology team in view of shock. What is the absolute contraindication?
    a. Severe MR
    b. Aortic valve insufficiency
    c. VSD
    d. Peripheral vascular disease

20. A 40-year-old male admitted with fever with cough since last 4 days. On arrival to ICU patient conscious but confused. On examination HR 130/min and sinus, BP 80/40 mm Hg and extremities cold. Patient was treated as LRTI with severe sepsis and after resuscitation of 2 hours BP was still 80/40 mm Hg with Injection Noradrenaline IV and patient has received around 2.5L of IV fluids. RR 24/min and chest clear and breathing spontaneously. The best modality to assess fluid responsiveness in this patient is:
    a. Passive leg raising test
    b. Stroke volume variation
    c. Central venous pressure
    d. IVC collapsibility

21. An elderly male, a known case of IHD with compromised LVEF (15%) is admitted with history of high-grade fever with cough and breathlessness. On examination patient conscious and oriented. HR 130/min, sinus rhythm and BP 70/40 mm Hg and cold extremities and empty neck veins and lactate elevated to 5.5 mmol/dL. RR 28/min and chest clear. Patient is having fever of 101°F. What is the next best step in resuscitation of this patient?
    a. IV dopamine
    b. IV noradrenaline with IV dobutamine
    c. IV fluids
    d. IV furosemide

22. An elderly male, a known case of IHD with compromised LVEF (35%) is admitted with history of high grade fever with cough and breathlessness. On examination patient conscious and oriented. HR 130/min, sinus rhythm and BP 70/40 mm Hg and cold extremities and empty neck veins and lactate elevated to 5.5 mmol/dL. RR 28/min and chest clear. Patient is having fever of 101°F. Despite resuscitation with IV fluids and IV vasopressors, BP now 110/70 mm Hg but lactates still 5.6 mmol/dL and urine output negligible. Passive leg raising test is done to assess fluid responsiveness. Regarding passive leg raising test which one of the following is false?

a. Can be performed in spontaneously breathing patient
b. Can be performed in patient with arrhythmias
c. > 10% increase in stroke volume of CO monitor suggests fluid responsiveness
d. Reliable even in patients with increased intra-abdominal pressure

23. An elderly male, a known case of IHD with compromised LVEF (35%) is admitted with history of high-grade fever with cough and breathlessness. On examination patient conscious and oriented. HR 130/min, sinus rhythm and BP 70/40 mm Hg and cold extremities and empty neck veins and lactate elevated to 5.5 mmol/dL. RR 28/min and chest clear. Patient is having fever of 101°F. Despite resuscitation with IV fluids and IV vasopressors, BP now 110/70 mm Hg but lactates still 5.6 mmol/dL and urine output negligible. On passive leg raising there is no further fluid responsiveness. Which of the following is best done next regarding resuscitation of this patient?
    a. Renal replacement therapy
    b. IV diuretics
    c. IV dobutamine if $ScvO_2$ < 70 mm Hg
    d. IABP insertion

24. A 46-year-old male was referred with sudden onset severe chest pain radiating to back. On arrival to ER patient is conscious and oriented. HR 110/min and BP 140/60 mm Hg. ECG was suggestive of ST depression in anterior leads and chest X-ray was suggestive of widening of mediastinum. CT angiogram done outside had diagnosed dissecting aneurysm of descending thoracic aorta. First drug of choice to lower BP in these patients is:
    a. IV hydralazine
    b. IV Nitroglycerine
    c. IV nitroprusside
    d. IV beta blockers

25. A 26-year-old female with 34 weeks pregnancy is admitted with complaints of severely increasing breathlessness since last 2 days. On arrival HR 100/min and BP 190/100 mm Hg and echocardiography done is suggestive of LVEF of 20%. Her investigation revealed high NT-pro BNP levels. Which of the following drugs is contraindicated in management of heart failure in the above case:
    a. Nitroglycerin
    b. ACE inhibitors
    c. Beta blockers
    d. Hydralazine

ANSWERS

1. **Ans. (d)**

   O'Gara PT, Kushner FG, Ascheim DD, et al. American College of Cardiology Foundation (ACCF)/American Heart Association Task Force on Practice Guidelines. 2013 Guideline for the management of ST-elevation myocardial infarction. Circulation. 2013;127(4):e362-425.

   Antiplatelet therapy though a part of management of acute STEMI, the definitive treatment in patients with STEMI remains revascularization (either IV thrombolysis or Primary PCI)

2. **Ans. (a)**

   O'Gara PT, Kushner FG, Ascheim DD, et al. American College of Cardiology Foundation (ACCF)/American Heart Association Task Force on Practice Guidelines. 2013 Guideline for the management of ST-elevation myocardial infarction. Circulation. 2013;127(4):e362-425.

   Illicit drug overdose induced myocardial ischemia is a common thing nowadays and should always be kept in mind. Benzodiazepines administered in such patients reduces the sympathetic drive and is the next best step in given clinical scenario. However, revascularization remains the best definitive therapy. IV beta blockers should be avoided in such patients as would result in unopposed alpha receptor activity.

3. **Ans. (d)**

   Ponikowski P, Voors AA, Anker SD, et al. 2016 ESC: Guidelines for the diagnosis and treatment of acute and chronic heart failure: The Task Force for the diagnosis and treatment of acute and chronic heart failure of the European Society of Cardiology (ESC). Developed with the special contribution of the Heart Failure Association (HFA) of the ESC. Eur J Heart Fail.2016;18(8):891-975.

   The above patient of acute heart failure fits in profile of wet and cold. In such cases, IV diuretics and IV vasodilators both combined give the best possible treatment benefit. Only IV vasodilators and IV diuretics shall not ameliorate the whole problem. Since the blood pressures are high IV dobutamine shall not add to any benefit.

4. **Ans. (c)**

   Konstantinides SV, Torbicki A, Agnelli G, et al. Task Force for the Diagnosis and Management of Acute Pulmonary Embolism of the European Society of Cardiology (ESC). 2014 ESC: Guidelines on the diagnosis and management of acute pulmonary embolism. Eur Heart J. 2014;35(43):3033-69, 3069a-3069k.

   Patient is a high probability candidate of pulmonary embolism. With neck veins engorged a possibility of sepsis as a differential diagnosis appears less likely. To establish a definitive diagnosis of pulmonary embolism, CT pulmonary angiography is the investigation of choice. But patient here is in definitive shock, fresh renal function tests are not known and shifting patient to CT console in such clinical condition is a huge transport risk. In such scenarios doing bedside echocardiography may help us in getting a presumptive diagnosis of pulmonary embolism and thereby initiating treatment promptly.

Chapter 15 Cardiovascular System

5. **Ans. (a)**
   Konstantinides SV, Torbicki A, Agnelli G, et al. Task Force for the Diagnosis and Management of Acute Pulmonary Embolism of the European Society of Cardiology (ESC). 2014 ESC: Guidelines on the diagnosis and management of acute pulmonary embolism. Eur Heart J. 2014;35(43):3033-69, 3069a-3069k.

   Clinical scenario best describes a high probability pulmonary embolism. IV anticoagulants may be given as stat doses pending investigation (bedside echocardiography and/or CT pulmonary angiography). Heparin and enoxaparin both are equally effective as anticoagulants, but in patients with shock SC dosing is less preferred due to erratic absorption. IV thrombolysis should not be initiated unless documented presumptive pulmonary embolism by echocardiography or by CT angiography. IV antibiotic is not the next best step given the clinical scenario.

6. **Ans. (c)**
   Konstantinides SV, Torbicki A, Agnelli G, et al. Task Force for the Diagnosis and Management of Acute Pulmonary Embolism of the European Society of Cardiology (ESC). 2014 ESC: Guidelines on the diagnosis and management of acute pulmonary embolism. Eur Heart J. 2014;35(43):3033-69, 3069a-3069k.

   IV heparin is the anticoagulant of choice. In patients with shock SC absorption of anticoagulants is erratic and hence SC enoxaparin and SC fondaparinux is not the first choice. Newer oral anticoagulants have not been studied well in massive pulmonary embolism with shock and oral absorption issues in shock patients are also there.

7. **Ans (d)**
   Konstantinides SV, Torbicki A, Agnelli G, et al. Task Force for the Diagnosis and Management of Acute Pulmonary Embolism of the European Society of Cardiology (ESC). 2014 ESC: Guidelines on the diagnosis and management of acute pulmonary embolism. Eur Heart J. 2014;35(43):3033-69, 3069a-3069k.

   A,b, and c options are absolute contraindications of thrombolysis. Menstruation is not an absolute contraindication and thrombolysis should not be withheld for the same.

8. **Ans (a)**
   Konstantinides SV, Torbicki A, Agnelli G, et al. Task Force for the Diagnosis and Management of Acute Pulmonary Embolism of the European Society of Cardiology (ESC). 2014 ESC: Guidelines on the diagnosis and management of acute pulmonary embolism. Eur Heart J. 2014;35(43):3033-69, 3069a-3069k.

   Newer oral anticoagulants have not been studied in pregnant patients and warfarin is teratogenic in pregnancy. Heparins are drug of choice for anticoagulation in pregnant patients.

9. **Ans (a)**
   Konstantinides SV, Torbicki A, Agnelli G, et al. Task Force for the Diagnosis and Management of Acute Pulmonary Embolism of the European Society of Cardiology (ESC). 2014 ESC: Guidelines on the diagnosis and management of acute pulmonary embolism. Eur Heart J. 2014;35(43):3033-69, 3069a-3069k.

Positive d-dimer is present in multiple medical conditions. D-dimer as a test for pulmonary embolism has good negative predictive value. Best investigation of choice for diagnosing pulmonary embolism is CT pulmonary angiography. Patients with pulmonary embolism may have normal echocardiography study and it should not be used to rule out a possibility of pulmonary embolism.

10. **Ans. (b)**

    American Heart Association (AHA). Guidelines for cardiopulmonary resuscitation and emergency cardiovascular care.

    Patient has become suddenly unresponsive. In this scenario, next best response should be to go back to basics of BLS and check for pulse.

11. **Ans. (d)**

    American Heart Association (AHA): Guidelines for cardiopulmonary resuscitation and emergency cardiovascular care.

    Call for help should be the first response in any cardiac arrest situation. Subsequently chest compression, IV adrenaline, and DC shock may follow as per ACLS protocol.

12. **Ans. (b)**

    National Institute for Health and Care Excellence. (2014) Diagnostics guidance on myocardial infarction (acute) — Early rule out using high-sensitivity troponin tests (Elecsys troponin T high-sensitive, ARCHITECT STAT high sensitive troponin-I and AccuTnI+3 assays). [online] Available from https://www.nice.org.uk/guidance/dg15. [Last accessed June, 2019].

    Patient is a high risk case for ACS. Also since patient has presented to hospital early and troponin was sent early; they may turn negative. Troponin usually starts rising 2–3 hours after myocardial injury. Hence repeating troponin T after another 6 hours shall be helpful. Once negative, subsequent work up may follow.

13. **Ans. (c)**

    O'Gara PT, Kushner FG, Ascheim DD, et al. American College of Cardiology Foundation (ACCF)/American Heart Association Task Force on Practice Guidelines. Guideline for the management of ST-elevation myocardial infarction. Circulation. 2013;127(4):e362-425.

    Primary PCI is the best step in management of STEMI. However in given clinical scenario the next best step or immediate best step would be giving sublingual nitrates. Morphine should be avoided unless pain in not responsive to nitrates. Since the patient is maintaining saturation > 94% supplemental oxygen therapy is not needed.

14. **Ans. (c)**

    ACC/AHA/SCAI. Primary percutaneous coronary intervention for patients with ST-elevation myocardial infarction, 2015 focused update (published 2016).

    O'Gara PT, Kushner FG, Ascheim DD, et al. American College of Cardiology Foundation (ACCF)/American Heart Association Task Force on Practice Guidelines. 2013 Guideline for the management of ST-elevation myocardial infarction. Circulation. 2013;127(4):e362-425.

Early revascularization is associated with better outcome in STEMI. Waiting till morning or referring patient to higher center without thrombolysis which is 6 hours away would be detrimental. In center where option of thrombolysis is available, patient should be thrombolysed and immediately shifted to higher center for further care.

15. **Ans. (c)**
    O'Gara PT, Kushner FG, Ascheim DD, et al. American College of Cardiology Foundation (ACCF)/American Heart Association Task Force on Practice Guidelines. 2013 Guideline for the management of ST-elevation myocardial infarction. Circulation. 2013;127(4):e362-425.

    Primary PCI is the best revascularization treatment plan for patient. Starting noradrenaline is as immediate best plan. IABP is not indicated at this juncture before initiation of vasopressors.

16. **Ans. (a)**
    American Heart Association (AHA): Guidelines for cardiopulmonary resuscitation and emergency cardiovascular care.

    DC shock is the best treatment for pulseless VT. Though in a patient with pulseless VT chest compression should be initiated until cardioverter is being readied.

17. **Ans. (c)**
    Ponikowski P, Voors AA, Anker SD, et al. 2016 ESC: Guidelines for the diagnosis and treatment of acute and chronic heart failure: The Task Force for the diagnosis and treatment of acute and chronic heart failure of the European Society of Cardiology (ESC). Developed with the special contribution of the Heart Failure Association (HFA) of the ESC. Eur J Heart Fail. 2016;18(8):891-975.

18. **Ans. (a)**
    Pinsky MR, Payen D. Functional hemodynamic monitoring. Crit Care. 2005;9(6):566-72.

    PPV > 13% is a dynamic parameter of fluid responsiveness and has been well validated in mechanically ventilated patients without arrhythmias. In spontaneously breathing patient it has not been useful and should not be used to judge fluid responsiveness. CVP and PAOP are static parameters and single values should not be used to judge fluid responsiveness.

19. **Ans. (b)**
    IABP is contraindicated in severe AR, aortic dissection, sepsis, bleeding diathesis and severe peripheral arterial disease that cannot be pretreated with stenting.

20. **Ans. (a)**
    Pinsky MR. Payen D. Functional hemodynamic monitoring. Crit Care. 2005;9(6): 566-72.

    SVV and IVC collapsibility index as a measure of preload or fluid responsiveness has been validated in mechanically ventilated patients. CVP is a static hemodynamic parameter and should not be used to assess fluid responsiveness.

21. **Ans (c)**

 Rhodes A, Evans LE, Alhazzani W, et al. Surviving Sepsis Campaign: International Guidelines for Management of Sepsis and Septic Shock: 2016. Intensive Care Med. 2017;43(3):304-77.

 Patient is a case of sepsis and fluid resuscitation should be first started as per surviving sepsis guidelines.

22. **Ans. (d)**

 Monnet X, Teboul JL. Passive leg raising: five rules, not a drop of fluid! Crit Care. 2015;19:18.

 In patient with increased intra-abdominal pressure, passive leg raising test may give false results due to compression of IVC impeding venous return.

23. **Ans. (c)**

 Rhodes A, Evans LE, Alhazzani W, et al. Surviving Sepsis Campaign: International Guidelines for Management of Sepsis and Septic Shock: 2016. Intensive Care Med. 2017;43(3):304-77.

 In the given clinical scenario there is still scope of optimization of hemodynamic status. If $ScvO_2$ < 70 especially in patients with reduced LVEF, a trial of inotropic agents may be helpful. IABP is not an option in sepsis. RRT or IV diuretics do not constitute a part of hemodynamic resuscitation.

24. **Ans (d)**

 In patients with dissecting aneurysm of aorta target BP that needs to be achieved is around 90-100 mmHg. In doing so first, HR should be controlled to decrease sheer stress over aortic wall. Hence beta blockers should be first choice in given condition.

25. **Ans. (b)**

 ACEI are contraindicated in pregnancy and should not be used

CHAPTER 16

Renal

SUNITHA BINU VARGHESE

QUESTIONS

1. Following urinary findings are suggestive of "prerenal "cause of kidney injury, *except*:
   a. Dipstick specific gravity (SG) is high (>1.018)
   b. Spot urine Na is low (< 20 mmol/L)
   c. Osmolality (>350 mOsm/l)
   d. FeNa is reduced >1%.

2. Following features are suggestive of rhabdomyolysis, *except*:
   a. Urinalysis positive for 'blood'
   b. High serum creatine phosphokinase (CPK)
   c. Low calcium and high phosphate
   d. High calcium and low phosphate

3. Among the following preferences which is the last choice for insertion of a dialysis catheter as per recommendations put forward by KDIGO guidelines:
   a. Right internal jugular vein
   b. Femoral vein
   c. Left internal jugular vein
   d. Subclavian vein with preference for the patient's dominant side

4. A 40-year-old diabetic lady has been in ICU for 2 days. On admission, she was confused, sweaty, tachycardia (HR—130/min), RR—40/min, BP—100/40 mm Hg. She was aggressively fluid resuscitated and started on dopamine infusion. Her urine output was 1–1.5 mL/kg/hr on the day of admission and her urea and creatinine were 100 mg/ dL and 0.9 mg/dL, respectively. After 48 hours her urine output has dropped to 0.5 mL/kg/hr. Diagnosis on AKI can only be made if:
   a. Her serum creatinine has increased to ≥ 1.2 mg/dL
   b. Biopsy reveals necrosis of renal cortical tubules
   c. Her creatinine raises to 1.5 times her baseline value
   d. Her urine output drops to < 0.3 mL/kg/hr for 6 hours

5. Which one of the following is most likely the false statement about RENAL oliguria?
   a. Urine osmolality of 280 mOsm
   b. Urine Na concentration > 20 mmol/L
   c. Fractional excretion of sodium of 3%
   d. BUN: Creatinine ratio of > 20:1

6. All the following measures have been suggested for prevention of CI-AKI in high-risk patients *except*:
   a. Oral NAC, together with IV isotonic crystalloids
   b. IV volume expansion with isotonic sodium chloride
   c. IV volume expansion with sodium bicarbonate solution
   d. Oral fluids with IV NAC

7. Which of the following anticoagulation is preferred for patients on CRRT?
   a. Regional citrate anticoagulation
   b. Unfractionated heparin
   c. Low molecular weight heparin
   d. Direct thrombin inhibitors

8. All the following are true with regards to nutritional management of critically ill patients with AKI, *except*:
   a. Patient should be started on insulin therapy targeting plasma glucose 110–149 mg/dL.
   b. A total energy intake of 20–30 kcal/kg/d has been suggested in patients with any stage of AKI.
   c. Protein intake should be restricted with the aim of preventing or delaying initiation of RRT.
   d. We suggest administering 1.0–1.5 g/kg/d in patients with AKI on RRT

9. In staging the severity of AKI, urine output of < 0.3 mL/kg/hr for 24 hours or anuria for 12 hours is:
   a. Stage 3 of AKIN, Class F of RIFLE
   b. Stage 3 of AKIN, Class I of RIFLE
   c. Stage 2 of AKIN, Class F of RIFLE
   d. Stage 2 of AKIN, Class I of RIFLE

10. All the following causes of "renal oliguria "are associated with high FeNa, *except*:
    a. Interstitial nephritis
    b. Rhabdomyolysis
    c. Aminoglycosides
    d. Renal artery obstruction

11. Which of the following statements comparing dialysis with filtration are false?
    a. Dialysis depends on diffusion whereas filtration depends on convection
    b. Filtration is more effective than dialysis at removing small molecules
    c. Filtration in more effective than dialysis at removing cytokines
    d. Dialysis is not as effective as filtration at removing water

12. All the following are indications for RRT in an ICU patient with AKI, *except*:
    a. Fluid overload (refractory to diuretics)
    b. Severe metabolic acidosis (pH < 7.1)
    c. Phenytoin overdose
    d. Metformin overdose

13. Which of the following biomarkers has been recommended at present for evaluation of renal function in patients of AKI?
    a. S creatinine and urine output
    b. Fractional excretion of sodium
    c. Urine output and NGAL
    d. Neutrophil gelatinase–associated lipocalin (NGAL)

14. Which among the following statements regarding the pathologies associated with urinary sediment examination is false:
    a. Muddy brown casts are associated with acute tubular necrosis
    b. Red cell casts are associated with glomerulonephritis
    c. Eosinophils are associated with interstitial nephritis
    d. Urate crystals are associated with tubular injury

15. As per KDIGO guidelines 2012, all the following are true regarding dose of RRT in AKI, *except*:
    a. The dose of RRT to be delivered should be prescribed before starting each session of RRT
    b. Provide RRT to achieve the goals of electrolyte, acid-base, solute, and fluid balance that will meet the patient's needs.
    c. When using intermittent or extended RRT in AKI the recommendation is to deliver a Kt/V of 5.9 per week
    d. We recommend delivering an effluent volume of 20–25 mL/kg/h for CRRT in AKI

ANSWERS

1. **Ans. (d)**
   In "prerenal" disease, the urinary macroscopic appearance is concentrated, the dipstick specific gravity (SG) is high (>1.018), as is the osmolality (> 350 mOsm/L); the spot urine Na is low (< 20 mmol/L), and the fractional excretion of sodium (FeNa) is reduced (<1%). These indices become unreliable once the patient has received diuretic therapy and may also be confounded by endogenous osmolar substances such as glucose or urea.

2. **Ans. (d)**
   The urinary changes suggest the presence of myoglobin in the urine (urinalysis positive for "blood" but no red cells on microscopy). Muscle necrosis is also suggested by the relatively high creatinine. Serum creatine phosphokinase (CPK) is rapidly measured and, although the test may not be immediately available, urine may be tested for the presence of myoglobin. Due to muscle destruction, a serum pattern may be evident—serum potassium (and phosphate) is usually unexpectedly high and calcium is low.

3. **Ans. (d)**
   The following preferences have been recommended in the KDIGO guidelines for insertion of a dialysis catheter:
   - *First choice:* Right internal jugular vein
   - *Second choice:* Femoral vein or left internal jugular vein
   - *Last choice:* Subclavian vein with preference for the patient's dominant side.

4. **Ans. (c)**
   AKI is defined as any of the following (not graded):
   - Increase in S. creatinine by 0.3 mg/dL within 48 hours; or
   - Increase in S. creatinine to 1.5 times baseline, which is known or presumed to have occurred within the prior 7 days; or
   - Urine volume < 0.5 mL/kg/h for 6 hours.

5. **Ans. (d)**
   BUN: Creatinine ratio of < 10:1 is suggestive of renal. BUN:Cr ratio of > 20:1 is suggestive of prerenal.

   Intrinsic renal failure: Renal damage causes reduced reabsorption of BUN, therefore lowering the BUN: Cr ratio.

6. **Ans. (d)**
   KDIGO AKI guidelines 2012 for prevention of CI-AKI
   - We recommend IV volume expansion with either isotonic sodium chloride or sodium bicarbonate solutions, rather than no IV volume expansion, in patients at increased risk for CI-AKI. (1A)
   - We recommend not using oral fluids alone in patients at increased risk of CI-AKI. (1C)
   - We suggest not using theophylline to prevent CI-AKI. (2C)
   - We recommend not using fenoldopam to prevent CI-AKI. (1B)

7. **Ans. (a)**
   KDIGO AKI Guidelines 2012

   For anticoagulation in CRRT, we suggest using regional citrate anticoagulation rather than heparin in patients who do not have contraindications for citrate. (2B). For anticoagulation during CRRT in patients who have contraindications for citrate, we suggest using either unfractionated or low-molecular-weight heparin, rather than other anticoagulants. (2C)

8. **Ans. (c)**
   KDIGO AKI Guidelines 2012

   We suggest achieving a total energy intake of 20–30 kcal/kg/d in patients with any stage of AKI. (2C). We suggest to avoid restriction of protein intake with the aim of preventing or delaying initiation of RRT. (2D). We suggest administering 0.8–1.0 g/kg/d of protein in noncatabolic AKI patients without need for dialysis (2D), 1.0–1.5 g/kg/d in patients with AKI on RRT (2D), and up to a maximum of 1.7 g/kg/d in patients on continuous renal replacement therapy (CRRT) and in hypercatabolic patients. (2D). We suggest providing nutrition preferentially via the enteral route in patients with AKI. (2C)

9. **Ans. (a)**
   Classification/staging system for acute kidney injury:

System	Class/stage	Serum creatinine criteria	Urine output criteria
RIFLE	Class R	Serum creatinine increase to 1.5-fold or GFR decrease > 25% from baseline	< 0.5 mL kg/hour for 6 hours
	Class I	Serum creatinine increase to 2.0-fold or GFR decrease > 50% from baseline	<0.5 mL/kg/hour for 12 hours
	Class F	Serum creatinine increase to 3.0-fold. GFR decrease > 75% from baseline or serum creatinine ≥ 354 µmol/l (> 4.0 mg/dL) with an acute increase of at least 44 µmol/l (0.5 mg/dL	< 0.3 mL/kg/hour for 24 hours or anuria for 12 hours
AKIN	Stage 1	Serum creatinine increase ≥ 26.4 µmol/L (> 0.3 mg/ dL) or increase to 1.5-fold to 2.0-fold from baseline	< 0.5 mL/kg/hour for 6 hours
	Stage 2	Serum creatinine increase > 2.0-fold to 3.0-fold from baseline	< 0.5 mL/kg/hour for 12 hours
	Stage 3	Serum creatine increase >3.0-fold from baseline or serum creatinine ≥ 354 µmol/L (> 4.0 mg/dL) with an acute increase of at least 44 µmol/L (0.5 mg/dL)	< 0.3 mL/kg/hour for 24 hours or anuria for 12 hours.
		Need for RRT	

10. **Ans. (a)**
    Not all causes of renal oliguria result in a high FeNa. Interstitial nephritis, acute glomerulonephritis, and uric acid nephropathy have been reported in association with low FeNa.

11. Ans. (b)

How the choice of RRT can be determined by goal of treatment

What do you want to remove?	Size of molecule (Daltons)	Example	Preferred type of RRT
Small molecules electrolytes	< 500	Urea, creatine, K$^+$, H$^+$,	Dialysis or filtration
Middle molecules	500–5,000	Large drugs, e.g. vancomycin	Filtration better than dialysis
Low molecular weight proteins	5,000–50,000	Cytokines, complement	Filtration
Water	18		Filtration better than dialysis

12. Ans. (c)

Indications for RRT in ICU patients with AKI are:
- Fluid overload (refractory to diuretics)
- Hyperkalemia (K$^+$ > 6.5 mEq/l)
- Severe metabolic acidosis (pH <7.1)
- Rapidly climbing urea/creatinine (or urea > 30 mmol/l)
- *Symptomatic uremia:* Encephalopathy, pericarditis, bleeding, nausea, and pruritus
- Oliguria/anuria.
- Examples of drugs/toxins that are either removed or not removed by RRT:

Removed	Not removed
Lithium	Digoxin
Methanol	Tricyclics
Ethylene glycol	Phenytoin
Salicylates	Gliclazide
Barbiturates	Beta-blockers (except atenolol)
Metformin	Benzodiazepines
Aminoglycosides and metronidazole carbapenems, cephalosporins and most penicillins	Macrolide and quinolone antibiotics Warfarin

13. Ans. (a)

14. Ans. (d)

Kanbay M, Kasapoglu B, Perazella MA. *Acute tubular necrosis and pre-renal acute kidney injury: utility of urine microscopy in their evaluation—a systematic review. Int Urol Nephrol. 2010;42(2):425-33.*

It is recommended that urinary biochemistry and microscopy be performed in patients with AKI, if they are unresponsive to fluid and/or hemodynamic therapy and to exclude primary renal disease.
- Muddy brown casts are associated with acute tubular necrosis.
- Red cell casts are associated with glomerulonephritis. Eosinophils are associated with interstitial nephritis.

- Crystals may be urate crystals associated with tumor lysis syndrome and uric acid nephropathy.

All the following are true regarding replacement fluid, *except*:
- It is recommended to use bicarbonate, rather than lactate, as a buffer in dialysate and replacement fluid for RRT in patients with AKI and circulatory shock
- Predilution may increase the incidence of filter clotting
- Predilution reduces clearance of solute
- Predilution is more commonly used.

KDIGO guidelines 2012:
- We suggest using bicarbonate, rather than lactate, as a buffer in dialysate and replacement fluid for RRT in patients with AKI. (2C)
- We recommend using bicarbonate, rather than lactate, as a buffer in dialysate and replacement fluid for RRT in patients with AKI and circulatory shock. (1B)
- We suggest using bicarbonate, rather than lactate, as a buffer in dialysate and replacement fluid for RRT in patients with AKI and liver failure and/or lactic acidemia. (2B)

The replacement fluid may either be added to the circuit before the hemofilter (predilution) or mixed with the blood in the venous drip chamber (postdilution). Predilution may reduce the incidence of filter clotting and hence anticoagulation requirements, but reduces clearance of solute; therefore, postdilution is more commonly used.

15. **Ans. (c)**

KDIGO guidelines 2012:

We recommend delivering a Kt/V of 3.9 per week when using intermittent or extended RRT in AKI. (1A)

CHAPTER 17

Toxicology

OMENDER SINGH, ANISH GUPTA, DEVEN JUNEJA

QUESTIONS

1. Which of the following substance is not well adsorbed by activated charcoal?
   a. Quinine
   b. Phenobarbital
   c. Iron
   d. Theophylline

2. The indications of whole bowel irrigation (WBI) are:
   a. Iron poisoning
   b. Lithium poisoning
   c. Body packing
   d. All of the above

3. Oxygen saturation gap is seen in which of the following poisoning:
   a. Carbon monoxide poisoning
   b. Cyanide toxicity
   c. Dyshemoglobinemia
   d. All of the above

4. Urinary alkalinization may be helpful in all of the following poisonings *except*:
   a. Salicylates
   b. Quinidine
   c. Phenobarbital
   d. Chlorpropamide

5. Which of the following substance can cause an elevated osmolal gap?
   a. Ethanol
   b. Amphetamine
   c. Dextromethorphan
   d. Organophosphorus

6. Which of the following statements about paracetamol poisoning is false?
   a. The maximum benefit is achieved if N-acetylcysteine (NAC) is administered within 8 hours of ingestion
   b. Intravenous NAC is preferred over oral NAC therapy
   c. The Rumack-Matthew nomogram has a 25% safety margin
   d. Acetaminophen is a dialyzable drug

CHAPTER 17 Toxicology

7. A 28-year-old female presents to emergency room with an alleged history of consumption of 25 tablets of 500 mg of paracetamol. On examination, she is drowsy and has a heart rate of 110/minute, blood pressure of 90/60 mm Hg, and a respiratory rate of 26/minute. Her initial arterial blood gas (ABG) analysis is suggestive of metabolic acidosis. Serum paracetamol levels are sent and NAC is initiated. Which of the following statements regarding the role of extracorporeal therapies is not true regarding paracetamol overdose?
   a. Extracorporeal toxin removal (ECTR) is indicated in the management of severe paracetamol overdose
   b. Initial presentation with altered sensorium and metabolic acidosis is an indication for ECTR even if NAC is administered
   c. Dose of NAC has to be increased if ECTR is initiated
   d. Continuous renal replacement therapy (CRRT) is the mode of choice for initiating ECTR

8. All the following statements regarding management of corrosive ingestion are true *except*:
   a. Upper gastrointestinal (GI) endoscopy should be performed, preferably within the first 24 hours in all patients
   b. Gastrointestinal perforation is an absolute contraindication for performing endoscopy
   c. Zargar score is an endoscopic classification which may aid in prediction of subsequent clinical progression
   d. Systemic steroids are indicated to prevent stricture formation

9. A 45-year-old female suffering from depression was brought to the ER after she consumed 50 tablets of aspirin. On examination, she was confused, agitated with heart rate—120/minute, blood pressure—124/70 mm Hg and respiratory rate (RR)—35/minute. Systemic examination was unremarkable. Her ABG on admission was suggestive of respiratory alkalosis. Which of the following statements is false?
   a. Alkalinization is key to management
   b. Glucose should be administered to all patients with altered sensorium
   c. Early endotracheal intubation is advisable to reduce work of breathing
   d. Hemodialysis is an effective treatment modality

10. A 22-year-old foreign national was brought to the ER after he developed a seizure at the airport. On admission, he was agitated, febrile (T—43°C), tachycardic and tachypneic. Pupils were dilated with normal reaction. In ER, he suddenly complained of chest pain and an electrocardiogram (ECG) was done which was suggestive of ST elevation MI in anterior chest leads. He was shifted to the catheterization laboratory for an urgent angiogram which was suggestive of normal coronaries. Which of the following substance can cause the above toxidrome?
    a. Lysergic acid diethylamide (LSD)
    b. Cocaine
    c. Amphetamine
    d. Ecstasy

11. Which of the following statements about cocaine intoxication is false?
    a. Benzoylecgonine is the major metabolite of cocaine
    b. Benzodiazepines are the first-line agent to manage cardiovascular symptoms
    c. Aspirin should be administered to all patients with acute coronary syndrome secondary to cocaine
    d. Beta-blockers are central to management of cocaine-induced myocardial infarction

12. A 65-year-old male presents with a history of alleged overdose of amitriptyline. He is complaining of dry mouth, blurring of vision, and altered mental status. On examination, he has a heart rate of 138/minute, blood pressure of 90/60 mm Hg and a respiratory rate of 20/minute. An urgent ECG is obtained which is suggestive of broad complex tachycardia with a prominent R wave in aVR. Which of the following medications is used for the management?
    a. Amiodarone
    b. Lignocaine
    c. Sodium bicarbonate
    d. Magnesium sulfate

13. A 25-year-old female from a farmer family was brought to a tertiary care hospital with an alleged history of ingestion of some liquid substance used for killing weeds in their farms, paraquat, around 12 hours before presentation. Her presenting complaints were melena and hematemesis, progressive respiratory distress (type 1 respiratory failure) requiring oxygen supplementation and noninvasive ventilation. Regarding oxygen supplementation in paraquat poisoning which statement is true:
    a. Target SpO_2 >95%
    b. Target SpO_2 ~88–92%
    d. Give 100% O_2 to wash off poison from lungs
    e. No O_2 supplementation at all

14. Which of the following is not an indication for hemodialysis in methanol poisoning?
    a. Metabolic acidosis
    b. Visual changes
    c. Elevated methanol levels
    d. Acute kidney injury

15. A 40-year-old male working in a paint factory was brought to the triage with fever, altered behavior and cyanosis. On examination, he was tachycardic, hypotensive and tachypneic. SpO_2 on room air was 85%. ABG was suggestive of hypoxemia with methemoglobin levels of 40%. He was G6PD deficient. Which of the following should be used for the treatment of methemoglobinemia?
    a. Methylene blue
    b. Vitamin C
    c. Cimetidine
    d. All of the above

16. The indications of DigiFab include all of the following *except*:
    a. Arrhythmias
    b. Hyperkalemia
    c. Hemodynamic instability
    d. Hypokalemia

17. A 45-year-old male patient presents with acute warfarin overdose. On day 4, his international normalized ratio (INR) is found to be 8. There is no evidence of bleeding at any site. What is the most appropriate treatment for him?
    a. Discontinuation of warfarin
    b. Intravenous vitamin K
    c. Oral vitamin K
    d. Fresh frozen plasma (FFP) transfusion

18. In the same patient, INR was found to be 11 on day 5, but still there is no evidence of bleeding and patient is stable. What would be the most appropriate treatment at this juncture?
    a. Intravenous vitamin K
    b. Oral vitamin K
    c. 4-factor prothrombin complex concentrate
    d. 3-factor prothrombin complex concentrate

19. The advantages of prothrombin complex concentrate over FFP to manage life-threatening bleeding in a patient of warfarin toxicity include all *except*:
    a. No need of thawing or blood group typing hence rapid availability
    b. Less risk of infectious disease transmission and volume overload
    c. Rapid reversal of coagulopathy
    d. No risk of thromboembolic events

20. All the following are indications for the administration of anti-snake venom *except*:
    a. Swelling after bites on fingers and toes
    b. Swelling involving less than half of the bitten limb
    c. Rapid extension of the swelling
    d. Enlarged tender lymph nodes

21. All of the following drug characteristics make it amenable for elimination using extracorporeal toxin removal (ECTR) *except*:
    a. Low protein binding
    b. High lipid solubility
    c. Low volume of distribution
    d. Low endogenous clearance

22. All the following statements regarding lipid emulsion therapy (LET) are true *except*:
    a. It is recommended to be used during cardiopulmonary resuscitation (CPR) in a patient with suspected local anesthetic systemic toxicity (LAST)
    b. A bolus dose of 1.5 mL/kg of 20% lipid emulsion intravenously is recommended

c. It can also be used in the management of severe poisonings other than LAST, like angiotensin-converting enzyme (ACE) inhibitors
d. The maximum dose should not exceed 12 mL/kg, in the management of LAST

23. All the following statements regarding carbon monoxide poisoning are true *except*:
    a. Neurological symptoms are first to appear
    b. "Cherry red" skin color is pathognomonic and early sign of carbon monoxide toxicity
    d. Serum carboxyhemoglobin levels may not correlate with clinical severity
    e. Pregnancy is an indication for initiating hyperbaric oxygen (HBO)

24. Which of the following statement regarding botulinum toxicity is false?
    a. Patient may present with type 2 respiratory failure due to intercostal muscle involvement
    b. Bulbar palsy may be a presenting feature of the illness
    c. Cognitive and sensory functions are invariably affected
    d. Antibiotics play a role only in cases of wound botulism

25. A 50-year-old male is recently diagnosed as sputum positive pulmonary tuberculosis. He is a nonsmoker and nonalcoholic with no other comorbidities. He has presented to the ER with a history of generalized tonic-clonic seizure after administration of isoniazid 600 mg and rifampicin 450 mg. On arrival, vitals were stable and physical examination revealed no abnormality. Which of the following statement concerning this patient is false?
    a. Isoniazid toxicity can manifest as generalized tonic-clonic seizures and metabolic acidosis
    b. Phenytoin is the antiepileptic of choice
    c. Intravenous pyridoxine 5 g is administered in suspected cases of isoniazid toxicity
    d. Isoniazid acts by blocking the enzyme pyridoxal 5'-phosphate

26. Which of the following factors is not inhibited by warfarin?
    a. Protein S
    b. Factor II
    c. Factor VIII
    d. Factor X

27. All the following statements regarding direct-acting oral anticoagulants (DOACs) are true *except*:
    a. Prothrombin time (PT), and activated partial thromboplastin time (aPTT) can be used routinely to adjust their doses
    b. In comparison to warfarin, the chances of fatal intracranial bleeding with DOACs are clearly lower
    c. Hemodialysis may be used to remove active dabigatran from circulation
    d. Antidote can reverse the anticoagulant effects of apixaban and rivaroxaban within minutes of its administration

28. Which of the following is not a component of King's College criteria for liver transplantation in acetaminophen-induced liver function?
    a. Lactate
    b. pH
    c. Creatinine
    d. Bilirubin

29. In carbon monoxide poisoning, hyperbaric oxygen therapy is indicated in the following conditions *except*:
    a. Unconscious patient
    b. Blood pH <7.1
    c. Pregnancy with COHb >25%
    d. Carbon monoxide level >25%

ANSWERS

1. **Ans. (c)**

   Levine M, Brooks DE, Truitt CA, et al. Toxicology in the ICU: Part 1: general overview and approach to treatment. Chest. 2011;140(3):795-806.

   Singh O, Nasa P, Juneja D. Approach to a poisoned patient. In: Singh O, Juneja D (Eds). Principles and Practice of Critical Care Toxicology, 1st edition. New Delhi, India: Jaypee Brothers Medical Publishers (P) Ltd; 2019. pp. 6-9.

   Activated charcoal is used for gastric decontamination. Efficacy is greatest when administered within 1 hour of toxin ingestion. It adsorbs systemic toxins and prevents their systemic absorption. Single-dose activated charcoal (SDAC) is used for ingestions with dapsone, carbamazepine, quinine, phenobarbital and theophylline. Iron, lithium and alcohols are not adsorbed by activated charcoal.

2. **Ans. (d)**

   Levine M, Brooks DE, Truitt CA, et al. Toxicology in the ICU: Part 1: general overview and approach to treatment. Chest. 2011;140(3):795-806.

   Singh O, Nasa P, Juneja D. Approach to a poisoned patient. In: Singh O, Juneja D (Eds). Principles and Practice of Critical Care Toxicology, 1st edition. New Delhi, India: Jaypee Brothers Medical Publishers (P) Ltd; 2019. pp. 6-9.

   Whole bowel irrigation refers to the administration of osmotically balanced solutions (polyethylene glycol solution) to induce diarrhea and expel unabsorbed toxins from the gut. The indications of WBI are toxicities with iron, lithium, sustained-release preparations and body packing.

3. **Ans. (d)**

   Akhtar J, Johnston BD, Krenzelok EP. Mind the gap. J Emerg Med. 2007;33(2):131-2.

   Oxygen saturation gap is the difference between the oxygen saturation as measured by pulse oximetry (SpO_2) and calculated from an arterial blood gas (SaO_2). A difference of greater than 5 is significant and signifies the presence of abnormal hemoglobins (carboxyhemoglobin, methemoglobin, sulfhemoglobin).

4. **Ans. (b)**

   Singh O, Nasa P, Juneja D. Approach to a poisoned patient. In: Singh O, Juneja D (Eds). Principles and Practice of Critical Care Toxicology, 1st edition. New Delhi, India: Jaypee Brothers Medical Publishers (P) Ltd; 2019. pp. 1-18.

   Bagai S, Khullar D. Approach to toxin induced renal failure. In: Singh O, Juneja D (Eds). Principles and Practice of Critical Care Toxicology, 1st edition. New Delhi, India: Jaypee Brothers Medical Publishers (P) Ltd; 2019. pp. 257-63.

   Urinary alkalinization has been shown to enhance excretion of certain drugs and hence may prove to be beneficial in the management of overdose of drugs like lithium, salicylates, sulfonamides, phenobarbital, methotrexate and chlorpropamide. Excretion of drugs which are primarily excreted by the kidneys, and have high volume of distribution and protein binding, may be enhanced by urinary alkalinization. Urine alkalinization may be achieved using sodium bicarbonate solution and target urine pH of 7.5–8.5 should be maintained. On the other hand, urinary acidification has been tried, using agents like ammonium chloride or ascorbic acid to enhance elimination of certain poisons such as amantadine, amphetamines, quinidine and phencyclidine.

5. **Ans. (a)**
Lynd LD, Richardson KJ, Purssell RA, et al. An evaluation of the osmole gap as a screening test for toxic alcohol poisoning. BMC Emerg Med. 2008;8:5.
Kraut JA, Xing SX. Approach to the evaluation of a patient with an increased serum osmolal gap and high-anion-gap metabolic acidosis. Am J Kidney Dis. 2011;58(3):480-4.

Osmolal gap is the difference between measured and calculated serum osmolality. The normal osmolal gap is less than 10. It signifies the presence of unmeasured solutes (apart from sodium, glucose and urea) in the blood. Toxic alcohols like ethanol, methanol, ethylene glycol, propylene glycol and isopropanol generally elevate the measured osmolality and thus the osmolal gap.

6. **Ans. (b)**
Schwarz E, Cohn B. Is intravenous acetylcysteine more effective than oral administration for the prevention of hepatotoxicity in acetaminophen overdose? Ann Emerg Med. 2014;63(1):79-80.
Gupta A, Juneja D. Acetaminophen (paracetamol) poisoning. In: Singh O, Juneja D (Eds). Principles and Practice of Critical Care Toxicology, 1st edition. New Delhi, India: Jaypee Brothers Medical Publishers (P) Ltd; 2019. pp. 203-9.

After acute paracetamol ingestion, it is best to initiate therapy with NAC as early as possible with maximal benefit if administered within 8 hours of ingestion. The Rumack-Matthew nomogram is used to predict the risk of hepatotoxicity by plotting serum acetaminophen levels measured at 4 hours postingestion on the nomogram. A value above the nomogram is suggestive of risk of hepatotoxicity and mandates administration of NAC. The nomogram line has a 25% safety margin to compensate for difference in laboratory techniques. NAC is the specific antidote for paracetamol (acetaminophen) poisoning. There are two regimens (oral and intravenous) which are USFDA approved. There is no difference with respect to efficacy between oral and intravenous NAC. Acetaminophen is a dialyzable drug and dialysis is recommended in cases with severe metabolic acidosis, altered mentation, hyperlactatemia and unavailability/allergic reaction to NAC.

7. **Ans. (d)**
Gosselin S, Juurlink DN, Kielstein JT, et al. Extracorporeal treatment for acetaminophen poisoning: recommendations from the Extrip workgroup. Clin Toxicol (Phila). 2014;52(8):856-67.
Juneja D, Singh O. Extracorporeal therapies: specific poisons. In: Singh O, Juneja D (Eds). Principles and Practice of Critical Care Toxicology, 1st edition. New Delhi, India: Jaypee Brothers Medical Publishers (P) Ltd; 2019. pp. 274-87.

N-acetylcysteine is the mainstay of therapy in patients with paracetamol overdose. However, ECTR may be indicated in cases where NAC is not available or there is evidence of massive ingestion. Altered mental status, metabolic acidosis, and elevated serum lactate levels are indicative of massive overdose and are associated with poor outcomes. Hence, ECTR is indicated if serum paracetamol levels are above 900 mg/L, even if NAC is administered. As NAC is also dialyzable, its dose must be increased when ECTR is initiated. Because of its ease of availability, low cost and good safety profile, intermittent hemodialysis has been recommended as the modality of choice for performing ECTR. Other alternative modalities include CRRT and hemoperfusion using resin or activated charcoal filters.

8. **Ans. (d)**

   Raghu R, Naik R, Vadivelan M. Corrosive poisoning. Indian J Clin Pract. 2012;23(3):131-4.

   Deepak D. Corrosive ingestion: acids and alkalis. In: Singh O, Juneja D (Eds). Principles and Practice of Critical Care Toxicology, 1st edition. New Delhi, India: Jaypee Brothers Medical Publishers (P) Ltd; 2019. pp. 218-26.

   It is recommended that upper GI endoscopy should be performed in all patients with suspected corrosive ingestion to evaluate the extent of involvement and predict subsequent clinical progression. It should be performed within the first 24–48 hours of ingestion. Scores like Zargar and Kikendall have been developed to grade esophageal injury. The absolute contraindications to performing endoscopy are GI perforation, hemodynamic instability and unprotective airway or respiratory distress. Presence of uncorrected airway and time to ingestion beyond 72 hours are relative contraindications. Systemic steroids have been tried to prevent formation of strictures, but are currently not indicated because of unproven benefit and chances of increased infectious complications.

9. **Ans. (c)**

   Gupta A, Singh O. NSAID overdose. In: Singh O, Juneja D (Eds). Principles and Practice of Critical Care Toxicology, 1st edition. New Delhi, India: Jaypee Brothers Medical Publishers (P) Ltd; 2019. pp. 210-7.

   Greenberg MI, Hendrickson RG, Hofman M. Deleterious effects of endotracheal intubation in salicylate poisoning. Ann Emerg Med. 2003;41(4):583-4.

   Stolbach AI, Hoffman RS, Nelson LS. Mechanical ventilation was associated with acidemia in a case series of salicylate-poisoned patients. Acad Emerg Med. 2008;15(9):866-9.

   From the history, the patient is a case of salicylate poisoning. Alkalinization of serum and urine is central to management as salicylate is a weak acid and in steady state, it exists as salicylate and hydrogen ion. Alkalemia increases dissociation of salicylic acid to salicylate and hydrogen ion thus alleviating the toxic effects. Glucose should be supplemented in all patients as neuroglycopenia is seen in aspirin-poisoned patients despite normal glucose levels. Hemodialysis is an effective modality to remove salicylate and correct electrolyte imbalance. Endotracheal intubation in an aspirin-poisoned patient is deleterious and can lead to worsening of clinical condition and even death.

It is advisable to intubate the patient only in cases of hypoventilation, respiratory failure and depressed level of consciousness. Aspirin stimulates the medullary respiratory center causing an increase in minute ventilation by increasing both the RR and tidal volume (TV). This leads to respiratory alkalosis by decreasing carbon dioxide levels ($PaCO_2$). Alkalosis is a protective mechanism as salicylic acid dissociates to salicylate and hydrogen ion in alkaline medium thus trapping the salicylate ions in the blood. During endotracheal intubation, the administration of sedative and neuromuscular blockers will blunt this protective response and lead to respiratory acidosis. As a result, there is redistribution and crossover of unionized salicylate back into the brain with subsequent increase in toxicity. Some schools of thought advise sodium bicarbonate administration prior to intubation so as to maintain an alkalotic pH (7.45–7.5). The ventilatory settings should be adjusted to maintain a high minute ventilation either by maintaining a high respiratory rate (preferably patient's preintubation rate) and/or a high TV.

10. **Ans. (b)**

Afonso L, Mohammad T, Thatai D. Crack whips the heart: a review of the cardiovascular toxicity of cocaine. Am J Cardiol. 2007;100:1040-3.

Lange RA, Cigarroa RG, Yancy CW Jr, et al. Cocaine-induced coronary-artery vasoconstriction. N Engl J Med. 1989;321(23):1557-62.

Singh O, Gupta A. Cocaine intoxication. In: Singh O, Juneja D (Eds). Principles and Practice of Critical Care Toxicology, 1st edition. New Delhi, India: Jaypee Brothers Medical Publishers (P) Ltd; 2019. pp. 93-8.

The patient has presented with neurological and cardiovascular manifestations of an unknown poison. Amongst the options cocaine intoxication can lead to the described toxidrome. The specific pointer is cardiovascular manifestation as cocaine can lead to STEMI with normal coronaries. Cocaine leads to coronary vasoconstriction which is responsible for the cardiovascular manifestations. Seizures, hyperthermia, tachypnea and tachycardia can be seen with all the above-mentioned poisons.

11. **Ans. (d)**

Hoffman RS. Cocaine and beta-blockers: should the controversy continue? Ann Emerg Med. 2008;51(2):127-9.

Richards JR, Hollander JE, Ramoska EA, et al. β-blockers, cocaine, and the unopposed α-stimulation phenomenon. J Cardiovasc Pharmacol Ther. 2017;22(3):239-49.

Singh O, Gupta A. Cocaine intoxication. In: Singh O, Juneja D (Eds). Principles and Practice of Critical Care Toxicology, 1st edition. New Delhi, India: Jaypee Brothers Medical Publishers (P) Ltd; 2019. pp. 93-8.

Beta-blockers are contraindicated in cocaine-induced myocardial infarction especially when cocaine abuse is within less than 24 hours. Beta-blockers can lead to unopposed alpha-adrenergic stimulation, which can cause hypertension and coronary arterial vasoconstriction, further exacerbating myocardial ischemia. The use of combined alpha-/beta-blockers (e.g. labetalol) is controversial with inconclusive evidence with regard to their safety and efficacy. Some authors believe that labetalol with mixed alpha- and beta-blocking properties (beta:alpha = 3:1 for oral and 7:1 for intravenous preparation) may be useful.

Aspirin should be given to patients with acute coronary syndrome (ACS) except in cases of aortic dissection. Benzodiazepines play a central role in management of cardiovascular symptoms as they reduce sympathetic flow and reduce tachycardia and hypertension. Cocaine is metabolized into various metabolites, i.e. benzoylecgonine, ecgonine methyl ester, norcocaine, meta-hydroxy BE (mOH-BE) and para-hydroxy-BE (p-OH-BE). The major metabolite of cocaine is benzoylecgonine.

12. **Ans. (c)**

Juneja D, Singh O. Sodium channel blockers. In: Singh O, Juneja D (Eds). Principles and Practice of Critical Care Toxicology, 1st edition. New Delhi, India: Jaypee Brothers Medical Publishers (P) Ltd; 2019. pp. 185-93.

Zima AV, Qin J, Fill M, et al. Tricyclic antidepressant amitriptyline alters sarcoplasmic reticulum calcium handling in ventricular myocytes. Am J Physiol Heart Circ Physiol. 2008;295(5):H2008-16.

Tricyclic antidepressants (TCAs) are commonly prescribed antidepressants. However, they have a similar effect on heart conduction as Class Ia antiarrhythmic agents like quinidine and procainamide. These effects are mainly attributed to sodium channel blockade and alteration in handling of calcium by the cardiac myocytes. Sodium bicarbonate is the drug of choice for TCA toxicity. It helps improve hypotension and QRS duration by sodium loading. It induces an alkalosis which may help by increasing protein binding of the drug and thereby reducing its effective concentration and also alter the charge of the TCA-receptor complex. The exact initial dose is unclear. Sodium bicarbonate is administered at 2 mEq/kg every few minutes until QRS duration shortens to less than 100 ms, hypotension resolves or seizures abort. Once hemodynamically stable, it is continued to maintain a pH of 7.5–7.55 and frequent monitoring with ABG and ECG (for QRS duration—target <100 ms).

13. **Ans. (b)**

Goel A, Singh O. Herbicides poisoning: paraquat and diquat. In: Singh O, Juneja D (Eds). Principles and Practice of Critical Care Toxicology, 1st edition. New Delhi, India: Jaypee Brothers Medical Publishers (P) Ltd; 2019. pp. 312-9.

O'Driscoll BR, Howard LS, Earis J, et al. British Thoracic Society guideline for oxygen use in adults in healthcare and emergency settings. BMJ Open Resp Res. 2017;4:e000170.

Lungs are the most affected organs in paraquat poisoning as they take up poison against a concentration gradient. Alveolar epithelium, especially type II pneumocytes in lungs, suffers maximum cell damage. The manifestations are acute alveolitis and diffuse alveolar collapse. The lung involvement has two phases: inflammation leading to acute alveolitis in 1–3 days and subsequent to this is secondary fibrosis. Patient typically presents with worsening respiratory functions due to decreased gas exchange in the next 3–7 days.

Ultimately in next 4–5 weeks severe hypoxia occurs due to ongoing fibrosis, leading to death. As oxidative stress and generation of free radicals is the mainstay of toxicity in paraquat poisoning and oxygen supplementation may further worsen oxidative stress, so it should be avoided in mild to moderate hypoxia and a SpO_2~88–92% should be accepted.

14. **Ans. (c)**
    Barceloux DG, Bond GR, Krenzelok EP, et al. American Academy of Clinical Toxicology practice guidelines on the treatment of methanol poisoning. J Toxicol Clin Toxicol. 2002;40(4):415-46.

    Hemodialysis is an effective modality to remove alcohol and their toxic metabolites. The typical indications for hemodialysis are high anion gap metabolic acidosis, visual changes and renal failure. Drug levels are not done routinely; results may not be available in time and hence is not a classic indication for dialysis. Patients who are nonacidemic are treated with fomepizole or ethanol to alleviate methanol toxicity.

    There is no data correlating blood levels of methanol and the need for dialysis. Hemodialysis is recommended when there is coma, seizures, high anion gap metabolic acidosis or new visual deficits.

15. **Ans. (b)**
    Rosen PJ, Johnson C, McGehee WG, et al. Failure of methylene blue treatment in toxic methemoglobinemia. Association with glucose-6-phosphate dehydrogenase deficiency. Ann Intern Med. 1971;75(1):83-6.

    The patient is a case of aniline dye exposure with consequent methemoglobinemia. The treatment of methemoglobinemia is methylene blue at a dose of 1–2 mg/kg over 5 minutes by intravenous route. However, this patient is G6PD deficient and methylene blue could lead to fatal hemolysis and hence is contraindicated. Vitamin C or ascorbic acid at a dose of 1 g 6 hourly is used in cases of methemoglobinemia with G6PD deficiency. Cimetidine has a role in the management of methemoglobinemia secondary to dapsone but has no routine use.

16. **Ans. (d)**
    Al-Khatib SM, Stevenson WG, Ackerman MJ, et al. 2017 AHA/ACC/HRS Guideline for management of patients with ventricular arrhythmias and the prevention of sudden cardiac death: executive summary: a report of the American College of Cardiology/American Heart Association Task Force on Clinical Practice Guidelines and the Heart Rhythm Society. J Am Coll Cardiol. 2018;72(14):1677-749.
    Singh O, Gupta A. Antidotes. In: Singh O, Juneja D (Eds). Principles and Practice of Critical Care Toxicology, 1st edition. New Delhi, India: Jaypee Brothers Medical Publishers (P) Ltd; 2019. p. 40.

    DigiFab is a commercial preparation of digoxin-specific antibody fragment. Each vial contains 40 mg of Fab fragments which binds to 0.5 mg of digoxin. It lacks the Fc portion of the antibody and hence allergic reactions are uncommon. It is used for the treatment of digitalis poisoning associated with life-threatening arrhythmias, hemodynamic instability and hyperkalemia.

17. **Ans. (a)**

    Holbrook A, Schulman S, Witt DM, et al. Evidence-based management of anticoagulant therapy: Antithrombotic Therapy and Prevention of Thrombosis, 9th ed: American College of Chest Physicians Evidence-Based Clinical Practice Guidelines. Chest. 2012;141(2 Suppl):e152S-84S.

    Witt DM, Nieuwlaat R, Clark NP, et al. American Society of Hematology 2018 guidelines for management of venous thromboembolism: optimal management of anticoagulation therapy. Blood Adv. 2018;2(22):3257-91.

    In cases of acute warfarin ingestion, if INR is ≤9, then the risk of bleeding has not been found to be very high. If no further warfarin exposure is expected, then nothing more needs to be done apart from discontinuing warfarin. If there is any other factor which makes these patients prone to high risk of bleeding, then oral vitamin K_1 in the dose of 1-2.5 mg can be given. FFP transfusion should be reserved for patients with active bleeding.

18. **Ans. (b)**

    Holbrook A, Schulman S, Witt DM, et al. Evidence-based management of anticoagulant therapy: Antithrombotic Therapy and Prevention of Thrombosis, 9th ed: American College of Chest Physicians Evidence-based Clinical Practice Guidelines. Chest. 2012;141(2 Suppl):e152S-84S.

    Witt DM, Nieuwlaat R, Clark NP, et al. American Society of Hematology 2018 guidelines for management of venous thromboembolism: optimal management of anticoagulation therapy. Blood Adv. 2018;2(22):3257-91.

    Dezee KJ, Shimeall WT, Douglas KM, et al. Treatment of excessive anticoagulation with phytonadione (vitamin K): a meta-analysis. Arch Intern Med. 2006;166(4):391-7.

    If INR >10, then oral vitamin K_1 (phytomenadione or phytonadione) in the dose of 2.5-5 mg should be preferred over intravenous vitamin K_1. Oral vitamin K_1 has very good bioavailability and is recommended when there is no life-threatening bleeding. Intravenous vitamin K_1 carries significant risk of anaphylaxis and therefore should be used cautiously. It should be reserved for those with severe or life-threatening bleeding. Prothrombin complex concentrate (PCC) should be used only when there is life-threatening bleeding.

19. **Ans. (d)**

    Sarode R, Milling TJ Jr, Refaai MA, et al. Efficacy and safety of a 4-factor prothrombin complex concentrate in patients on vitamin K antagonists presenting with major bleeding: a randomized, plasma-controlled, phase IIIb study. Circulation. 2013;128(11):1234-43.

    Dentali F, Marchesi C, Giorgi Pierfranceschi M, et al. Safety of prothrombin complex concentrates for rapid anticoagulation reversal of vitamin K antagonists. A meta-analysis. Thromb Haemost. 2011;106(3):429-38.

    Because patients being treated with vitamin K antagonist (VKA) therapy have an underlying risk of or a diagnosed thromboembolic disease state, administration of prothrombin complex concentrate (PCC) may predispose the patient to a thromboembolic complication. Benefits of reversing VKA therapy should be weighed against the potential risk of a thromboembolic event.

20. Ans. (b)

Senthilkumaran S, Subramanian PT. Envenomation: snake, scorpion, and spider. In: Singh O, Juneja D (Eds). Principles and Practice of Critical Care Toxicology, 1st edition. New Delhi, India: Jaypee Brothers Medical Publishers (P) Ltd; 2019. pp. 348-52.

The indications of anti-snake venom are a confirmed or suspected snakebite with signs and symptoms of envenomation.

The features of envenomation are divided into systemic and local envenomation.

Systemic envenomation	Local envenomation
Hematological: • Spontaneous systemic bleeding • Coagulopathy [whole blood clotting time (WBCT) >20 minutes or prolonged prothrombin time/deranged INR], or thrombocytopenia (platelets <100,000/mm³) *Neurological:* Ptosis, external ophthalmoplegia and muscle paralysis *Cardiovascular:* Hypotension, shock, arrhythmias *Renal:* Acute kidney injury • Hemoglobinuria, myoglobinuria • Rhabdomyolysis	• Swelling involving more than half of the limb (in the absence of a tourniquet) within 48 hours of the bite • Swelling after bites on the digits • Rapid extension of swelling within a few hours of bite • Enlarged tender lymph node draining the bitten limb

21. Ans. (b)

Juneja D, Singh O. Extracorporeal therapies: general principles. In: Singh O, Juneja D (Eds). Principles and Practice of Critical Care Toxicology, 1st edition. New Delhi, India: Jaypee Brothers Medical Publishers (P) Ltd; 2019. pp. 264-73.
Roberts DM, Buckley NA. Pharmacokinetic considerations in clinical toxicology: clinical applications. Clin Pharmacokinet. 2007;46(11):897-939.

Extracorporeal toxin removal is being increasingly used in the management of severe poisonings. However, not all poisonings can be managed with ECTR. Certain characteristics make some substances amenable for removal through ECTR. These include small molecular weight, low volume of distribution, low protein binding, low endogenous clearance and low lipid solubility. These basic characteristics also determine which mode of ECTR will be more beneficial.

22. Ans. (c)

Singh O, Juneja D. Lipid emulsion therapy. In: Singh O, Juneja D (Eds). Principles and Practice of Critical Care Toxicology, 1st edition. New Delhi, India: Jaypee Brothers Medical Publishers (P) Ltd; 2019. pp. 60-7.
Neal JM, Mulroy MF, Weinberg GL, et al. American Society of Regional Anesthesia and Pain Medicine checklist for managing local anesthetic systemic toxicity: 2012 version. Reg Anesth Pain Med. 2012;37(1):16-8.

Lipid emulsion therapy has been recommended by the American Society of Regional Anesthesia (ASRA) in the management of patients with severe LAST as an adjunct to airway management and good CPR. A bolus dose is recommended, 1.5 mL/kg of 20% lipid emulsion intravenously over 1 minute, which should be followed by a maintenance dose at a rate of 0.25 mL/kg/minute. It is recommended to be used for at least 60 minutes, but it has been used for longer periods. However, the total maximum dose should not exceed 12 mL/kg. Although there is a probable role of LET in the management of severe toxicities associated with cardiac toxic drugs like beta-blockers and calcium channel blockers, and there are several reports of its successful use in such patients, presently, there is no role of LET in management of ACE inhibitor overdose.

23. **Ans. (b)**

Guzman JA. Carbon monoxide poisoning. Crit Care Clin. 2012;28(4):537-48.
Bhalla A, Suri V, Nayer J. Carbon monoxide poisoning. In: Singh O, Juneja D (Eds). Principles and Practice of Critical Care Toxicology, 1st edition. New Delhi, India: Jaypee Brothers Medical Publishers (P) Ltd; 2019. pp. 162-6.

Neurological symptoms are first to appear, and headache is the most common presenting symptom. "Cherry red" color is classically associated with carbon monoxide toxicity, but it is rarely present in clinical practice. Although serum carboxyhemoglobin (COHb) levels are often necessary to make a diagnosis, they may not correlate with clinical severity.

Supplementation with 100% oxygen is the treatment of choice, as it reduces the half-life of COHb from 4–5 hours to 30 minutes. HBO has been used traditionally in the management of severe CO poisoning; however, its role remains controversial. Patients with severe neurological or cardiovascular complications and those with very high COHb levels (>25%) should be considered for therapy with HBO. In addition, CO-poisoned pregnant women should also be considered for HBO because of its potential benefit to the mother and the fetus.

24. **Ans. (c)**

Chaudhari A, Juneja D. Botulism. In: Singh O, Juneja D (Eds). Principles and Practice of Critical Care Toxicology, 1st edition. New Delhi, India: Jaypee Brothers Medical Publishers (P) Ltd; 2019. pp. 128-32.
Centers for Disease Control and Prevention (CDC). Botulism: information and guidance for clinicians. CDC; 2008. Last accessed 15/05/2019.
American Academy of Pediatrics. Botulism and infant botulism (Clostridium botulinum). In: Kimberlin DW, Brady MT, Jackson MA, Long SS (Eds). Red Book: 2015 Report of the Committee on Infectious Diseases, 30th edition. Elk Grove Village, IL: American Academy of Pediatrics; 2015. p. 294.

Botulism presents with a constellation of neurological symptoms that begin with the involvement of ocular muscles resulting in diplopia, ptosis and paralysis of facial muscle, muscles of mastication and swallowing with eventual involvement of the larger groups of muscles of limbs. However, cognitive and sensory functions are usually spared. It is a classical descending type of symmetrical flaccid paralysis and many patients present with signs of bulbar palsies to emergency room. If the illness goes undiagnosed and untreated, it may involve intercostal muscles with other muscles of respiration including the diaphragm resulting in respiratory failure and need for mechanical ventilation. The bulbar palsy presents with motor involvement of cranial nerves with signs and symptoms of blurring of vision, diplopia, nystagmus, dilated pupils, sore throat, dysphagia, dysphonia, and diminished gag reflexes. Treatment consists of general supportive measures and antitoxin administration. Antibiotic use may be recommended in case of wound botulism (although not proven by clinical trials so far). Recommended antibiotics include penicillin G (3 million units intravenous 4th hourly) or metronidazole (500 mg intravenous 8th hourly).

25. **Ans. (b)**
    Chaudhari D, Chaudhari A, Singh O. Toxin-induced seizures. In: Singh O, Juneja D (Eds). Principles and Practice of Critical Care Toxicology, 1st edition. New Delhi, India: Jaypee Brothers Medical Publishers (P) Ltd; 2019. pp. 109-14.
    Sharma AN, Hoffman RJ. Toxin-related seizures. Emerg Med Clin North Am. 2011;29(1):125-39.
    Chen HY, Albertson TE, Olson KR. Treatment of drug-induced seizures. Br J Clin Pharmacol. 2016;81(3):412-9.

    Isoniazid is an antitubercular agent known to cause seizures. Acute toxicity may result in high anion gap metabolic acidosis and even coma. Hydrazines like isoniazid block the enzyme pyridoxal 5'-phosphate, which is a cofactor in the synthesis of GABA, resulting in its deficiency. Thus, pyridoxine (vitamin B_6) is the treatment of choice in seizures of hydrazine toxicity with a possible role in theophylline toxicity as well. Empirically dose of 5 g intravenously (70 mg/kg in pediatric) is given if the ingested dose of isoniazid is unknown. However, if the amount of drug ingested is known, then pyridoxine should be replaced in equal quantities to the dose of administered isoniazid. Role of phenytoin in drug-induced seizures is questionable. Studies have shown that phenytoin does not effectively terminate seizures caused by a number of drugs and toxins and its use is contraindicated in seizures induced by theophylline, lidocaine, or TCAs.

26. **Ans. (c)**
    Hanley JP. Warfarin reversal. J Clin Pathol. 2004;57:1132-9.
    Butler AC, Tait RC. Management of oral anticoagulant-induced intracranial haemorrhage. Blood Rev. 1998;12:35-44.
    Pindur G, Mörsdorf S. The use of prothrombin complex concentrates in the treatment of hemorrhages induced by oral anticoagulation. Thromb Res. 1999;95:S57-61.
    Coagulation factors II, VII, IX and X along with anticoagulation factors protein C and protein S are inhibited by warfarin.

27. **Ans. (a)**
    Miyares MA, Davis K. Newer oral anticoagulants: a review of laboratory monitoring options and reversal agents in the hemorrhagic patient. Am J Health Syst Pharm. 2012;69(17):1473-84.

Frontera JA, Lewin JJ 3rd, Rabinstein AA, et al. Guideline for reversal of antithrombotics in intracranial hemorrhage: a statement for healthcare professionals from the Neurocritical Care Society and Society of Critical Care Medicine. Neurocrit Care. 2016;24(1):6-46.

Amin P, Amin V. Overdose of newer anticoagulants. In: Singh O, Juneja D (Eds). Principles and Practice of Critical Care Toxicology, 1st edition. New Delhi, India: Jaypee Brothers Medical Publishers (P) Ltd; 2019. pp. 236-41.

The DOACs are being used increasingly in clinical practice as they require no routine monitoring. Routine coagulation tests like thrombin time (TT), PT, and aPTT should not be performed to adjust their doses, but only to corroborate their anticoagulation effect. These agents are also considered to be safer than warfarin and chances of fatal intracranial hemorrhage (ICH) are lower in patients on DOAC. In patients with DOAC-induced severe bleeding, several general measures have been tried, which include antifibrinolytic agents like tranexamic acid and epsilon-aminocaproic acid, FFP and PCC.

Patients on dabigatran may benefit from hemodialysis, as it has been shown to be dialyzable. Idarucizumab, a monoclonal antibody fragment, has been developed which specially targets and reverses the effect of dabigatran. More recently, Andexanet has been approved by FDA, and it has been reported to reverse the anticoagulant effects of apixaban and rivaroxaban, within a few minutes of its administration.

28. Ans. (d)

O'Grady JG, Alexander GJ, Hayllar KM, et al. Early indicators of prognosis in fulminant hepatic failure. Gastroenterology. 1989;97(2):439-45.

The King's College criteria are used to list patients with acetaminophen-induced acute liver failure for liver transplantation. The following are the parameters, i.e. arterial lactate, blood pH levels (acidosis), coagulopathy, hepatic encephalopathy and serum creatinine levels. Bilirubin is not a component of the criteria.

29. Ans. (c)

Kao LW, Nañagas KA. Carbon monoxide poisoning. Emerg Med Clin North Am. 2004;22(4):985-1018.

The role of hyperbaric oxygen therapy (HBOT) in carbon monoxide poisoning is limited with no clear guidelines. If it has to instituted, it should be started within 6 hours. The indications for HBOT include: carbon monoxide level >25%, pregnancy with carbon monoxide level >20%, unconscious state, severe metabolic acidosis (pH <7.1), evidence of end-organ ischemia.

CHAPTER 18

Obstetric Critical Care

Prasanna Pradip Murudwar

QUESTIONS

1. About physiological adaptations in pregnancy, which of the following is incorrect?
   a. Anemia of pregnancy is due to decrease in circulating erythropoietin levels
   b. Anemia of pregnancy leads to decreased viscosity of blood, is favorable adaptation leading to improvement in placental circulation
   c. Disproportionate rise in blood volume to that of red cell mass stabilize by end of second trimester
   d. Maternal requirement of iron increases to 5–6 mg/day

2. A 32-year-old primigravida at 34 weeks of gestation, shifted to ICU for control of blood pressure. She was on tablet Labetalol 200 mg TDS. On examination in ICU she was complaining of headache, blurred vision. Her BP was 180/130 mm Hg. Which medical strategy for control of BP is correct?
   a. Intravenous labetalol along with oral *nifedipine* till her BP is controlled i.e. < 140/90 mm Hg
   b. Intravenous enalaprilat can be used
   c. Magnesium sulfate is used as an antihypertensive in this situation
   d. Target BP should be < 140/90 mm Hg in patients without end-organ involvement

3. A pregnant patient with long-standing asthma at 26 weeks of gestation presents with acute exacerbation. Most inappropriate statement of the following is:
   a. Short-acting β_2 agonist with inhaled corticosteroids are main drugs in management
   b. Oral corticosteroids are contraindicated in pregnancy
   c. Noninvasive ventilation can be tried prior to invasive mechanical ventilation
   d. Respiratory alkalosis of pregnancy can lead to misinterpretation of severity of exacerbation

4. A 36-year-old primigravida at 33 weeks of gestation was admitted in ward with features of preeclampsia. She was on tablet labetalol 100 mg TDS, shifted to ICU for control of blood pressure. In ICU, it was controlled with IV labetalol. Her laboratory reports before 48 hours were normal. After 2 hours she complained of frontal headache, blurred vision, generalized abdominal pain. Labs s/o:
   Hb – 14.6 g%, TLC – 15,500/mm³, Platelets – 60,000/mm³ Blood urea – 50 mg%, serum creatinine – 1.5 mg%
   ALT – 470U/L, AST – 380U/L, Serum Bilirubin – 4.3 mg%
   PT – 14 sec, INR – 1.2, LDH 620 IU/L, Sr. Haptoglobin 200 mg/dL

What is your diagnosis?
a. Cholestasis of pregnancy
b. Acute fatty liver of pregnancy
c. HELLP syndrome
d. Viral hepatitis

5. **Regarding renal system in pregnancy, find the incorrect statement:**
   a. Decreased renal clearance of drugs
   b. Pregnancy predisposes to urinary tract infection
   c. Glycosuria is normal in pregnancy
   d. Serum creatinine and blood urea nitrogen are reduced in pregnancy

6. **A 30-year-old primigravida at 34 weeks of gestation was admitted in ICU with nausea, vomiting, encephalopathy, jaundice, marked elevation of liver enzymes, coagulopathy, renal dysfunction. She is having persistent hypoglycemia. Likely diagnosis is:**
   a. HELLP syndrome
   b. Acute fatty liver of pregnancy
   c. Intrahepatic cholestasis of pregnancy
   d. Viral hepatitis

7. **A 37-year-old G3P2L2A0 at 36 weeks of gestation, admitted to ICU with severe shortness of breath. No previous comorbid conditions. On examination HR 120/min, BP 100/60 mm Hg, S3+, chest bilateral rales, requiring high flow oxygen, raised JVP, bilateral lower limb pedal edema. 2D echo shows LVEF 40%, Fractional shortening < 30%, no RA/RV dilatation. Likely diagnosis is:**
   a. Pulmonary embolism
   b. Amniotic fluid embolism
   c. Peripartum cardiomyopathy
   d. Acute respiratory distress syndrome (ARDS)

8. **A 34-year-old G3P2L2A0 otherwise healthy patient was shifted to ICU in respiratory distress, hypotension, hypoxia following induction of labor. Investigation revealed low platelet count, fibrinogen, high INR, X-ray s/o bilateral infiltrates. There is no per-vaginal bleed. Likely diagnosis is:**
   a. Abruptio placentae
   b. Myocardial infarction
   c. Septic shock
   d. Amniotic fluid embolism (AFE)

9. **All of the following statements are correct about resuscitation as per AHA guidelines for cardiac arrest in pregnancy *except*:**
   a. Chest compression at the rate of 100–120/min with depth of 2 inches (5 cm)
   b. Patient in supine position with continuous left uterine displacement in which uterus is palpated at or above umbilicus
   c. Place hands at center of chest i.e. lower half of sternum
   d. Place patient in slight left lateral tilt of 27–30° using firm wedge while chest compressions are going on

10. A 28-year-old female, G2P1L1A0, nil comorbid conditions, at 24 weeks of gestation referred to tertiary care center for management of preterm labor. She has received tablet ritodrine and MgSO$_4$. She complained of palpitations, shortness of breath. Likely cause is:
    a. Aspiration pneumonitis
    b. Peripartum cardiomyopathy
    c. Tocolytic therapy
    d. Myocardial infarction

11. In the diagnosis of preeclampsia all is included *except*:
    a. Proteinuria > 300 mg/day alone
    b. Gestational hypertension, visual disturbances
    c. Gestational hypertension, systolic BP > 140 mm Hg
    d. Gestational hypertension, proteinuria > 300 mg/day

12. A 28-year-old healthy female patient, primigravida, following hysterectomy for PPH developed shock. She was shifted to ICU on stiff vasopressors. She has acute kidney injury, severe metabolic acidosis. All of the following statements regarding management are correct except:
    a. Intubation and mechanical ventilation
    b. Thromboelastographic guided blood products transfusion
    c. Urgent 2D echo, inotropic agents if required, invasive hemodynamic monitoring
    d. Recombinant activated factor VII has no role in this situation

13. A 27-year-old female at 32 weeks of gestation, admitted to ICU for management of severe ARDS. Decision of intubation was taken. Which is the incorrect statement of the following:
    a. Consider smaller diameter endotracheal tube
    b. Rapid sequence intubation with etomidate and succinylcholine
    c. High dose benzodiazepine with vecuronium as preferred anesthetic drugs for intubation
    d. Laryngoscopy and intubation may be difficult

14. A 33-year-old multigravida at the 38th week of gestation was admitted to nursing home with complaints of headache. On evaluation, she was found to have Preeclampsia, baby delivered by LSCS. Postoperative day 3 she complained of severe headache, blurring of vision. Developed seizures. BP was 190/110 mm Hg. MRI brain images obtained after neurology consultation revealed hyperintense and FLAIR signal lesions extending beyond the occipital lobes and involved both cerebellar hemispheres. Likely diagnosis is:
    a. Posterior reversible encephalopathy syndrome (PRES)
    b. Cerebral venous sinus thrombosis (CVST)
    c. Eclampsia
    d. Intracerebral hemorrhage

15. A 37-year-old female pregnant patient, diagnosed to have mitral stenosis at 10 weeks of gestation with atrial fibrillation. She was started on tablet metoprolol and anticoagulation. At 25 weeks she complained of dyspnea with minimal exertion, on asking she revealed h/o orthopnea, paroxysmal nocturnal dyspnea. On examination she was having B/L pedal edema, raised JVP, HR 130/min with Afib, BP 138/80 mm Hg; 2decho findings–the size of the left atrium increased with worsening of pulmonary hypertension. Incorrect statement about the management is:
    a. Continue anticoagulation
    b. Increase dose of beta-blocker
    c. Add digoxin with furosemide
    d. Ideal timing for intervention (percutaneous mitral valvuloplasty) is 26–30 weeks in this situation

16. Which among the following is an early sign of magnesium sulfate toxicity?
    a. Depression of deep tendon reflexes
    b. Respiratory depression
    c. Cardiac arrest
    d. Decreased urine output

17. All of the following drugs can be used for acute and emergency management of hypertension in pregnancy *except*:
    a. Intravenous labetalol
    b. Telmisartan
    c. Intravenous hydralazine
    d. Intravenous sodium nitroprusside, nitroglycerine

ANSWERS

1. **Ans. (a)**
   Anemia of pregnancy is physiological adaptation that helps to decrease viscosity of blood leading to improved perfusion to placenta. This hemodilution is at its peak at 30th to 34th weeks of gestation. In pregnancy, erythropoietin levels are increased under estrogen and progesterone. Increase in plasma volume is 30–50% while that of red cell mass is 15–20%. This disproportionate rise in blood volume stabilizes by second trimester and by third trimester hematocrit may increase. This increase in red cell mass depends on appropriate iron supplementation during pregnancy. Iron requirement increases during pregnancy to 5–6 mg/day. Developing fetus utilizes maternal stores of iron.

2. **Ans. (a)**
   Obstetricians and gynecologists have classified hypertension of pregnancy into two categories: (1) pre-existing or (2) gestational with preeclampsia superimposed on either gestational or pre-existing chronic hypertension. In 2015, the American College of Obstetricians and Gynecologists Committee on Obstetrics defined a hypertensive obstetric emergency as acute-onset, severe hypertension persistent for 15 minutes or longer. Gestational hypertension, including preeclampsia, occurs de novo after 20 weeks of gestation. Chronic hypertension is defined as blood pressure > 140/90 mm Hg either pre-existing before the pregnancy or manifesting before the 20th week of gestation. In normal pregnancy there is fall in blood pressure maximum by second trimester. But significant elevation of blood pressure by second trimester is associated with increased risk of preeclampsia. Targets of blood pressure treatment are acute, treatment is required if (1) Blood pressure is more than 160/110 mm Hg or (2) if the SBP is more than 30 mm Hg greater than the baseline value or the DBP is more than 15 mm Hg greater than the baseline. For women with pre-existing chronic hypertension, a blood pressure of more than 160/100 should be targeted. If blood pressure is more than 140/90 mm Hg with end-organ involvement, it should be reduced. Medications used for urgent reduction of blood pressure during pregnancy include intravenous hydralazine and labetalol. Intravenous nitroglycerin and sodium nitroprusside can be used but convincing data is lacking. Oral medications alpha-methyldopa, labetalol, and nifedipine are supplemented with intravenous for urgent control of blood pressure along with fetal monitoring, once target is achieved can be switched to orals. ACE inhibitors and ARBs should not be used due to increased risk of mortality. Magnesium sulfate is not recommended as an antihypertensive agent but is the drug of choice for seizure prophylaxis in severe preeclampsia and for controlling seizures in eclampsia.

3. **Ans. (b)**
   Initial evaluation of asthma exacerbation in the emergency department or labor and delivery should be the same as for acute asthma in the nonpregnant state: measurement of PEFR and comparison with predicted or previously recorded best. Oxygen should be given and oxygen saturation kept higher than 95%. Asthma exacerbation in pregnancy

should be treated as in nonpregnant patient. Give supplemental oxygen to maintain oxygen saturation above 95%, nebulization with salbutamol (2.5 mg in 2.5 mL normal saline)/levosalbutamol (1.25 mg) driven by oxygen every 20 minutes, maximum 3 doses in first hour. If no improvement, give oral or intravenous corticosteroids (Methylprednisolone IV or prednisone PO 40–80 mg/d in 1 or 2 divided doses until PEFR reaches 70% of predicted or personal best). Inhaled corticosteroids have limited role in acute settings. Initial noninvasive ventilation can be tried if patients' mental status is good enough to prevent aspirationas exhaustion or CO_2 retention are suggestive of impending respiratory failure and contraindication for NIV. Those are refractory all treatment modalities, delivery of fetus should be considered as therapeutic option. Tidal volume is increased during pregnancy almost about 40% due to circulating progesterone which acts on respiratory center. Arterial blood gas measurements shows respiratory alkalosis compensated by metabolic acidosis that results in a relatively normal pH. $PaCO_2$ usually ranges from 28 to 32 mm Hg. This respiratory alkalosis may result in confusion in the assessment of severity of asthma.

4. **Ans. (c)**
From history patient is known case of preeclampsia. Her investigations prior to 48 were normal, and now symptoms and laboratory reports were suggestive of low platelet count, evidence of hemolysis by increased LDH and haptoglobin levels, elevated liver enzymes. HELLP typically presents between 28 and 36 weeks of gestation. Patients with preeclampsia complaints of headache, epigastric pain, blurring of vision with elevated blood pressure after 20 weeks of gestation. Right hypochondriac pain may be due to hepatomegaly stretching Glisson's capsule. Liver injury results as a consequence of vasoconstriction and fibrin precipitation in the liver. Cholestasis of pregnancy is associated with intense itching on palms and soles mainly developed in second or third trimester. There are increased blood levels of bile acids. Jaundice is rarely seen and this condition usually resolves after delivery of fetus. If jaundice is the presenting symptom, further evaluation for alternative explanations is necessary. Fat malabsorption can result in fat-soluble vitamin deficiencies requiring supplementation. First-line therapy for IHCP is UDCA at 10–15 mg/kg maternal body weight. Acute fatty liver of pregnancy is life-threatening condition characterized by microvesicular fatty infiltration of liver, leading to liver failure.

5. **Ans. (a)**
Under hormonal influence blood flow to the uterus, breast and kidney is preferentially increased in pregnancy, resulting in increased renal clearance of drugs. Renal length and weight increases results in widening of renal pelvis and ureter, leading to stasis of urinary and predisposition for urinary tract infection. Sodium excretion is also increased in pregnancy. Serum creatinine and blood urea levels are reduced proportionately to increased GFR. Glycosuria may appear normally due to increased GFR and reduced tubular absorption of glucose. There is significant water and sodium retention during pregnancy, leading to cumulative retention of almost a gram of sodium, and a hefty

increase in total body water by 6–8 liters including up to 1.5 liters in plasma volume and 3.5 liters in the fetus, placenta, and amniotic fluid. This disproportionate water retention compared to Sodium results in mild reduction in serum sodium concentration and serum osmolality than nonpregnant.

6. **Ans. (b)**
Acute fatty liver of pregnancy is life-threatening condition characterized by microvesicular fatty infiltration of liver leading to acute liver failure. There is strong link with abnormalities in fatty acid oxidation. Mostly diagnosed in third trimester. Though, presenting symptoms are nonspecific like nausea, vomiting, and persistent abdominal pain. Laboratory tests reveal elevated bilirubin and liver enzymes. Patient may develop signs of liver failure like hepatic encephalopathy, persistent hypoglycemia, coagulopathy. Decreased levels of antithrombin III are a common finding in AFLP. There may be associated renal failure and pancreatitis. Diagnosis is by clinical measures, laboratory, and imaging tests. The "Swansea Criteria" combine symptoms and laboratory derangements. After maternal stabilization, fetus is delivered as soon as possible. Pre- and post-partum treatment should be supportive in a critical care environment with appropriate monitoring and treatment of complications such as hypoglycemia, coagulopathy, renal failure, encephalopathy, diabetes insipidus, and acute pancreatitis. Plasmapheresis may be considered in cases where liver failure continues to worsen despite delivery. In extremis, orthotopic liver transplant may be required.

7. **Ans. (c)**
Peripartum cardiomyopathy is a rare condition usually affected in third trimester, requires ICU admission for ventilation, hemodynamic management. Associated risk factors include multiparity, old maternal age, associated preeclampsia/eclampsia, etc. These patients present with signs of cardiac failure within last month of pregnancy or first 5 months after delivery. After evaluation there will be no identifiable causes for heart failure, absence of prior heart disease, reduced left ventricular function. It may be associated with pulmonary embolism but associated with specific echocardiographic changes. Management of peripartum cardiomyopathy includes minimally invasive hemodynamic monitoring, preload optimization with diuretics, salt restriction, afterload reduction with vasodilators, inotropic and vasopressor agent, mechanical ventilation depending on severity. Early involvement of senior obstetric assistant and fetal monitoring is essential. Amniotic fluid embolism is usually postinduction delivery that results in sudden onset breathlessness, hypoxia, crepts in chest, coagulopathy may be DIC. ARDS is diagnosed based on Berlins definition, absence of cardiogenic pulmonary edema.

8. **Ans. (d)**
It is catastrophic, uncommon, unique to pregnancy, thought to be developed due to exposure of amniotic fluid to maternal circulation mostly at the time of labor. Risk factors include induction of labor, grandmultiparity, advanced age, placenta previa and abruptio placentae. The classical clinical picture of AFE involves acute development of severe hypoxia, cardiovascular collapse, and disseminated intravascular coagulation. Other features may include sweating, shivering, dyspnea, cyanosis,

bronchospasm, and fetal compromise. Hypoxia may be secondary to ventilation perfusion mismatching, pulmonary vasospasm, pulmonary edema following acute left ventricular dysfunction, bronchospasm. Initially cardiogenic and distributive shock develops progressing to disseminated intravascular coagulation and hemorrhage. Management is mainly supportive involving multidisciplinary approach, initially by obstetrician, anesthesiologist till intensive care team approaches. Mortality is as high as 30% in first hour.

9. **Ans. (d)**
Cardiac arrest during pregnancy demands some modifications, priorities being high quality CPR and prevention of aorto-caval compression. Rate and depth of chest compression, hand position, quality indicators of good CPR remain same as in nonpregnant patient. As per 2015 AHA guidelines in supine position if uterus height is above umbilicus, there should be manual left uterine displacement. This is modified statement as compared to 2010 AHA guidelines on CPR. Explanation given was with left lateral tilt there is impact on high quality CPR. Other modification in 2015 AHA guidelines, in case of nonsurvivable maternal condition such as trauma or prolonged pulseless resuscitation, there is no reason to delay performing perimortem cesarean delivery (PMCD). PMCD should be considered at 4 minutes after onset of maternal cardiac arrest or resuscitative efforts (for the unwitnessed arrest) if there is no maternal ROSC.

10. **Ans. (c)**
Under influence of circulating hormones there is relaxation of lower esophageal sphincter so chances of aspiration pneumonitis are high in pregnant patient during intubation or receiving general anesthesia. But our patient has not received any anesthetic drug. Regarding peripartum cardiomyopathy, mostly seen around 36 weeks of gestation. Tocolytic therapy she received can lead to pulmonary edema and such kind of clinical picture. Drugs like beta agonists like salbutamol, terbutaline, ritodrine, magnesium sulfate, nitroglycerine; calcium channel blockers e.g. nifedipine; cyclo-oxygenase enzyme inhibitors e.g. indomethacin; oxytocin hormone inhibitors e.g. atosiban, can also be used during preterm labor. But their use has decreased dramatically in view of lack of evidence and side effects. Management includes supplemental oxygenation, fluid restriction diuretics. Symptoms usually resolves 12 hours of cessation.

11. **Ans. (a)**
Obstetricians and gynecologists have classified hypertension of pregnancy into two categories: (1) pre-existing or (2) gestational with preeclampsia superimposed on either gestational or pre-existing chronic hypertension. National High Blood Pressure Education Working Group on High Blood Pressure in Pregnancy classified hypertension as (1) chronic hypertension, (2) preeclampsia-eclampsia, (3) preeclampsia superimposed on chronic hypertension, and (4) gestational hypertension. Gestational hypertension: It is said to be present when BP > 140/90 mm Hg for first time during pregnancy after 20 weeks, but no proteinuria. This is transient hypertension and blood pressure returns to normal by 12 weeks postpartum. Preeclampsia: It is defined as new hypertension presenting after 20 weeks with significant proteinuria [more than 300 mg per 24 hours, or persistent

30 mg/dL (1+ on dipstick)] in random urine samples. Patient may have visual disturbances, epigastric and right hypochondriac pain, headache, pedal edema, thrombocytopenia, increased proteinuria > 2 g/day, serum creatinine more than 1.2 mg%, BP may be more than 160/110 mm Hg indicating severe preeclampsia.

12. **Ans. (d)**
Obstetric hysterectomy is done in extremes of cases in whom medical and surgical management of postpartum hemorrhage has failed. Also, it can be considered in patients in whom they have completed their family or limitations in transfusion (presence of antibodies or patient refusal). Principles of management includes activation of blood bank for massive transfusion, point of care testing of coagulation parameters like thromboelastography, reducing work of breathing by intubation and mechanical ventilation, invasive hemodynamic monitoring like invasive arterial blood pressure, cardiac output monitor, using dynamic parameters of preload assessment. 2D echo can guide about left ventricular function, if there is requirement of inotropy or not. Recombinant activated factor VII can be used in this situation. It is not recommended in bleeding surgical patients unless definitive correction of bleeding has been done.

13. **Ans. (c)**
There are certain airway related changes during pregnancy that may cause endotracheal intubation difficult. All obstetric patients should be considered as having potential difficult airways until proven otherwise. Weight gain and increased breast size during pregnancy leads difficulty in obtaining optimum position of head and neck. As pregnancy advances, oropharyngeal diameter reduces due to mucosal edema of upper airway, false cords, glottis, arytenoids; it is recommended to use smaller diameter endotracheal tube. Pregnant patients after 14 weeks of gestation are considered at high risk for aspiration due to anatomic and physiologic changes under circulating hormones. So during intubation use short-acting agent, cardio stable agents like thiopentone, etomidate and succinylcholine, perform rapid sequence intubation. Avoid benzodiazepine as it can cause fetal respiratory depression. Oxygen reserves are less in pregnancy with increased demand so they develop early hypoxia after apnea.

14. **Ans. (a)**
PRES can occur along with preeclampsia, eclampsia, with CVST or isolated. It is a cliniconeuroradiological syndrome associated with various clinical conditions, presenting with headache, encephalopathy, seizures, cortical visual disturbances or blindness. Seizures, visual disturbances are common in eclampsia, what differentiates is the neuroimaging. Multiple theories have been proposed on the pathophysiology of PRES, the most accepted being the vasogenic edema. Cerebral autoregulation maintains a constant blood flow to the brain despite alterations in the systemic pressures. Once this mechanism gets disrupted, increased perfusion pressure is sufficient to overcome the blood-brain barrier, allowing extravasation of fluid, macromolecules and even red blood cells. So, PRES represents vasogenic rather than cytotoxic edema in the majority of cases. CT brain shows edema as bilateral

symmetrical hypodensities involving the white matter typically in the parieto-occipital regions. Magnetic resonance imaging shows high signal intensity on T2-weighted and fluid attenuated inversion recovery (FLAIR) sequences. Clinical improvement is seen with control of blood pressure and removal of offending agent. Magnesium therapy should be initiated as soon as eclampsia or PRES in pregnancy is suspected, as it treats both seizures and hypertension.

15. **Ans. (b)**
Managing pregnant patient with mitral stenosis is really a challenge. As pregnancy advances, physiological adaptions like fluid retention, puts the patient on risk for decompensation.

Mitral stenosis results in resistance for blood to flow from left atrium to left ventricle resulting enlargement of left atrium, stasis of blood, predisposition for thrombus formation, atrial fibrillation, pulmonary hypertension, embolic stroke. If the patient is already diagnosed mitral stenosis, usually on digoxin, beta blocker, anticoagulation (warfarin, newer oral anticoagulation). It is necessary to convert to heparin or low molecular heparin during first trimester, LMWH is preferred. From second trimester onwards, warfarin can be restarted with INR monitoring but to change to heparin after 36 weeks of gestation. Those patients who gets evaluated during pregnancy for increased breathlessness out of proportion exertion and diagnosed as mitral stenosis, cardiology consultation is mandatory. They may be started on beta blocker like metoprolol, anticoagulation and diuretics depending on 2D echo findings. In our patient she was diagnosed as having mitral stenosis at 10 weeks of gestation. As pregnancy advanced, she decompensated and presented with heart failure. Anticoagulation should be continued. If atrial fibrillation with increased heart rate, it should be controlled with either beta blocker or digoxin. Beta blockers are contraindicated in active heart failure. Diuretics can be added. Regarding surgical intervention, if patient is diagnosed early in the pregnancy and symptoms could not be controlled with medical management, intervention like percutaneous mitral valvuloplasty, percutaneous mitral commissurotomy is delayed at least up to 12–14 weeks to avoid adverse fetal effects. If patient decompensates despite of optimum medical management after 20 weeks, best time of intervention is 26–30 weeks of gestation. Surgical procedures are better avoided due to adverse effects on fetus.

16. **Ans. (a)**
Magnesium sulfate is used for prophylaxis and management of seizures in pregnancy. It is used in high dose with infusion. Plasma concentration to be monitored. Patellar reflex – starts diminishing at plasma concentration of 4mEq/L and disappears when plasma magnesium level reaches 10 mEq/L; warning impending Mg toxicity), Rate and depth of respiration (depressed at level above 10 mEq/L), respiratory paralysis and arrest occurs above 12 mEq/L), Urine output (Mg is cleared totally by renal excretion, when there is renal insufficiency, plasma magnesium level needs to be checked periodically and dosage adjusted accordingly). Toxic levels may depress uterine contractions. Treatment of toxicity is stop the MgSO4 infusion, inj. calcium gluconate 1gm iv slowly, intubation and mechanical ventilation if respiratory depression has occurred.

17. **Ans. (b)**

   American College of Obstetricians and Gynecologists Committee on Obstetric Practice. Committee opinion no. 623: emergent therapy for acute-onset, severe hypertension during pregnancy and the postpartum period. Obstet Gynecol. 2015;125(2):521-5.

   Medications used for urgent reduction of blood pressure during pregnancy include intravenous hydralazine and labetalol. Intravenous nitroglycerin, and sodium nitroprusside can be used but convincing data is lacking. Oral medications alpha-methyldopa, labetalol, and nifedipine are supplemented with intravenous for urgent control of blood pressure along with fetal monitoring, once target is achieved can be switched to orals. ACE inhibitors and ARBs should not be used due to increased risk of mortality.

CHAPTER 19

End-of-Life/Ethics/Transplant

JIGNESH SHAH, MOTURU DHARANINDRA

QUESTIONS

1. Which of the following is not a prerequisite criterion that should be excluded before testing for brainstem function?
   a. Hypothermia
   b. Effect of sedatives, hypnotics, muscle relaxants
   c. Hypothyroidism
   d. Hypernatremia

2. Non-heart-beating donor (NHBD) transplantation is banned in which country?
   a. Germany
   b. India
   c. USA
   d. Canada

3. Mr Suresh, 30-year-old male suffered major road traffic accident (RTA) with severe traumatic brain injury following which he was assessed as brain dead (BD). His family consented for organ donation, the local transplant coordinator was informed. As preparations for organ retrieval were on going, he suddenly has a cardiac arrest. The Surgical team decides to go ahead with organ retrieval. Which class of the Maastricht NHBD categories, he belongs to?
   a. Category 1
   b. Category 2
   c. Category 3a
   d. Category 4

4. Warm ischemia time is the longest in which of the following Maastricht NHBD categories?
   a. Category 1
   b. Category 2
   c. Category 3a
   d. Category 4

5. In some countries, it is assumed that you want to donate your organs after death. If you do not, then you have to register this wish to "opt out", such policy was first started in which country?

a. Belgium
b. France
c. United Kingdom
d. Australia

6. What is a "conditional organ donation"?
   a. Removing organs from patients who have no comorbidities
   b. Acceptance of organ donation from relatives of NHBD patient for financial gains
   c. Family accepts organ retrieval on condition that organ is given only to a particular person belonging to a religion, community, ethnicity
   d. Organ donation consent given by relatives when patients living will was against organ donation

7. The compensatory mechanisms that contribute to the development of hepatorenal syndrome include all of the following *except*:
   a. Increased activation of RAAS
   b. Increased activation of ADH
   c. Increased activation of sympathetic nervous system
   d. Prostaglandin-mediated reversal of renal vasoconstriction

8. A 58-year-old cirrhotic patient underwent liver transplantation, and shifted to the ICU post-transplantation for further management. He is hemodynamically stable, with adequate urine output, his coagulation status has stabilized. When is the best time to extubate this patient?
   a. 3–6 hours
   b. 12–24 hours
   c. More than 24 hours
   d. 48 hours

9. A 44-year-old male underwent orthotopic liver transplantation. Predictors of failure to meet extubation criteria post-liver transplantation include all except:
   a. Body mass index (BMI) more than 34
   b. Perioperative encephalopathy
   c. High United Network for Organ Sharing (UNOS) score
   d. Intraoperative transfusion of more than 6 units of blood

10. What do you understand by the meaning of public health service increased risk donors?
    a. A donor who accepts monetary benefit for organ donation
    b. A donor who is not related to the recipient
    c. A donor who is involved in high-risk sexual activity
    d. A donor who has pre-existing medical comorbidities

11. Which of the following action is an example of doctrine of double effect?
    a. Administering a medication having agonist and antagonist properties
    b. A single intervention achieving two therapeutic goals
    c. Giving opioid sedation/analgesia to a terminally ill patient
    d. Withholding vasopressor support to terminally ill patient

12. A 34-year-old patient with no history of liver disease starts to develop progressive jaundice after paracetamol poisoning. 10 hours following admission, you found him to have bleeding from nose previously through which Ryle's tube was inserted for gastric lavage. He starts becoming drowsy, his laboratory test results are as follows: hemoglobin (Hb)—10.1 g/dL, international normalized ratio (INR)—6.0, platelets—125,000, white blood cell (WBC) count—16,000. The hepatologist decides to enlist him for transplantation and asks you to calculate his Model for End-stage Liver Disease (MELD) score, which of the following is not a part of MELD score?
    a. Encephalopathy
    b. Coagulopathy—INR
    c. Serum creatinine
    d. Serum bilirubin

13. A 58-year-old patient, post-liver transplant surgery comes to the intensive care unit (ICU). He was planned for extubation after the hemodynamics and coagulopathy stabilizes. You notice that there is a stroke volume variation and pulse pressure variation, the end-expiratory occlusion test also comes positive, which of the following is the best to use?
    a. Crystalloids
    b. Hydroxyethyl starch
    c. Albumin and blood
    d. Norepinephrine and dopamine

14. On day 2 of liver transplantation you review a patient for extubation, the patient is hemodynamically stable with the Richmond Agitation-Sedation Scale (RASS) of zero (0), you decided to review his labs before extubation and the labs come back after an hour, elevation in which of the following variables is considered benign?
    a. Coagulation profile—PT, INR, APTT
    b. Serum indirect bilirubin
    c. Serum lactate
    d. Serum procalcitonin

15. A 40-year-old female underwent orthotopic liver transplantation, 5 months back which of the following organisms is more likely to cause infections now?
    a. Herpes simplex virus (HSV) pneumonia
    b. Wound infections with *Staphylococcus aureus*
    c. Infected biloma
    d. Urinary tract infection

16. An 88-year-old patient with dementia, hypertension, type 2 diabetes mellitus and known case of ischemic heart disease with ejection fraction of 35%, develops massive intracranial bleed with midline shift, the neurosurgeon opines that he may have a poor neurological outcome despite surgical management, the family decides to undergo surgery, postoperatively the patient is in ICU and weaned progressively from ventilator. He continuously to be bed bound dependent on nursing care. In general, which of the following patient factors in intensive care are NOT triggers for palliative care?

a. Brain injury with global cerebral ischemia
   b. Carcinomatosis and unresectable malignancy
   c. Any disease with median survival less than 4 months
   d. Psychiatric disorder with extreme dependence and antipsychotic poisoning
17. A 40-year-old patient with acute appendicitis is admitted to the ICU in view of peritonitis. Sepsis bundles were followed and hemodynamics was stabilized. His neurological status was normal with GCS 15/15, oriented to time, place and person. He is being posted for open appendicectomy by a surgical fellow. But the patient rejects to give consent for the surgery and says that he wants to get operated by the consultant through laparoscopic surgery even though it means delay by 6 hours. The right that patient excised now is called:
    a. Liberty
    b. Law of self-doctrine
    c. Law of double effect
    d. Autonomy
18. The following should be general principles regarding patient confidentiality and the management of confidential information:
    a. Once an adult has died, his next of kin has the right to full access of the patient's medical records
    b. When a patient suffering from a genetically heritable disease has refused consent to disclosure, it is illegal to inform their next of kin
    c. Permission from the next of kin authorizes disclosure of a patient's confidential medical records after their death
    d. Caldicott Guardians can authorize a treatment when the patient has refused to consent
19. A 75-year-old patient after suffering a high speed motor vehicle collision is being offered palliative care because of severe head injury in the form of diffuse axonal injury, which of the following statement regarding palliative care delivery is false?
    a. It can be offered simultaneously with medical treatments aimed at extending life
    b. Integrative palliative model integrates palliative care practices into everyday critical care routines
    c. The consultative model relies on palliative care consultants to provide care for selected ICU patients with highest risk of poor outcomes
    d. Proactive ICU palliative care increases length of stay in the ICU
20. You are called to give a talk on patient rights to general public and you want to stress on the important aspects of patient rights, which of the following is not a true medical tenet?
    a. Autonomy
    b. Beneficence
    c. Nonmaleficence
    d. Double effect

21. An 84-year-old male, resident of old age home having diabetic, hypertensive, chronic kidney disease (on conservative management) comes with the chief complaint of bilateral lower limb pain and edema. On lower limb examination, he is found to had bilateral multiple ulcerations and cellulitis and subtotal occlusion of popliteal vein on compression Doppler. Meanwhile he develops sepsis-induced acute kidney injury, and goes on intermittent hemodialysis. Surgical opinion suggested extensive debridement. The patient denied further surgical treatment and family endorsed patient's views. Treating team discusses about patient's autonomy being important ethical consideration but doubts about legality of not intervening in current scenario. Which of the following option is recently dealt with in Supreme Court of India judgment?
    a. Passive euthanasia
    b. Physician-assisted suicide
    c. Advanced directives
    d. Forgoing of life-sustaining treatment (FLST)

22. A 70-year-old patient suffering from multiorgan failure secondary to sepsis in a case of Guillain-Barré syndrome has been assigned for forgoing of life-sustaining treatments. You as senior resident were assigned to end-of-life (EOL) family conference. Your head of the department asks you to follow a standardized approach to your counseling and you decide to follow the VALUE approach. Which one of the following is not a part of the "VALUE" approach?
    a. Appreciate and value what the family says
    b. Acknowledge the family member's emotions
    c. Listen to their concerns
    d. Ask questions to the family members

23. You are asked by your senior ICU staff member to get to know more about an 80-year-old patient with respiratory failure. He has failed therapy for myelodysplastic syndrome and is on palliative care in the process. You want to know about the patient's spiritual beliefs, you plan to obtain the ancillary details using mnemonic "SPIRIT". Which of the following is not a part of the SPIRIT questionnaire?
    a. Spiritual belief system
    b. Integration with a spiritual community
    c. Ritualized practices and restrictions
    d. Medical event planning

24. You and your ICU team are at the end of swine flu season with almost 52 cases of acute respiratory distress syndrome (ARDS) in 3 months with a high mortality rate. Medical social worker raises the concern of "Compassion fatigue" amongst ICU consultants on round. Which of the following person is most likely to develop compassion fatigue?
    a. The senior consultant who is responsible for declaring the death of patients in all your units
    b. The senior nursing staff managing your high-acuity ICU
    c. The Junior critical care fellows and students
    d. The fresher nursing staff who started working 2 weeks back in your unit

25. A 58-year-old chronic alcoholic with established cirrhosis and a Child-Pugh class C with failed several alcohol abstinence trials is admitted in ICU for refractory septic shock and acute kidney injury not responding to steep doses of vasopressors. After thorough discussions about goals of care, family accepts outcomes and asks for forgoing of life-sustaining treatment. Which of the following is not part of withdrawal of life-sustaining ICU treatment?
    a. Document decision and rationale for withdrawal of life support
    b. Discuss the withdrawal plan with interdisciplinary ICU team
    c. Explain the family the process and expected duration of the process based on patient's clinical context
    d. Continue renal replacement therapy

26. A 50-year-old diabetic, hypertensive, ischemic heart disease patient with metastatic cervical cancer now admitted in your unit with refractory septic shock and acute kidney injury. The ICU team and palliative team discuss regarding EOL care with the patient attenders. Which of the following is not a part of "ABCD" approach of EOL care?
    a. Attitudes
    b. Behaviors
    c. Patient characteristics
    d. Dialogue

27. A 55-year-old software engineer suffering from advanced pancreatic cancer who is already counseled regarding the outcome of the disease, asks the intensivist and palliative care physician about the Physician Orders for Life-Sustaining Treatment (POLST) advance care planning which he witnessed being offered to an elderly relative with terminal condition when he was abroad. Which of the following is not part of POLST?
    a. Advance care planning
    b. Informed shared decision making
    c. Ensuring patient treatment wishes are honored
    d. Trying out experimental therapy for rare noncurable cancers

28. A patient on EOL plan is progressively getting life supports removed, as soon as the ventilator is disconnected, he develops breathlessness and has respiratory distress. The consultant on call instructs you to give injection fentanyl 100 μg. You tell him that it may hasten the dying process and feel that it may amount to legal consequences. Senior consultant questions about the doctrine of double effect, which means:
    a. Doing an act out of good intention causing nonforeseeable side effect
    b. Injecting a drug in good intention which leads to an adverse drug reaction
    c. Relieving distress of a terminally ill patient leading to sedation and apnea, predictable shortening of life span
    d. Unintentional death of a patient with normal therapeutic intervention

29. A 75-year-old male with hypertensive, diabetic, chronic obstructive pulmonary disease (COPD) and a history of ischemic stroke comes with chief complaint of breathlessness and altered sensorium. He is functionally dependent on others for daily activities. Now he is diagnosed to have community-acquired pneumonia requiring invasive

ventilation. On day 2 of ICU, he develops septic shock and acute kidney injury. The nephrologist advises renal replacement therapy. ICU team discusses treatment options and the family suggests a time-limited trial. Which of the following statement about time-limited trial is false?
   a. Explicit goals have to be set
   b. Helps in giving time for taking difficult EOL decisions
   c. A time-limited trial is an agreement between clinicians and a patient family to use certain medical therapies over a defined period of time to see if he improves
   d. It is an example of double effect

30. A 78-year-old male with end-stage COPD presented to the emergency with shortness of breath. He is tachypneic, but is awake and alert. Initial working diagnosis was acute infective exacerbation with pneumonia. His condition worsened in the ICU with impending respiratory failure, though he remains awake and alert. He had expressed to treating doctors in previous admission that he does not want invasive ventilation. No surrogate decision maker is available. Which of the following is the next best thing to do?
   a. The presence of a living will or other advance directive obviates the responsibility to involve a competent patient in medical decision making
   b. If the patient has remained awake and alert, his living will is irrelevant to his current medical decision making
   c. The potential risks and benefits of mechanical ventilation need not be presented to the patient because of the presence of a valid living will
   d. Even if the patient refuses mechanical ventilation therapy, his wishes need not be honored because he is in the emergency room

ANSWERS

1. **Ans. (d)**
   Pandit RA, Zirpe KG, Gurav SK, et al. Management of potential organ donor: Indian Society of Critical Care Medicine: position statement. Indian J Crit Care Med. 2017;21:303-16.
   Wijdicks EF. The diagnosis of brain death. N Engl J Med. 2001;344:1215-21.

   Hypernatremia is commonly seen after brainstem death; it is an effect rather than a prerequisite for brain death assessment. Hyponatremia, hypothermia, sedatives, hypnotics and muscle relaxants do interfere with diagnosis of brainsteam death and skew findings.

2. **Ans. (a)**
   Bardale R. Issues related to non-heart beating organ donation. Indian J Med Ethics. 2016;7(2):104-6.

   Countries like Germany ban NHBD. The shortage of organs from heart-beating, brainstem death (BSD) donors has resulted in renewed interest in donors who have been declared dead using (the more usual) cardiopulmonary criteria, rather than neurological criteria—"non-heart-beating donors/donation" (NHBD). The use of NHBD constituted the only donor source at the beginning of the transplant era. Apart from a significantly higher incidence of delayed graft function, the short- and long-term results of NHBD kidney transplantation are equal. Transplantation of Human Organs Act 1994 allows cadaveric donations.

3. **Ans. (d)**
   Thuong M, Ruiz A, Evrard P, et al. New classification of donation after circulatory death donors definitions and terminology. Transpl Int. 2016;29:749-59.

   Category 4: "Cardiac arrest while BD". Patients with unexpected cardiac arrest in the process of or after being diagnosed brain dead but before arriving in the OR.

   Maastricht NHBD Categories
   Category 1: "Dead on arrival". Patients declared dead outside the hospital, without attempt to resuscitate either outside of the hospital or after accident and emergency (A&E) department admission (example: RTA victims found dead at the scene).
   Category 2: "Unsuccessful resuscitation". Patients brought into A&E while being resuscitated but where resuscitation attempts proved to be unsuccessful and therefore discontinued (example: RTA victims, myocardial infarction patients unsuccessfully resuscitated by volunteers, ambulance crew).
   Category 3: "Awaiting cardiac arrest".
   3a: Hospitalized patients with obviously irreversible brain damage but not meeting all brain death criteria. These patients may or may not be ventilator-dependent (example: patients with severe neurotrauma, or with primary brain tumors in a terminal stage, who will not be resuscitated).
   3b: Hospitalized, ventilated patients with cardiopulmonary arrest after ventilatory support are withdrawn intentionally.
   Category 4: "Cardiac arrest while BD". Patients with unexpected cardiac arrest in the process of or after being diagnosed brain dead but before arriving in the OR.

4. **Ans. (a)**
   Thuong M, Ruiz A, Evrard P, et al. New classification of donation after circulatory death donors definitions and terminology. Transpl Int. 2016;29:749-59.

   Warm ischemia time is more in category 1 and category 2 Maastricht NHBD categories as the patients are dead on arrival at the casualty.

5. **Ans. (a)**
   Belgium was the first country to introduce optional opt out for organ transplantation where in every medically eligible patient was considered for organ retrieval unless and until "opted out" by the person himself while he was alive.

6. **Ans. (c)**
   Wilkinson TM. What's not wrong with conditional organ donation? J Med Ethics. 2003;29:163-4.

   Conditional organ donation is the one which the family of the deceased donor directs whom the organs can be given based on factors like religion, race, cast and community. Unlike donation from a living donor (a situation in which the donation is typically for a specific and well-identified receiver), donation from dead donors (both BSD and NHBD) is always free and without limits. Conditional donation is refused by protocols and is illegal in many countries.

7. **Ans. (d)**
   Wolf AD, Martin P, Tan HH. Liver disease: epidemiology, pathophysiology, and medical management. In: Pretto EA Jr (Ed). Oxford Textbook of Transplant Anaesthesia and Critical Care, 1st edition. Oxford, UK: Oxford University Press. 2015. p. 183.

   Patients with cirrhosis have a hyperdynamic circulation, sometimes called hyperdynamic circulatory syndrome, i.e. peripheral vasodilation, reduced arterial blood flow increased heart rate and cardiac output. In hepatorenal syndrome, the compensatory mechanism to this hyperdynamic circulatory state occurs with the production of RAAS, ADH—arginine vasopressin pathway and sympathetic nervous system activation which leads to renal, coronary and cerebral vasoconstriction. This is apparent in kidneys and leads to HRS. Prostaglandin-mediated protective mechanism is activated but fails to cause reversal of renal vasoconstriction.

8. **Ans. (a)**
   Vizzini S, Johri A, Anis F. Critical care of liver transplant recipient. In: Pretto EA Jr (Ed). Oxford Textbook of Transplant Anaesthesia and Critical Care, 1st edition. Oxford, UK: Oxford University Press. 2015. p. 239.

   Early discontinuation of mechanical ventilation in the postoperative period is not only beneficial for patient pulmonary status but also for graft viability. Positive pressure ventilation increases intrathoracic pressures, decreases venous return and increases venous congestion which in turn decreases splanchnic blood flow. Splanchnic blood flow is obviously critical for graft survival and compromise of this factor at a crucial time when the graft is recovering from ischemic reperfusion injury may lead to early graft failure increased morbidity and mortality.

9. **Ans. (c)**
   Vizzini S, Johri A, Anis F. Critical care of liver transplant recipient. In: Pretto EA Jr (Ed). Oxford Textbook of Transplant Anaesthesia and Critical Care, 1st edition. Oxford, UK: Oxford University Press. 2015. p. 239.

   Although it is being demonstrated that early extubation is beneficial, it cannot be done with all patients especially those with BMI more than 24, uncontrolled preoperative encephalopathy, more than 6 red blood cell transfusions intraoperatively and also no correlation has been found with UNOS score, Child-Turcotte-Pugh score, age or alcoholic liver disease.

10. **Ans. (c)**
    Movahedi B, Martins P, Nagy S. Critical care of liver transplant recipients. In: Irwin RS, Lilly CM, Mayo PH, Rippe JM (Eds). Irwin and Rippe's Intensive Care Medicine, 8th edition. Philadelphia: Wolters Kluwer; 2017.

    Some donors engage in behaviors that put them at increased risk for infections that can be transmitted by blood or body fluids. These infections include human immunodeficiency virus (HIV), hepatitis B virus (HBV) and hepatitis C virus (HCV). Donors with these risk behaviors are referred to as public health service increased risk donors. These high-risk behaviors include sexual (vaginal, anal, oral), injection drug users, history of sexually-transmitted infections (syphilis, gonorrhea, chlamydia or genital ulcers).

11. **Ans. (c)**
    Flavin K, Morkane C, Marsh S. Withdrawal of treatment and end-of-life care on the ICU. In: Flavin K, Morkane C, Marsh S (Eds). Questions for the Final FFICM Structured Oral Examination. Cambridge UK: Cambridge University Press; 2018. p. 506.

    One act can embrace two effects an intended good effect and unintended bad effect. The doctrine or principle of double effect distinguishes consequences that are intended from those that are foreseeable though unintended. For example, the management of a terminally ill patients pain with an opiate (an otherwise legitimate act) may also cause an effect that the physicians normally be obliged to avoid (sedation and a shortened life). Given these effects were not the intention, the action of pain relief is ethically justified.

12. **Ans. (a)**
    Movahedi B, Martins P, Nagy S. Critical care of liver transplant recipients. In: Irwin RS, Lilly CM, Mayo PH, Rippe JM (Eds). Irwin and Rippe's Intensive Care Medicine, 8th edition. Philadelphia: Wolters Kluwer; 2017.

    The severity of illness and prognosis of patients with chronic liver disease can be estimated by a variety of scoring models including the Child-Pugh-Turcotte score and MELD score. The MELD score is widely used in the United States for allocation of organs. It is used to predict 3-month mortality for patients awaiting liver transplant and uses three laboratory values to generate a score that determines priority for liver transplantation. The three laboratory values used were serum bilirubin, serum creatinine and INR.

13. **Ans. (c)**
    Movahedi B, Martins P, Nagy S. Critical care of liver transplant recipients. In: Irwin RS, Lilly CM, Mayo PH, Rippe JM (Eds). Irwin and Rippe's Intensive Care Medicine, 8th edition. Philadelphia: Wolters Kluwer; 2017.

Most liver transplant recipients have a reduced intravascular volume as a result of insufficient correction of intraoperative bleeding, ongoing postoperative hemorrhage and/or fluid shifts through third spacing. Hypovolemia should be corrected using volume resuscitation. In contrast to nontransplant critical care patients, liver transplant recipients may benefit from more blood transfusions and albumin. The osmotic effect of blood and colloids promotes the shift of fluids from extravascular space into the circulation, thereby improving organ perfusion while reducing graft congestion.

14. **Ans. (b)**
Movahedi B, Martins P, Nagy S. Critical care of liver transplant recipients. In: Irwin RS, Lilly CM, Mayo PH, Rippe JM (Eds). Irwin and Rippe's Intensive Care Medicine, 8th edition. Philadelphia: Wolters Kluwer; 2017.

The patient who rapidly awakens from anesthesia and whose mental status progressively improves likely has a well-functioning graft. Laboratory values that corroborate good function include normalization of lactate, coagulation profile and resolution of hypoglycemia. Bilirubin levels may rise for a few days before trending down.

15. **Ans. (c)**
Movahedi B, Martins P, Nagy S. Critical care of liver transplant recipients. In: Irwin RS, Lilly CM, Mayo PH, Rippe JM (Eds). Irwin and Rippe's Intensive Care Medicine, 8th edition. Philadelphia: Wolters Kluwer; 2017.

The infections that can occur posthepatic transplantation usually can happen in the following chronology:

First 30 days after transplant
- Nosocomial infections (bacterial and fungal)
- Wound infections—superficial, deep, organ space infections
- Urinary tract infections
- Pneumonia
- Biliary tract infections
- Invasive fungal infections
- Donor derived infections—lymphocytic choriomeningitis virus (LCMV), rabies, West Nile virus, HIV, *Trypanosoma cruzi*.

Between 1 month and 6 months
Biliary tract complications—infected bilomas, cholangitis, hepatic abscess
Reactivation of latent viral infections
Reactivation or acquisition of opportunistic infections
Community-acquired infection
Reactivation of latent infections.

Later than 6-months post-transplant
Community-acquired infections, late-onset viral infections, reactivation or acquisition of opportunistic infections—including fungal pathogens.

16. **Ans. (d)**
Movahedi B, Martins P, Nagy S. Critical care of liver transplant recipients. In: Irwin RS, Lilly CM, Mayo PH, Rippe JM (Eds). Irwin and Rippe's Intensive Care Medicine, 8th edition. Philadelphia: Wolters Kluwer; 2017.

The following are triggers for palliative care in the ICU:

Clinical triggers:
1. Age more than 80 years
2. Severe brain injury or global cerebral ischemia
3. Status postcardiac arrest
4. Stage 4 malignancy
5. Pre-ICU admission length of stay more than 10 days
6. Intracerebral hemorrhage requiring mechanical ventilation
7. Multiorgan failure more than 3 organs
8. Advanced stage dementia
9. Death likely during this hospital admission.

Surgical ICU triggers:
1. Greater than three admissions to the ICU during index hospitalization
2. Length of surgical ICU stay more than 1 month
3. Multiorgan failure more than three organ systems in a patient over 60 years
4. Any disease with median survival less than 4 months
5. GCS less than 8 for more than 1 week
6. Carcinomatosis/unresected malignancy.

17. **Ans. (d)**

    Integrating palliative care and ethical issues in intensive care unit. In: Irwin RS, Lilly CM, Mayo PH, Rippe JM (Eds). Irwin and Rippe's Intensive Care Medicine, 8th edition. Philadelphia: Wolters Kluwer; 2017.

    The patient utilized the law of autonomy. In medical practice, autonomy is defined as right of competent adults to make informed decisions about their own medical care, the principle underlies the requirement to seek the consent or informed agreement of the patient before any investigation or treatment takes place. The principle is perhaps seen at its most forcible when patient exercises their autonomy by refusing life-sustaining treatments.

18. **Ans. (b)**

    Corporate Information Governance. (2018). Confidentiality Policy. [online] Available from https://www.england.nhs.uk/wp-content/uploads/2016/12/confidentiality-policy-v4.pdf [Last accessed June, 2019].

    Duty of confidentiality continues after the patient dies. Personal information can be disclosed in specific circumstances but the next of kin has no rights to access the patient's records. Genetic information about a patient might, at the same time, also be information about others with whom the patient shares genetic links. If the patient refuses consent to disclose information which may benefit others (help them get prophylaxis or other preventative treatments or interventions), there is a balance between the need to respect patient confidentiality and the duty to protect others from serious harm. In certain circumstances, the duty to others may override the duty to the patient and the information can be legally disclosed. The next of kin is not able to authorize disclosure of confidential information about a patient, whether the patient is dead or alive, unless they have been authorized to make decisions on behalf of, or if they are appointed to support and represent a mentally incapacitated patient. The Caldicott Committee (chaired by Dame Fiona Caldicott) produced a report on the review of patient-identifiable information in 1997. They identified six key principles: (1) justify the purpose of using confidential information, (2) do not use patient-identifiable information unless absolutely necessary, (3) use the minimum necessary patient-identifiable information that is required, (4) access to patient-identifiable information should be on a strict need-to-know basis, (5) everyone with access to patient-identifiable information should be aware of their responsibilities and (6) understand and comply with the law.

19. **Ans. (d)**
Integrating palliative care and ethical issues in intensive care unit. In: Irwin RS, Lilly CM, Mayo PH, Rippe JM (Eds). Irwin and Rippe's Intensive Care Medicine, 8th edition. Philadelphia: Wolters Kluwer; 2017.
An important feature of palliative care is that it can be offered simultaneously with medical treatments aimed at extending life and does not require a distinct choice between treatment focused critical care and comfort care. There are two approaches to palliative care delivery in the ICU. (1) The integrative model—integrates palliative care practices into everyday critical care routine for all ICU patients. (2) Consultative model—focuses on increasing the involvement and effectiveness of palliative care consultants for the care of ICU patients and their families, especially those at risk of poorest outcomes. Typically, the consultative model can only accommodate a subset of most challenging or symptomatic patients rather than all patients in the ICU, owing to workforce shortage of palliative care providers and lack of round the clock on site coverage, as a practical matter many ICUs will function best with a hybrid model that offers advantages of both integrative and consultative models, Proactive palliative care decreases the length of ICU stay.

20. **Ans. (d)**
Ethics and palliative medicine. In: Berg SM, Bittner EA (Eds). Massachusetts General Hospital Review of Critical Care Medicine, 1st edition. Philadelphia: Wolters Kluwer; 2014.
The key medical tenets are:
  Autonomy: The right to self-govern
  Beneficence: The obligation to promote good and to prevent or remove harm
  Justice: The goal to promote the greatest benefit to the largest number of individuals while inflicting the least amount of harm
  Nonmaleficence: The need to refrain from inflicting harm

Patient autonomy, the respect for an individual's right to make decisions about their medical care is a highly valued ethical principle in medicine. Autonomy is best preserved by involving the patient in medical decision making, whenever possible. Using the principle of substituted judgment, a surrogate (typically a family member or healthcare proxy) will make decisions for a patient when he or she cannot. The surrogate is to make the decision that the patient would make given the situation; this decision may even differ from the surrogate's wishes. If the surrogate does not know what the patient would decide, he or she should make the decision he or she feels is in the best interest of the patient and which best reflects the patient's previously voiced beliefs and personality.

21. **Ans. (c)**

The Supreme Court of India. (2018). Writ petition (civil) no. 215 of 2005. [online] Available from: https://www.livelaw.in/5judges-said-recognizing-passive-euthanasia-living-wills-advance-directives/ [Last accessed June, 2019].

The word euthanasia is derivative from the Greek words eu and thanatos which literally means good death. It is otherwise described as mercy killing. The death of a terminally ill patient is accelerated through active or passive means in order to relieve such patient of pain or suffering.

Active euthanasia involves taking specific steps such as injecting the patient with a lethal substance, e.g. sodium thiopental which causes the person to go in deep sedation, apnea. It amounts to killing a person by positive act in order to end suffering of a person in terminal illness. Active euthanasia is illegal and a crime under section 302 or 304 of the IPC. Physician-assisted suicide is also a crime under section of 306 IPC (abetment of suicide). The core point of distinction from active and passive euthanasia as noted by Supreme Court is that in active euthanasia, something is done to end the patient life while in passive euthanasia something is not done that would have preserved the life. Passive euthanasia is further classified into voluntary and nonvoluntary. In nonvoluntary euthanasia, the consent is unavailable on account of the condition of the patient, for example, when he is in coma.

Forgoing of life support (FLST) decision is for stopping life-sustaining therapy when there is a low probability of survival, a very high probability of severely impaired cognitive function and recognition that patients would not want to continue life support in such situations if they could speak for themselves.

Passive euthanasia and living will/advance directives are legal according to a landmark judgment delivered by the honorable Supreme Court of India in 2018. The judgment was delivered by the bench (group of judges), it has also laid down the principles relating to the procedure for execution of advance directives and where there is none, in exercise of the power under article 142 of the constitution. Advance directives are an individual's healthcare decisions or to identify persons who will take those decisions for the said individual in the event he is unable to communicate to doctor.

22. **Ans. (d)**

Cook D, Rocker G. Dying with dignity in the intensive care unit. N Engl J Med. 2014;370:2506-14.
Lautrette A, Darmon M, Megarbane B, et al. A communication strategy and brochure for relatives of patients dying in the ICU. N Engl J Med. 2007;356:469-78.

In the "VALUE" mnemonic "E" stands for eliciting questions and not asking. The mnemonic "VALUE" framed the five objectives of the proactive family conference: (1) **V**alue and appreciate what family members say, (2) **A**cknowledge the family member's emotions, (3) **L**isten to their concerns, (4) **U**nderstand who the patient was in active life by asking questions and (5) **E**licit questions from the family members. In one study, family members of 126 dying patients in 22 ICUs were randomly assigned to participate in a standard EOL family conference or to participate in proactive family conference and received a brochure on bereavement. Patients who were assigned to the proactive conference group were treated with significantly fewer nonbeneficial interventions after the family conference than were those family members who were assigned standard conference group.

23. **Ans. (d)**

    Cook D, Rocker G. Dying with dignity in the intensive care unit. N Engl J Med. 2014;370:2506-14.
    Medical event planning is NOT a part of "SPIRIT" questionnaire. Clinicians should be able to pose questions about spiritual beliefs that may bear on experiences with respect to illness. A useful mnemonic for obtaining ancillary details is SPIRIT, although it is unrealistic to expect that clinicians will be familiar with the views of all the world religions regarding death, they should be cognizant of how belief systems influence EOL care.

24. **Ans. (a)**

    Cook D, Rocker G. Dying with dignity in the intensive care unit. N Engl J Med. 2014;370:2506-14.
    Often the physician who heads the patient communication in the team is susceptible to have compassion fatigue. Dying patients and their families in the ICU are not alone in their suffering. For some clinicians' views about suitability of advanced life support that diverges from those of the patients or family can be a source of moral distress. Clinicians who detect physical or psychic pain and other negative symptoms may suffer indirectly yet deeply. Vicarious traumatization results from repeated empathic engagement with sadness and loss, particularly when predisposing characters amplify clinician's response to workplace stress. Clinician should be aware of how their emotional withdrawal or lability and compassion fatigue can jeopardize the care of dying patients and their families. Informal debriefing or case-based rounds local meetings with other professionals, modified work assignments and other strategies may help clinicians to cope with distress.

25. **Ans. (d)**

    Mani RK, Amin P, Chawla R, et al. Guidelines for end-of-life and palliative care in Indian intensive care units: ISCCM consensus Ethical Position Statement. Indian J Crit Care Med. 2012;16(3):166-81.

    If process for withdrawal of life-sustaining treatment has been initiated, it should adhere to expected standards of quality medical care including appropriate documentation, attention to detail, an explicit plan and interdisciplinary implementation. ISCCM position statement on EOL care in Indian intensive care gives an idea of sequence of steps to be followed during withdrawal of life-supporting therapy.

26. **Ans. (c)**

    Cook D, Rocker G. Dying with dignity in the intensive care unit. N Engl J Med. 2014;370:2506-14.
    Knowing patient characteristics is not part of "ABCD" of EOL care and dignity conserving care. The "ABCDs" of EOL critical care are: **Attitudes, Behaviors, Compassion and Dialogue**. This approach is likely to vary as determined by specific patient-centered palliative measures. This ABCD approach helps in eliciting the values of the patient.

27. **Ans. (d)**

    Palliative care and withholding or withdrawing of life sustaining therapy. In: Hall JB, Schmidt GA, Wood LH (Eds). Principles of Critical Care, 4th edition. New York, NY: McGraw-Hill Education, 2015. National POLST Paradigm. [online] Available from https://www.polst.org [Last accessed June, 2019].

    Trying out experimental therapy is not part of POLST. The National POLST Paradigm is an approach to EOL planning that emphasizes patients' wishes about the medical treatments they receive. The POLST Paradigm emphasizes advance care planning conversations between patients, healthcare professionals and loved ones, informed shared decision-making between a patient and his/her healthcare professional about the treatment the patient would like to receive at the end of his/her life; and ensuring patient treatment wishes are honored. The decisions from these conversations may be documented as actionable medical orders on a POLST form. A POLST form is a tool that helps ensure patient treatment wishes are known and will be followed by healthcare professionals during a medical crisis, when the patient cannot speak for him/herself. The POLST decision-making process and resulting medical orders are intended for patients who are considered to be at risk for a life-threatening clinical event because they have a serious life-limiting medical condition, which may include advanced frailty. For these patients, their current health status indicates the need for standing medical orders. For healthy patients, an advance directive is an appropriate tool for making future EOL care wishes known to loved ones.

28. **Ans. (c)**
End of life care. In: Bersten AD, Soni N (Eds). Oh's Intensive Care Manual, 7th edition. Oxford: Elsevier; 2014.

The doctrine (or principle) of double effect is often invoked to explain the permissibility of an action that causes a serious harm, such as the death of a human being, as a side effect of promoting some good end.

29. **Ans. (d)**
End of life care. In: Joseph LA, Yu M; Andrea G, Wood KE (Eds). Civetta, Taylor and Kirby's Critical Care Medicine, 5th edition. Philadelphia: Lippincott Williams & Wilkins; 2017.

Time limited trial is not an example of double effect. A time-limited trial is an agreement between clinicians and patient family to use certain medical therapies over a defined period of time to see if the patient improves or deteriorates according to the agreed on clinical outcomes, time-limited trials may help advance the discussion when there is an uncertainty between shifting to full comfort care measures and proceeding with potentially burdensome treatment.

30. **Ans. (b)**
University of Washington School of Medicine. Ethics in medicine: Advance directives—case 1 discussion. [online] Available from: http://depts.washington.edu/bioethx/topics/advdird1.html [Last accessed June, 2019].

If the patient has remained awake and alert, his living will be irrelevant to medical decision making. Advanced directives or living will has been accepted by Supreme Court of India in a recent judgment of 2018. However, process laid down is tedious. The potential risks and benefits of mechanical ventilation need to be presented to the patient. If he refuses this therapy with an understanding of the consequences, his wishes should be honored. If he opts for mechanical ventilation, it should be instituted when it becomes medically necessary. The presence of a living will or other advance directive does not obviate the responsibility to involve a competent patient in medical decision making.

CHAPTER 20

Oncology

DEVEN JUNEJA, ANISH GUPTA, OMENDER SINGH

QUESTIONS

1. All the following may suggest presence of multiple myeloma *except*:
   a. Renal dysfunction
   b. Hypercalcemia
   c. Polycythemia
   d. Bone lesions.

2. All the following statements regarding management of anemia in cancer patients are correct *except*:
   a. Therapy with erythropoiesis-stimulating agents (ESAs) is recommended in patients with symptomatic anemia, on chemotherapy, with hemoglobin levels less than 10 g/dL
   b. Therapy with ESA is not routinely recommended in patients not on chemotherapy
   c. Target hemoglobin is a stable level above 12 g/dL, without any need for blood transfusions
   d. Iron treatment should be initiated only after completion of ESA therapy

3. All the following statements regarding delirium in critically ill oncology patients are true *except*:
   a. Presence of brain or meningeal metastasis are recognized risk factors for delirium
   b. Infection may precipitate delirium
   c. All the cancer patients should be screened for presence of delirium, on a daily basis, using scores like Memorial Delirium Assessment Scale (MDAS) and Delirium Rating Scale (DRS)
   d. Presence of delirium is associated with increased mortality

4. Which one of the following statements is true regarding tumor lysis syndrome?
   a. It can occur only after initiation of chemotherapy
   b. Patients may develop hyperkalemia, hyperphosphatemia, and hypercalcemia
   c. Most common in patients with solid organ malignancies
   d. Patients may develop life-threatening arrhythmias

5. A 69-year-old male, with acute myeloid leukemia (AML), on chemotherapy, develops acute respiratory failure (ARF). He has not shown good response to chemotherapy and his estimated survival is only 1 year. Which one of the following statements regarding his further management is not appropriate?

a. He should be immediately shifted to intensive care unit (ICU) and full-code management should be offered
b. Computed tomography (CT) scan of chest should be done as early as possible
c. Bronchoscopy with bronchoalveolar lavage (BAL) should be performed to aid in diagnosis
d. Trial of noninvasive ventilation (NIV) is warranted

6. All the following statements regarding methotrexate (MTX) toxicity are true *except*:
   a. Leukopenia is an early manifestation of toxicity
   b. Urinary alkalization may enhance MTX elimination
   c. Leucovorin is antidote of choice for MTX toxicity
   d. Use of intravenous contrast can also induce MTX toxicity.

7. As per Cairo Bishop definition, all the following are parameters of clinical tumor lysis syndrome *except*:
   a. Seizure
   b. Creatinine > 1.5 times ULN
   c. Sudden cardiac death
   d. Symptomatic hypocalcemia

8. One of the intrinsic tumor risk factors for tumor lysis syndrome is large tumor burden. The term "Large tumor burden" refers to all of the following *except*:
   a. Tumor size > 10 cm
   b. WBC count > 100,000/µL
   c. Organ infiltration
   d. Bone marrow involvement

9. Leukostasis refers to:
   a. Elevated WBC count (>50,000 cells/µL)
   b. Elevated blast cells
   c. Decreased tissue perfusion
   d. All of the above

10. The initial treatment of choice for symptomatic leukostasis is:
    a. Hydroxyurea + Hydration + Allopurinol
    b. Cytoreduction + Hydration + Allopurinol
    c. Hydration + Allopurinol
    d. Leukapheresis

11. Which malignancy is most commonly associated with superior vena cava (SVC) syndrome?
    a. Small cell lung carcinoma
    b. Nonsmall cell lung carcinoma
    c. Hodgkin's lymphoma
    d. Non-Hodgkin's lymphoma

12. Which of the following statements regarding SVC syndrome is false?
    a. Intrathoracic malignancy is responsible for 60–85% cases
    b. The most common presenting symptom is neurological symptoms

c. Venography is the diagnostic modality of choice in cases with life-threatening symptoms
d. Glucocorticoids may reverse SVC syndrome in cases of lymphomas

13. The following are the mechanisms of hypercalcemia in malignancy:
    a. Parathyroid hormone-related protein (PTHrP) secretion by tumor
    b. Osteolytic metastasis
    c. Tumor production of 1,25-dihydroxyvitamin D
    d. All of the above

14. The most common neurological emergency of malignancy is:
    a. Spinal cord compression
    b. Cerebral metastasis
    c. Status epilepticus
    d. Stroke

15. Which of the following statements regarding spinal cord compression secondary to malignancy is false?
    a. Dorsal cord is the most common site
    b. Tumor spread is by hematogenous route
    c. Most frequent primary malignancies involved are breast and prostate
    d. Presenting features include paraplegia and incontinence

16. As per IDSA, fever in neutropenic patients is defined as:
    a. Single oral temperature > 100.4°F for more than 1 hour
    b. Single oral temperature > 100.4°F for more than 2 hours
    c. Single core body temperature (rectal) > 100.4°F for more than 1 hour
    d. Single core body temperature (rectal) > 100.4°F for more than 1 hour

17. A 24-year-old female with acute myeloid leukemia (AML) presented to the ER with fever of 101°F, 10 days after receiving chemotherapy. On examination, she was hemodynamically stable. Her Multinational Association for Supportive Care in Cancer (MASCC) score was 23. Which of the following statements are true?
    a. Treat the patient on outpatient basis
    b. Administer fluoroquinolone and amoxicillin + clavulanic acid, the 1st dose of antibiotic should be given in the clinic, hospital
    c. Admit the patient if fever does not subside after 2–3 days
    d. All of the above

18. What is the duration of empirical antibiotic therapy in febrile neutropenic patients?
    a. Depends on the organism and the site of infection
    b. Till absolute neutrophil counts >500
    c. Till the duration of neutropenia
    d. Until marrow recovery
    e. All of the above

19. A 40-year-old male patient of non-Hodgkin's lymphoma was admitted with fever, cough and difficulty in breathing for 2 days. On examination, his pulse rate was 126 beats/min, BP: 80/60 mm Hg. Respiratory examination was suggestive of bronchial breathing and crepitations. ABG was suggestive of metabolic acidosis with lactates of 8. He has a chemoport in situ and has received chemotherapy 10 days back. Provisional blood culture is suggestive of *Pseudomonas aeruginosa* with a differential time to positivity of 150 minutes between chemoport and peripheral samples. Which of the following statement is false?
    a. Administer fluids @ 30 mL/kg
    b. Remove chemoport
    c. Administer a carbapenem or beta-lactam/beta-lactam inhibitor
    d. Start antifungal prophylaxis

20. In cases of CLABSI with which of the following organism the catheter may be retained?
    a. MRSA
    b. *Pseudomonas aeruginosa*
    c. Mycobacteria
    d. Coagulase negative staphylococci

21. With respect to thromboembolism in cancer patients select the incorrect statement:
    a. Venous thromboembolism (VTE) is the second most common cause of death after surgery
    b. Antithrombotic prophylaxis should be administered for at least 4 weeks after surgery in cancer patients
    c. LMWH is administered for a minimum of 3–6 months in hemodynamically stable patients with confirmed acute VTE
    d. VKA is superior to LMWH to reduce risk of VTE events

22. A 30-year-old male with germ cell tumor received bleomycin-based chemotherapy. After 2 months of therapy he developed cough, dyspnea, and chest pain. Chest X-ray was suggestive of bilateral interstitial infiltrates. A diagnosis of bleomycin-induced interstitial pulmonary fibrosis was made. Which one of the following statement is false?
    a. For hypoxemic patients the target oxygen saturation is 94–98%
    b. Prednisolone is administered at 1 mg/kg
    c. NIV may help reduce work of breathing
    d. Discontinue bleomycin

23. A 35-year-old male with acute myeloid leukemia underwent allogenic hematopoietic stem cell transplant (HSCT). Which of the following infections is commonly seen in the first 3 weeks post-transplant?
    a. Mucor
    b. Nocardiosis
    c. *Clostridium difficile*
    d. Neisseria

ANSWERS

1. **Ans. (c)**
   Moreau P, San Miguel J, Sonneveld P, et al. Multiple myeloma: ESMO Clinical Practice Guidelines for diagnosis, treatment and follow-up. Ann Oncol. 2017;28 (Suppl 4):iv52-iv61.

   Multiple myeloma is a plasma cell proliferative disorder which causes end-organ damage exhibiting as hypercalcemia (serum calcium > 1 mg/dL), renal dysfunction (creatinine clearance < 40 mL/min or serum creatinine > 2 mg/dL), anemia (<10 g/dL) and bone lesions (one or more osteolytic lesions on skeletal radiography, CT or PET-CT). Presence of these signs/symptoms should raise a suspicion of presence of multiple myeloma. Presence of one or more biomarkers of malignancy, like clonal bone marrow plasma cells or involved/uninvolved serum-free light chain ratio > 100, may also suggest presence of multiple myeloma. However, to make a definitive diagnosis, bone marrow biopsy is warranted.

2. **Ans. (d)**
   Aapro M, Beguin Y, Bokemeyer C, et al. Management of anaemia and iron deficiency in patients with cancer: ESMO Clinical Practice Guidelines. Ann Oncol. 2018;29 (Suppl 4): iv96-iv110.

   In cancer patients on chemotherapy or combined radio- and chemotherapy, with symptomatic anemia, ESA therapy is recommended if hemoglobin (Hb) levels are below 10 g/dL. However, in asymptomatic patients, ESA therapy should be initiated only when the Hb levels fall below 8 g/dL. Currently, it is not recommended to initiate ESA in patients who are not on chemotherapy. The recommended endpoints of ESA therapy is a stable Hb of 12 g/dL with no requirement for blood transfusions. Iron therapy should be initiated before or during ESA therapy in patients with functional iron deficiency. In patients with severe anemia related symptoms, and Hb below 7-8 g/dL, red blood cell transfusion may be justified, in order to improve Hb and related symptoms, immediately.

3. **Ans. (c)**
   Kim SY, Kim SW, Kim JM, et al. Differential associations between delirium and mortality according to delirium subtype and age: a prospective cohort study. Psychosom Med. 2015;77:903-10.
   Bush SH, Lawlor PG, Ryan K, et al. Delirium in adult cancer patients: ESMO Clinical Practice Guidelines. Ann Oncol. 2018;29 (Suppl 4):iv143-iv165.

   Several risk factors have been recognized, which can predispose cancer patients for developing delirium. These factors can be broadly classified as cancer related, treatment related, and indirect factors related to physical complications or underlying comorbidities. Cancer related factors include primary central nervous system (CNS) cancer, brain/meningeal metastasis or para-neoplastic neurological syndromes. Presence of any infection may precipitate delirium in these patients. However, daily routine screening for presence of delirium is currently not recommended and patient should be evaluated by a trained healthcare professional if there is presence of any change in cognitive or emotional

CHAPTER 20 Oncology

behavior or psychomotor activity suggestive of delirium. Presence of delirium is associated with increased risk of mortality and, hence, it should be recognized and treated early.

4. **Ans. (d)**
   Gupta A, Moore JA. Tumor lysis syndrome. JAMA Oncol. 2018;4(6):895.
   Mirrakhimov AE, Voore P, Khan M, et al. Tumor lysis syndrome: A clinical review. World J Crit Care Med. 2015;4(2):130-8.

   Tumor lysis syndrome is the most common oncological emergency and patients generally present with hyperkalemia, hyperphosphatemia, hypocalcemia, and hyperuricemia. It is generally associated with the initiation of cytotoxic chemotherapy; however, it may occur spontaneously or after radiation therapy too. High-risk tumors include acute lymphocytic leukemia, acute myeloid leukemia with a high WBC count, B-cell acute lymphoblastic leukemia and Burkitt lymphoma. Solid organ tumors are considered to be low-risk. It may be associated with high mortality rates and acute kidney injury (AKI) and arrhythmias are the common life-threatening complications.

5. **Ans. (c)**
   Kiehl MG, Beutel G, Böll B, et al. Consensus statement for cancer patients requiring intensive care support. Ann Hematol. 2018;97(7):1271-82.
   Azoulay E, Soares M, Darmon M, et al. Intensive care of the cancer patient: recent achievements and remaining challenges. Ann Intensive Care. 2011;1(1):5.

   Recent years have witnessed improved outcomes in critically ill cancer patients. Patients with acute deterioration should be managed in ICU and full-code management should be offered to patients in remission or those with an estimated survival of 1 year or more. Cancer patients who have poor performance status and are not eligible for further anti-cancer therapy, or dying patients, along with those who reject critical care treatment, may not be admitted to the ICU.

   It is also recommended that all cancer patients with ARF should undergo CT scan of chest, as soon as clinically feasible, to determine the cause of ARF. However, bronchoscopy and BAL should only be carried out if other noninvasive diagnostic modalities fail to make a diagnosis and it can be performed without causing any clinical worsening. It is also recommended that NIV should be attempted first to avoid intubation in immunocompromised patients, if there is no contraindication to its use.

6. **Ans. (a)**
   Howard SC, McCormick J, Pui CH, et al. Preventing and managing toxicities of high-dose methotrexate. Oncologist. 2016;21(12):1471-82.
   Singh A, Singh O. methotrexate and other chemotherapeutic drugs toxicity. In: Singh O, Juneja D (eds). Principles and Practice of Critical Care Toxicology, 1st edition. New Delhi: Jaypee Brothers Medical Publishers (P) Ltd.; 2019. pp. 374-85.

   Hematologic toxicity associated with MTX is dose related. In the initial phase, patients may develop thrombocytopenia, which is followed by a rapidly progressive leukoneutropenia. In most of the cases, leukopenia occurs after 1–3 weeks. The incidence of pancytopenia is higher in patients with advanced age, hypoalbuminemia, folic acid deficiency, concomitant infections, and underlying dehydration.

As MTX is primarily excreted by the kidneys, chances of MTX toxicity are higher in patients with impaired renal function or in those who receive renal toxic drugs including intravenous contrast. Such patients may develop MTX toxicity, even if they are receiving therapeutic doses.

Management of patients with MTX toxicity includes methods to enhance elimination, antidotal therapies and organ-specific care. Aggressive hydration and urinary alkalization may enhance its urinary excretion. Extracorporeal therapies using high-flux filters or hemadsorption columns may also be helpful in patients with severe toxicity and those with underlying renal dysfunction. Leucovorin (folinic acid) is the antidote of choice for managing MTX toxicity.

7. **Ans. (d)**
   Cairo MS, Bishop M. Tumour lysis syndrome: new therapeutic strategies and classification. Br J Haematol. 2004;127:3.

   The Cairo Bishop definition for tumor lysis syndrome (TLS) was proposed in 2004. As per the definition clinical TLS is defined as laboratory TLS plus one of the following parameters—increased serum creatinine concentration ≥1.5 times the upper limit of normal, cardiac arrhythmia/sudden death, or a seizure. Laboratory TLS is defined as two or more abnormal serum values of the following parameters—uric acid > 8 mg/dL, potassium > 6 mEq/L, phosphorus > 4.5 mg/dL (adults) and calcium < 7 mg/dL.

8. **Ans. (b)**
   Cairo MS, Coiffier B, Reiter A, et al. Recommendations for the evaluation of risk and prophylaxis of tumour lysis syndrome (TLS) in adults and children with malignant diseases: an expert TLS panel consensus. Br J Haematol. 2010;149:578.
   Howard SC, Jones DP, Pui CH. The tumor lysis syndrome. N Engl J Med. 2011;364:1844.

   The risk of tumor lysis syndrome is maximum in patients with hematological malignancies but there are certain tumor related factors which dictate the overall risk. These include: high tumor cell proliferation rate, chemosensitive tumors, large tumor burden—tumor size >10 cm or WBC count > 50,000/μL, organ infiltration, bone marrow involvement and serum lactate dehydrogenase (LDH) > 2 times ULN prior to commencing treatment.

9. **Ans. (d)**
   Porcu P, Cripe LD, Ng EW, et al. Hyperleukocytic leukemias and leukostasis: A review of pathophysiology, clinical presentation and management. Leuk Lymphoma. 2000;39:1.

   Leukostasis is a medical emergency characterized by elevated blast cells and decreased organ perfusion secondary to white cell plugs in the microvasculature. It is also called as symptomatic hyperleukocytosis and is commonly seen in patients of acute or chronic myeloid leukemia in blast crisis.

10. **Ans. (b)**
    Porcu P, Farag S, Marcucci G, et al. Leukocytoreduction for acute leukemia. Ther Apher. 2002;6:15.
    Bug G, Anargyrou K, Tonn T, et al. Impact of leukapheresis on early death rate in adult acute myeloid leukemia presenting with hyperleukocytosis. Transfusion. 2007;47:1843.

Leukostasis is associated with a high mortality to the tune of 20–40%. Cytoreduction or induction chemotherapy helps reduce the WBC count. Hydroxyurea is usually reserved for asymptomatic leukostasis. Hydration and allopurinol are started for all patients to prevent tumor lysis syndrome. The role of leukapheresis is controversial and is not usually recommended as initial therapy.

11. **Ans. (b)**
    Rice TW, Rodriguez RM, Light RW. The superior vena cava syndrome: clinical characteristics and evolving etiology. Medicine (Baltimore). 2006;85(1):37-42.

    The most common malignancy leading to SVC syndrome is nonsmall cell lung carcinoma accounting for about 50% cases. Small cell lung carcinoma accounts for about 25% cases followed by non-Hodgkin's lymphoma which accounts for about 10% cases.

12. **Ans. (b)**
    Rice TW, Rodriguez RM, Light RW. The superior vena cava syndrome: Clinical characteristics and evolving etiology. Medicine (Baltimore). 2006;85(1):37-42.
    Rowell NP, Gleeson FV. Steroids, radiotherapy, chemotherapy and stents for superior vena caval obstruction in carcinoma of the bronchus: A systematic review. Clin Oncol (R Coll Radiol). 2002;14(5):338-51.

    The most common cause of SVC syndrome is intrathoracic malignancy (nonsmall cell carcinoma is the most common cause). Irrespective of etiology, the most common presenting symptom is dyspnea. In life-threatening situations venography (CT venogram, MR venogram or SVC cavogram) is the diagnostic modality as it provides an accurate diagnosis and can help plan further management. In mild to moderate cases Doppler sonography or a contrast-enhanced CT can be performed as the initial investigation. Glucocorticoids have a role in steroid sensitive tumors (lymphoma/thymoma) wherein they help reduce tumor size and airway edema.

13. **Ans. (d)**
    Stewart AF. Clinical practice. Hypercalcemia associated with cancer. N Engl J Med. 2005;352(4):373-9.

    The mechanisms of hypercalcemia in patients with malignancy are secretion of parathyroid hormone related protein peptide by the tumor. This is the most common mechanism of hypercalcemia and is called humoral hypercalcemia of malignancy (HHM). It accounts for about 80% cases. The other mechanisms include production of 1,25 dihydroxyvitamin D by the tumor and osteolytic metastasis. Ectopic secretion of parathormone (PTH) has also been described but is a rare mechanism.

14. **Ans. (b)**
    Giglio P, Gilbert MR. Neurologic complications of cancer and its treatment. Curr Oncol Rep. 2010;12(1):50-9.

    The most common neurological emergency in cancer patients is cerebral metastasis. Spinal cord compression is the second most common neurological emergency. Seizures can occur secondary to brain metastasis while paraparesis can occur secondary to cord compression.

15. Ans. (b)

Giglio P, Gilbert MR. Neurologic complications of cancer and its treatment. Curr Oncol Rep. 2010;12(1):50-9.

Spinal cord compression is the second most common neurological emergency secondary to malignancy. It usually occurs secondary to extradural spread from vertebral metastasis. Hematogenous spread is rare. Primary malignancies involved with the spread include breast, lung, prostate and kidney. Depending upon site involved patients may present with quadriparesis, paraparesis and bowel bladder incontinence.

16. Ans. (a)

Freifeld AG, Bow EJ, Sepkowitz KA, et al. Clinical practice guideline for the use of antimicrobial agents in neutropenic patients with cancer: 2010 update by the Infectious Diseases Society of America. Clin Infect Dis. 2011;52(4):e56-93.

The Infectious Diseases Society of America (IDSA) defines fever in neutropenic patients as a single oral temperature of >100.4°F lasting for more than 1 hour. Even though rectal temperature reflects the core body temperature, oral and axillary measurements are acceptable as there is a risk of inducing infection with insertion of rectal thermometers in neutropenic patients.

17. Ans. (d)

Taplitz RA, Kennedy EB, Bow EJ, et al. Outpatient management of fever and neutropenia in adults treated for malignancy: American Society of Clinical Oncology and Infectious Diseases Society of America Clinical Practice Guideline Update. J Clin Oncol. 2018;36(14):1443-53.

As per the data given she has stable vitals and has an MASCC score above 21. She is a candidate for outpatient treatment as she is at low risk of complications. The 1st dose of antibiotic should be given in the ER, clinic or hospital in such patients. Recommended empirical antibiotic therapy is a fluoroquinolone and amoxicillin clavulanic acid. In cases of penicillin, allergy substitutes amoxicillin clavulanic acid with clindamycin.

18. Ans. (e)

Freifeld AG, Bow EJ, Sepkowitz KA, et al. Clinical practice guideline for the use of antimicrobial agents in neutropenic patients with cancer: 2010 update by the infectious diseases society of america. Clin Infect Dis. 2011;52(4):e56-93.

As per IDSA guidelines in neutropenic patients with documented infections the duration of antibiotic therapy depends upon the organism cultured and the site of infection. Antimicrobials are continued till neutropenia recovers or the ANC > 500 cells or even longer. In patients with fever and neutropenia, but without any documented infection, antimicrobials are to be continued till there are signs of marrow recovery or the ANC exceeds 500 cells/mm^3.

In patients who are neutropenic despite resolution of fever and no signs and symptoms of infection. Usually fluoroquinolone prophylaxis is given till marrow recovers.

19. **Ans. (d)**

    Freifeld AG, Bow EJ, Sepkowitz KA, et al. Clinical practice guideline for the use of antimicrobial agents in neutropenic patients with cancer: 2010 update by the infectious diseases society of america. Clin Infect Dis. 2011;52(4):e56-93.

    The patient seems to be in septic shock. As per the surviving sepsis campaign he should be administered fluids @ 30 mL/kg to correct hypotension and reverse tissue hypoperfusion. Broad spectrum antibiotics should be administered as soon as possible in such patients, preferably before cultures are sent, but within a maximum time of 1 hour. Since we have a positive culture of *Pseudomonas aeruginosa* with a DTP > 2 hours it is suggestive of CRBSI and should be removed. The usual recommended antibiotics are anti-pseudomonal beta-lactam such a cefepime or a carbapenem or piperacillin tazobactam. Antifungals are not started at the outset but are administered in patients with fever after 4–7 days of antibiotic therapy.

20. **Ans. (d)**

    Freifeld AG, Bow EJ, Sepkowitz KA, et al. Clinical practice guideline for the use of antimicrobial agents in neutropenic patients with cancer: 2010 update by the infectious diseases society of america. Clin Infect Dis. 2011;52(4):e56-93.

    For CLABSI caused by *S. aureus, P. aeruginosa*, fungi, or mycobacteria, catheter removal is recommended along with systemic antimicrobial therapy for at least 14 days (A-II). Catheter should also be removed for tunnel infection or pocket site infection, septic thrombosis, endocarditis, sepsis with hemodynamic instability, or bloodstream infection that persists despite > 72 hours of appropriate antibiotic therapy (A-II). For documented CLABSI caused by coagulase-negative staphylococci, the catheter may be retained using systemic therapy with or without antibiotic lock therapy (B-III).

21. **Ans. (d)**

    Zamorano JL, Lancellotti P, Rodriguez Muñoz D, et al. 2016 ESC Position Paper on cancer treatments and cardiovascular toxicity developed under the auspices of the ESC Committee for Practice Guidelines: The Task Force for cancer treatments and cardiovascular toxicity of the European Society of Cardiology (ESC). Eur Heart J. 2016;37(36):2768-801.

    The VTE is the second most common cause of death in cancer patients after surgery. Postsurgery all patients with cancer should receive antithrombotic prophylaxis for a minimum of 4 weeks. The role of prophylaxis in ambulatory patients with cancer is unclear. In cases of confirmed VTE with hemodynamic stability LMWH is recommended for a period of 3-6 months. This strategy is considered superior to VKA therapy with no difference in mortality or bleeding.

22. **Ans. (a)**

    British Thoracic Society. (2017). The BTS Guideline for oxygen use in adults in healthcare and emergency settings. [online] Available from: https://www.brit-thoracic.org.uk/document-library/clinical-information/oxygen/2017-emergency-oxygen-guideline/bts-guideline-for-oxygen-use-in-adults-in-healthcare-and-emergency-settings. [Last accessed June, 2019].

As per British Thoracic Society guidelines the target oxygen saturation in patients with bleomycin-induced lung injury and paraquat poisoning is 85–88%. Oxygen should not be administered to patients if they are not hypoxemic and have oxygen saturation > 88%. The evidence supporting this recommendation is not robust with a grade D recommendation.

Bleomycin can cause life-threatening interstitial pulmonary fibrosis, organizing pneumonia and hypersensitivity pneumonitis. Glucocorticoids are administered in cases with declining DLCO, hypoxemia and symptomatic patients. Noninvasive ventilation may help reduce respiratory load and reduce work of breathing. Bleomycin should be discontinued in all cases of toxicity.

23. **Ans. (c)**

Pagalilauan GL, Limaye AP. Infections in transplant patients. Med Clin North Am. 2013;97(4):581-600.

Post-HSCT the risk of infections is divided into three phases (pre-engraftment, early postengraftment and late postengraftment). The first 3 weeks post-HSCT corresponds to pre-engraftment phase. The risk of bacteremia, pneumonia, *Clostridium difficile* infection, *Candida* infection and reactivation of HSV infection is high during this phase. *Candida* and invasive mold infections are commonly seen during this phase. Mucor is not a common organism isolated during any of the three phases of HSCT. *Nocardia* and encapsulated bacteria like *Neisseria* are common infections during the late engraftment stage.

CHAPTER 21

Hematology

Abhijit Baheti

QUESTIONS

1. A 54-year-old female in a preoperative clinic is found to have CBC as—Hb 19 g/dL; red blood count $6.0 \times 10^{12}/L$ (3.9–5.6); WBC 6,000/mm³, platelets 350,000/mm³. Select the underlying medical condition which could explain the abnormalities in the CBC due to a physiologically appropriate rise in erythropoietin:
   a. Renal cell carcinoma
   b. Polycythemia vera
   c. COPD
   d. Cerebellar hemangioma
   e. Essential thrombocythemia

2. Erythropoietin is mainly synthesized by:
   a. Erythroid precursors
   b. Glomerular cells
   c. Hematopoietic stem cells
   d. Hepatocytes
   e. Peritubular interstitial cells of kidney

3. A 60-year-old, previously well, man presents via the casualty department with a few day history of progressive fatigue, dyspnea on exertion and yellow discoloration of skin. Which of the following would *not* be supportive of a diagnosis of autoimmune hemolytic anemia (AIHA)?
   a. Anemia with high reticulocyte count
   b. Positive DCT
   c. Raised haptoglobin level
   d. Raised LDH
   e. Generalized lymphadenopathy

4. Which *one* of the following transfusions is likely to cause intravascular hemolysis?
   a. Group O blood to group A recipient
   b. Group B blood to group O recipient
   c. Group O blood to group AB recipient
   d. Rh-positive blood to a Rh-negative recipient

5. Following are vitamin K-dependent coagulation factors *except*:
   a. Factor X
   b. Factor VII
   c. Protein C

    d. Protein S
    e. Factor VIII
6. A 36-year-old woman with SLE presents with the acute onset of lethargy and jaundice. On initial evaluation, she is tachycardic, hypotensive, appears pale, is dyspneic, and is somewhat difficult to arouse. On examination she had splenomegaly. Her initial hemoglobin is 6 g/dL, white blood cell count is 6,300/mm³, and platelets are 294,000/mm³. Her total bilirubin is 4 g/dL, reticulocyte count is 18%, and haptoglobin is not detectable. Renal function is normal, as is urinalysis. What would you expect on her peripheral blood smear?
    a. Macrocytosis and PMNs with hypersegmented nuclei
    b. Microspherocytes
    c. Schistocytes
    d. Sickle cells
    e. Target cells
7. A 39-year-old woman who is known to have a lupus anticoagulant presents with a large pulmonary embolus. As she is hemodynamically unstable, a decision is made to treat her with unfractionated heparin by continuous infusion. Her coagulation screen shows prothrombin time (PT) 15 sec (normal range 12–14) and APTT 48 sec (normal range 26–33) with a normal thrombin time. The most appropriate management is:
    a. Fixed dose of 20,000 units per day without monitoring
    b. Monitor with anti-Xa assay aiming for a heparin concentration of 0.3–0.7 IU/mL
    c. Monitor with APTT aiming for a ratio of about 2.0
    d. Monitor with APTT aiming for a ratio of about 4.0
    e. Monitor with APTT aiming for a ratio that indicates a heparin concentration of 0.2–0.4 IU/mL
8. A 64-year-old man has Hb of 6.7 g/dL following emergency aortic valve replacement surgery. He is short of breath and the cardiothoracic surgeons have requested four units of red cells to relieve his anemia. He is known to have chronic lymphocytic leukemia (Binet stage A) which has never been treated. The blood bank had difficulty cross-matching blood because of positive direct and positive indirect antiglobulin tests against all panel cells. His peripheral blood film confirms a normal platelet count and there are no significant morphological changes in the red cells. He has a normal bilirubin and LDH. Urgent transfusion is required, which is the most appropriate transfusion product?
    a. Irradiated packed red cells
    b. ABO/Rh/K matched, "least incompatible" packed red cells
    c. HLA matched packed red cells
    d. Washed packed red cells
    e. IgA-deficient packed red cells
9. A 62-year-old male is admitted to the casualty after a car accident. He is hemodynamically unstable. USG confirms a large intra-abdominal bleed with suspected spleen rupture. He had received tranexamic acid on site. He was taking regular aspirin. His blood reports are awaited.

What combination of blood products should this patient receive initially as part of the massive hemorrhage protocol?
a. 4 units red blood cells (RBC) + 2 units fresh frozen plasma (FFP) + intravenous tranexamic acid (IV TXA) infusion (1g)
b. 4 units RBC + 4 units FFP + IV TXA infusion (1 g)
c. 4 units RBC + 4 units FFP + IV TXA infusion (1 g)
d. 4 units RBC + 4 units FFP + IV TXA infusion (1 g) + 2 packs cryoprecipitate
e. 4 units RBC + 4 units FFP + IV TXA infusion (1 g) + 1 pool platelets

10. Which *one* of these statements is *true* concerning anemia of chronic disease?
a. The serum iron is low and the anemia usually responds to treatment with iron
b. Macrophages are deficient in iron which is released and bound to ferritin
c. Usually, the erythrocyte sedimentation rate is raised but the C-reactive protein level is low
d. Some cases may respond to treatment with erythropoietin

11. A patient is bleeding in casualty following a road traffic accident. The staff find a card saying the patient has anti-c red cell antibodies. They ask for your advice on urgent provision of red cells. Do you advise:
a. Using group O Rh D-positive
b. Arranging an urgent cross-match as only this will be safe
c. Ignoring the antibody since it is not clinically significant
d. Using group O Rh D-negative

12. A 64-year-old female presented with a hematemesis. She had been on regular hemodialysis with unfractionated heparin as an anticoagulant. A full blood count showed a platelet count of 103×10^9/L and Hb of 6 g/dL. D-Dimer was elevated (4 mg/L) and coagulation screen was normal. There was no previous history of thrombocytopenia. Her HIT antibody screen was negative. In the mean time she was transfused two units of packed red cells. A week later her platelet count was found to be 20×10^9/L and an urgent hematological consultation was requested. The most likely explanation of the platelet counts of 20×10^9/L is:
a. Chronic immune thrombocytopenia (ITP)
b. Disseminated intravascular coagulation (DIC)
c. Evans syndrome
d. Heparin-induced thrombocytopenia (HIT)
e. Post-transfusion purpura (PTP)

13. A 54-year-old woman with atrial fibrillation is anticoagulated with warfarin, 5 mg daily. She developed a urinary tract infection that her primary care physician has treated with ciprofloxacin, 250 mg orally twice daily for 7 days. She presents to the emergency room today complaining of blood in her urine and easy bruising. Her physical examination shows ecchymoses on her arms. Her urine is bloody in appearance, but no clots are present. After flushing the bladder with 100 mL of sterile saline, the urine returns with a slight pink hue only. A urinalysis shows 3–5 white blood cells per high power field and many red blood cells per high power field. There are no bacteria present. The

international normalized ratio (INR) is 7.0. What is the best approach to treatment of this patient's coagulopathy?
a. Administer vitamin K 10 mg IV
b. Administer vitamin K 2 mg SC
c. Administer vitamin K 1 mg sublingually
d. Hold further warfarin doses until the INR falls to 2.0
e. Transfuse four units of fresh-frozen plasma

14. A 53-year-old woman with relapsed leukemia is being regularly transfused with red cells and platelets. Ten minutes after starting a platelet transfusion she becomes severely dyspneic with wheeze and stridor and is found to be hypotensive. You suspect anaphylaxis. You have stopped the transfusion and are infusing normal saline. What should you do next?
a. Administer chlorphenamine
b. Administer inhaled salbutamol
c. Administer intramuscular epinephrine (adrenaline)
d. Administer intravenous epinephrine (adrenaline)
e. Administer 200 mg of hydrocortisone

15. A 75-year-old patient on warfarin for atrial fibrillation has a fall with a head injury. He is brought into the casualty where he is found to have an intracranial bleed on CT scanning with urgent neurosurgery indicated. Blood tests show that his INR is 3.5. What treatment options would you recommend in relation to his warfarin therapy?
a. Withhold warfarin only
b. Immediate transfusion with fresh frozen plasma and Vitamin K
c. Immediate treatment with prothrombin complex concentrate only
d. Immediate treatment with prothrombin complex concentrate and Vitamin K
e. Immediate treatment with Vitamin K only

16. An 85-year-old female patient who weighs 45 kg is found to have a hemoglobin concentration (Hb) of 7 g/dL. She has recently had an operation for a fractured neck of femur and is not acutely bleeding. She has given three units red transfusion and becomes acutely short of breath with bilateral pulmonary infiltrates.
The respiratory complications are most likely to be due to:
a. Acute chest infection
b. Anemia
c. Fat embolus
d. TRALI
e. TACO (transfusion associated circulatory overload)

17. Cryoprecipitate is used to replace which of the following coagulation factors in clinical practice?
a. II
b. VII
c. X

d. IX
e. Fibrinogen

18. Once removed from the blood fridge a transfusion of red cells must be completed within:
    a. 1 hr
    b. 4 hr
    c. 6 hr
    d. 12 hr
    e. 24 hr

19. Suitable plasma for transfusion of a group B Rh D positive woman would include:
    a. B Positive and AB Positive
    b. B negative and AB Negative
    c. O Positive
    d. O negative

20. A 23-year-old pregnant woman with no significant past medical history was found to have a platelet count of 54,000/mm³ at booking in her first pregnancy (14 weeks gestation). At 34 weeks gestation her platelet count was 48,000/mm³. She had required no treatment to maintain her platelet count during pregnancy. A platelet count on a cord blood sample taken from the neonate at delivery shows a platelet count of 15,000/mm³. The most likely explanation for the thrombocytopenia in the mother is:
    a. Gestational thrombocytopenia
    b. ITP
    c. HELLP
    d. TTP

21. A patient with a short history of easy bruising has a normal coagulation screen and a normal platelet count. It is thought that they probably have abnormal platelet function. Which drug is the most likely cause of this?
    a. Aspirin
    b. Dabigatran
    c. Rivaroxaban
    d. All the above

22. Coagulation factor synthesis occurs mainly in the:
    a. Bone marrow
    b. Liver
    c. Intestine
    d. Spleen

23. A man is found to have a prolonged prothrombin time but a normal aPTT. He is not taking any anticoagulant medication. His liver function is normal.
    a. Factor V mutation
    b. Factor VII deficiency
    c. Factor VIII deficiency
    d. Factor IX deficiency

24 A 49-year-old man is admitted with abdominal pain and fever. A CT scan shows a diverticular abscess. He was commenced on a prophylactic dose of low molecular weight heparin on admission. One day after admission he has deteriorated with signs of sepsis. The prothrombin time (PT) is 16 seconds (normal range 11.0–13.9), activated partial thromboplastin time (APTT) is 49 seconds (NR 26–34) and platelet count 67,000/mm^3. Fibrinogen concentration is 2.1 g/L. The most likely explanation for the coagulation results is:
a. Acquired hemophilia
b. Acute liver failure
c. DIC
d. LMWH related

CHAPTER 21 Hematology

ANSWERS

1. **Ans. (c)**

    Hoffman R, Benz E, Heslop H, et al. Pathobiology of the human erythrocyte and Its hemoglobins. In: Hematology, 6th edition. Philadelphia: Churchill Livingstone; 2012.

    In essential thrombocythemia, the main finding is an elevated platelet count and there should be no significant increase in erythropoiesis. A raised Hb, RBC, and hematocrit could be seen in all of the other medical conditions. In renal cell carcinoma and cerebellar hemangioma, the erythropoietin (Epo) is produced by the tumor and is thus inappropriate. Polycythemia vera is a primary myeloproliferative disorder and so Epo production from the kidney is suppressed. Chronic obstructive pulmonary disease with chronic hypoxia results in increased Epo production which is physiologically appropriate.

2. **Ans. (e)**

    Hoffman R, Benz E, Heslop H, et al. Pathobiology of the Human Erythrocyte and Its Hemoglobins. In: Hematology, 6th edition. Philadelphia: Churchill Livingstone; 2012.

    Mostly erythropoietin is synthesized is by renal peritubular interstitial cells with a minor component being from the liver.

3. **Ans. (c)**

    Hoffman R, Benz E, Heslop H, et al. Autoimmune Hemolytic Anemia. In: Hematology, 6th edition. Philadelphia: Churchill Livingstone; 2012.

    Anemia with a short duration of symptoms associated with jaundice should trigger investigation for hemolytic anemia. Hemolysis is confirmed by raised levels of bilirubin, raised levels of LDH (an intracellular enzyme released from the red cells), low haptoglobin (used to "mop up" the free hemoglobin released from the red cells) and characteristic blood film changes. The immune mechanism for the hemolysis is confirmed with a positive DAT (i.e. confirming that the red cells have bound antibody–autoantibodies in AIHA, maternal alloantibodies in hemolytic anemia of the newborn). Unless the individual has preexisting bone marrow failure there should be a brisk reticulocyte response (release of early red cells from the bone marrow). Generalized lymphadenopathy would raise the possibility of undiagnosed chronic lymphocytic leukemia or non-Hodgkin lymphoma, both of which are associated with an increased prevalence of AIHA.

4. **Ans. (b)**

    Hoffman R, Benz E, Heslop H, et al. Human Blood Group Antigens and Antibodies. In: Hematology, 6th edition. Philadelphia: Churchill Livingstone; 2012.

    Group B to O leads to major mismatch and causes intravascular hemolysis.

5. **Ans. (e)**

    Vitamin K is a fat-soluble vitamin that plays an essential role in hemostasis. It is absorbed in the small intestine and stored in the liver. It serves as a cofactor in the enzymatic carboxylation of glutamic acid residues on prothrombin-complex proteins. The three major causes of vitamin K deficiency are—(1) poor dietary intake, (2) intestinal malabsorption, and (3) liver disease. The prothrombin complex proteins (factors II, VII,

IX, and X and protein C and protein S) all decrease with vitamin K deficiency. Factor VII and protein C have the shortest half-lives of these factors and therefore decrease first. Therefore, vitamin K deficiency causes prolongation of the prothrombin time first. With severe deficiency, the activated partial thromboplastin time (APTT) will be prolonged as well. Factor VIII is not influenced by vitamin K.

6. Ans. (b)

Hoffman R, Benz E, Heslop H, et al. Autoimmune Hemolytic Anemia. In: Hematology, 6th edition. Philadelphia: Churchill Livingstone; 2012.

This patient's lupus and her rapid development of truly life-threatening hemolytic anemia are both very suggestive of autoimmune hemolytic anemia. Diagnosis is made by a positive Coombs test, but smear will often show microspherocytes, indicative of the damage incurred to the red cells in the spleen. Schistocytes are typical for microangiopathic hemolytic anemias such as hemolytic-uremic syndrome (HUS) or thrombocytopenic thrombotic purpura (TTP).

The lack of thrombocytopenia makes these diagnoses considerably less plausible. Macrocytosis and PMNs with hypersegmented nuclei are very suggestive of vitamin B12 deficiency, which causes a more chronic, nonlife-threatening anemia. Target cells are seen in liver disease and thalassemias. Sickle cell anemia is associated with aplastic crises, but she has no known diagnosis of sickle cell disease and is showing evidence of erythropoietin response based on the presence of elevated reticulocyte count.

7. Ans. (b)

Kitchen S, Gray E, Mackie I, et al. Measurement of non-coumarin anticoagulants and their effects on tests of Haemostasis: Guidance from the British Committee for Standards in Haematology. Br J Haematol, 2014;166, 830-10;841.

It has been suggested that if a patient is receiving at least 30,000 units of heparin per day monitoring may not be needed but a dose of 20,000 units would need to be monitored. In the presence of a prolonged baseline APTT as a result of a lupus anticoagulant, the APTT ratio cannot be used for monitoring and it is necessary to use an anti-Xa assay.

8. Ans. (b)

Hoffman R, Benz E, Heslop H, et al. Principles of Red Blood Cell Transfusion. In: Hematology, 6th edition. Philadelphia: Churchill Livingstone; 2012.

In the presence of positive antibody tests, it can be difficult to provide compatible red cell units. When there is symptomatic anemia, the risk of tissue hypoxia may be greater than the risk of hemolysis due to incompatible red cell transfusion. Ideally red cell alloantibodies should be excluded by absorbing out the autoantibody using autologous red cells. If the patient has been transfused during the preceding 3 months allogeneic cells of appropriate phenotype are chosen to absorb out autoantibody as the patient's own blood may contain transfused cells against which alloantibodies have been generated and attempts to "auto-absorb" would also remove the alloantibody. Absorption studies take time (4–8 hours) which may not be available in emergencies (e.g. ongoing bleeding in theater). In this case there would probably be time to absorb and screen. Ideally ABO Rh (cCDeE) and Kk matched "least incompatible" red cells can be issued by the blood bank. If the volume of red cells demanded and the urgency of the request does not allow this ABO and RhD matched red cells would be transfused. In this case, providing there was no active bleeding, a transfusion of two units would be reasonable followed by reassessment. In addition, if there was clear evidence of autoimmune hemolysis, which there is not in this case, specific treatment such as corticosteroids, would also be necessary. Washing red cells will remove plasma proteins, but not red cell antigens. HLA matching is not of benefit because the antibodies are directed against the red cell antigens, not HLA antigens. Gamma-irradiation protects against transfusion associated graft-versus-host disease, but this patient is not at risk. IgA-deficient red cells may be of benefit in IgA-deficient recipients who have previously reacted to non-IgA deficient blood products, but there is no indication that this is the case here.

9. **Ans. (e)**
Hunt B, Allard S, Keeling D, et al. A practical guideline for the haematological management of major haemorrhage. Br J Haematol. 2015;170:788-803.

The patient should receive a 1:1 ratio of FFP and RBC as his blood loss follows trauma. The use of cryoprecipitate will only be required if the fibrinogen level is <1.5 g/L and therefore cryoprecipitate is not part of the initial transfusion pack.

In trauma, an infusion of tranexamic acid of 1 g over 8 hours should always follow the administration of the 1 g bolus.

In view of the aspirin use, a pool of platelets should be considered. There is a low threshold for platelet transfusion in trauma patients.

10. **Ans. (d)**
Hoffman R, Benz E, Heslop H, et al. Anemia of Chronic Diseases. In: Hematology, 6th edition. Philadelphia: Churchill Livingstone; 2012.

11. **Ans. (a)**
O Rh D-negative blood is not suitable for all emergencies.
Hoffman R, Benz E, Heslop H, et al. Principles of Red Blood Cell Transfusion. In: Hematology, 6th edition. Philadelphia: Churchill Livingstone; 2012.

The patient is in urgent need of red cells and cannot wait for a cross-match. Anti-c is clinically significant, causing delayed transfusion reactions (and also hemolytic disease of the newborn). O Rh D-negative blood is Cde/Cde so would cause a reaction in this patient. O Rh D-positive emergency blood is selected to be suitable for this situation as it is CDe/CDe.

12. **Ans. (e)**
Araujo F, Sa JJ, Araujo V, et al. Post-transfusion purpura vs. heparin-induced thrombocytopenia: differential diagnosis in clinical practice. Transfus Med. 2000;10(4):323-4.

British Society for Haematology. BSH Guidelines in Haematology: Guidelines for the use of platelet transfusion. London: BSH; 2003.

The low platelet count on initial admission is unexplained but negative ELISA testing and low clinical probability for HIT makes HIT unlikely. The significant drop of platelet count occurring 1 week after blood transfusion raises the suspicion of the diagnosis of PTP. This was confirmed by demonstration of the presence of anti-HPA1-a antibodies. PTP is characterized by severe thrombocytopenia and bleeding following a blood component transfusion caused by alloimmunization to human platelet-specific antigens. The majority of affected patients are multiparous women who presumably have been previously sensitized during pregnancy. DIC and ITP are very unlikely with normal clotting screen and no previous history of thrombocytopenia.

13. **Ans. (c)**

    DA Garcia. The risk of hemorrhage among patients with warfarin-associated coagulopathy. J Am Coll Cardiol. 2006;47:804-8.

    J Ansell, Hirsh J, Poller L, et al. The pharmacology and management of the vitamin K antagonists: the Seventh ACCP Conference on Antithrombotic and Thrombolytic Therapy. Chest. 2004;126:204S.

    Warfarin accumulates in the liver when it undergoes oxidative metabolism by the CYP2C9 system. Multiple medications can interfere with the metabolism of warfarin by this system causing both over- and underdosing of warfarin. This patient has recently been treated with a fluoroquinolone antibiotic that is known to increase the prothrombin time and INR if the warfarin dose is not adjusted during treatment. When the INR is >6, there is a greater risk of development of bleeding complications. However, if no evidence of bleeding is present at presentation, it is safe to hold warfarin and allow the INR to fall gradually into the therapeutic range before reinstituting therapy. In this patient, however, there is evidence of minor bleeding complications warranting treatment. Thus, treatment of the elevated INR is indicated. In the absence of life-threatening bleeding, treatment with vitamin K is indicated. When the INR falls between 4.9 and 9, an oral dose of vitamin K, 1 mg, is usually adequate to correct the INR without conferring vitamin K resistance, evidenced by decreased sensitivity to oral warfarin for an extended period.

    When a more rapid correction of anticoagulation is needed, vitamin K can be given by the IV or IM route. However, there is a risk of anaphylaxis, shock, and death. This can be minimized by delivering the drug slowly. Additionally, fresh-frozen plasma is indicated to replete coagulation factors when there is significant bleeding in the setting of an elevated INR. While the SC route for delivery of vitamin K has long been a primary route of correction, a meta-analysis has shown the SC route to be no better than placebo and inferior to the oral and IV routes, which have similar efficacy

14. **Ans. (c)**

    Treat anaphylaxis with adrenaline. BMJ. 2003;327(7427).

    The patient may have anaphylaxis. She requires adrenaline (epinephrine) urgently. BSH guidelines advise that this be given intramuscularly. The other measures can be considered after adrenaline has been administered.

The correct route of administration and dose of adrenaline has been under debate. One study showed that subcutaneous administration of adrenaline was associated with a striking difference in the time of maximum plasma adrenaline concentrations of children compared with the intramuscular route (average time: intramuscular group, 8 minutes; subcutaneous group, 34 minutes). The average maximum plasma concentration was also significantly higher for the intramuscular group than for the subcutaneous group (grade B).

15. **Ans. (d)**

    British Committee for Standards in Haematology. BCSH Guidelines. [online] Available from http://www.bcshguidelines.com/documents/warfarin_4th_ed.pdf. [Last Accessed June, 2019].

    Warfarin is a coumarin oral anticoagulant drug, which reduces the level of the vitamin K-dependent coagulation factors II, VII, IX and X. The INR is a standardized laboratory test used for monitoring warfarin therapy.

    Patients on warfarin who have significant bleeding or need urgent surgery need immediate reversal of anticoagulation and the British Committee for Standards in Haematology (BCSH) guidelines recommend that prothrombin complex concentrate (PCC) be given. PCC containing all four clotting factors will bring about immediate correction but vitamin K 5 mg should also be given intravenously together with the PCC to maintain ongoing correction.

    Fresh frozen plasma produces suboptimal correction of oral anticoagulant therapy and should not be used first line when PCC is available.

16. **Ans. (e)**

    JPAC. Transfusion Guidelines. [online] Available from www.transfusionguidelines.org. [Last Accessed June, 2019].

    TACO is defined as acute or worsening pulmonary edema within 6 hours of transfusion with acute respiratory distress and evidence of fluid overload.

    Low weight patients, such as the frail and elderly, are at increased risk of receiving inappropriately high-volume and rapid blood transfusions, predisposing to TACO. Comprehensive pretransfusion assessment, with particular attention to the speed and volume of transfusion, fluid balance monitoring and use of diuretics if indicated may help prevent this complication.

    Single-unit transfusions should be given with further transfusion only if thought to be needed after repeat Hb check and further clinical assessment. The treatment of TACO involves stopping the transfusion and administering oxygen and diuretic therapy, with critical care support, as required.

    Given the above clinical history TRALI is less likely as a possible complication. The reference below gives more information on the different features of TACO and TRALI.

17. **Ans. (e)**

18. **Ans. (b)**

In order to reduce the risk of bacterial replication in the bag while at room temperature, blood transfusion must be completed within 4 hours. The transfusion should be started within 30 minutes of removal from the fridge

19. **Ans. (b)**
Hoffman R, Benz E, Heslop H, et al. Principles of Plasma Transfusion: Plasma, Cryoprecipitate, Albumin, and Immunoglobulins. In: Hematology, 6th edition. Philadelphia: Churchill Livingstone; 2012.

20. **Ans. (b)**
McCrae KR. Thrombocytopenia in Pregnancy, Platelet Disorders. Washington DC: Ash Education Book (Hematology); 2010. pp. 397-402.

Gestational thrombocytopenia: Mild, apparent in the mid-second to third trimester of pregnancy, less likely when the platelet count is $70,000/mm^3$. Occasionally presents as more severe thrombocytopenia in pregnancy not responsive to steroid therapy and resolving postpartum. The incidence of fetal or neonatal thrombocytopenia is no higher than that of non-thrombocytopenic women.

ITP: One-third first diagnosed during pregnancy; two-thirds in patients with preexisting disease. One of few causes of thrombocytopenia that may manifest in the first trimester. Approximately 30% require therapy. Thrombocytopenia, platelet count $100 \times 10^9/L$, in approximately 15% of the offspring of mothers with ITP. Platelet counts are below $50 \times 10^9/L$ in 10% of neonates and 4% are $20 \times 10^9/L$.

PET: Thrombocytopenia in up to 50%; severity parallels the preeclampsia. May precede other manifestations; preeclampsia must be considered in the differential diagnosis of isolated thrombocytopenia in the late second or third trimester. The syndrome of hemolysis, elevated liver function tests, and low platelets (HELLP) affects 0.5-0.9% of all pregnancies and develops in 10% of patients with preeclampsia. Thrombotic thrombocytopenic purpura (TTP) and HUS; not pregnancy-specific, more frequent in pregnancy. Greatest incidence during the mid-second trimester, and third trimester. The management of TTP during pregnancy is as in the nonpregnant patient, with plasma exchange yielding a response rate of approximately 80%.

21. **Ans. (a)**
Aspirin causes irreversible platelet dysfunction and is the likely the cause in this patient. Warfarin and unfractionated heparin prolong the prothrombin time and activated partial thromboplastin time, respectively. Low molecular weight heparin inhibits activated factor X. Dabigatran is a direct thrombin inhibitor. Other than aspirin, none of these drugs affects platelet function.

22. **Ans. (b)**
Coagulation factors are mainly synthesized in the liver.

23. **Ans. (b)**
A prolonged prothrombin time is characteristic of a patient taking a vitamin K antagonist such as warfarin. The prothrombin time is also a sensitive marker of liver disease.

In this patient the most likely cause is factor VII deficiency. Factor VIII and IX deficiency would result in a prolonged APTT and a normal prothrombin time (PT). Factor XII deficiency also causes a prolonged APTT (but patients are not at increased risk of bleeding).

Factor V Leiden is the most common inherited cause of thrombophilia and does not prolong the PT or APTT.

24. Ans. (c)

Hoffman R, Benz E, Heslop H, et al. Hematologic Problems in the Surgical Patient: Bleeding and Thrombosis. In: Hematology, 6th edition. Philadelphia: Churchill Livingstone; 2012.

Disseminated intravascular coagulation can be caused by many disorders including sepsis, obstetric emergencies, trauma and malignancy. Most patients will present with bleeding from a number of sites and will have a prolongation of the PT and APTT and a fall in platelet count. An increase in D dimer and a fall in the fibrinogen are often also usually noted. In this case the fibrinogen was normal but is an acute phase protein so can be normal even though fibrinogen is being consumed. Low molecular weight heparin does not cause prolongation of the coagulation tests. Acute liver failure can cause a widespread coagulopathy but there is nothing in this patient's history to suggest this diagnosis.

CHAPTER 22

Postoperative Critical Care

Sushma K Gurav

QUESTIONS

1. In a patient who is undergoing major surgery, which of the following is not the better site for accurate measures of core temperature?
   a. Tympanic membrane
   b. Nasopharynx
   c. Bladder or pulmonary catheter
   d. Groin/axilla/oral

2. During neurosurgery in the posterior cranial fossa done in sitting position, which of the following is correct statement about chances of pulmonary embolism?
   a. Positive end expiratory pressure (PEEP) of 10 cm H_2O prevents air entering the venous system
   b. Using PEEP makes pulmonary air embolism more likely
   c. Fluid loading should be avoided
   d. Continuous jugular venous compression should be used

3. A patient with history of ischemic heart disease awaits major surgery. He needs cardiopulmonary exercise testing. Which of the following statement is correct for quantifying risk of perioperative complications?
   a. Patients with an anaerobic threshold (AT) of >15 mL/min O_2 have a high relative risk of cardiopulmonary morbidity following major noncardiac surgery
   b. Cardiopulmonary exercise testing is strongly recommended in the presence of severe aortic stenosis
   c. 1 metabolic equivalent (MET) is roughly equivalent to climbing one flight of stairs
   d. The anaerobic threshold (AT) is the point at which oxygen supply exceeds demand

4. A 77-year-old man is admitted to the intensive care unit following emergency repair of a ruptured abdominal aortic aneurysm. Intraoperatively he received a 10-unit blood transfusion. He was shifted to critical care unit. He was ventilated with minimal oxygen requirements. Twenty-four hours later his oxygen requirement has begun to increase. His P/F ratio is 200 and his chest X-ray shows new bibasal interstitial shadowing. An echocardiogram demonstrates good right and left ventricular function with an ejection fraction of 55%. His stroke volume variation is 14%. The most likely diagnosis is:

a. Acute lung injury (ALI)
b. Acute respiratory distress syndrome (ARDS)
c. Ventilator-associated pneumonia
d. Transfusion-related acute lung injury

5. A 57-year-old man was admitted to the ICU following emergency left hemicolectomy for perforated diverticular disease 10 days previously. He has an ileus, and a nasogastric tube in situ is on free drainage. He is becoming agitated, tachycardic and hypertensive but does not pose a threat to staff. His tracheostomy is patent and his capnography trace is normal. ECG shows sinus tachycardia (rate 121), normal axis, QTc 460 ms. He has a fluctuating mental state, inattention and disorganized thinking, and a diagnosis of hyperactive delirium is made. What is the best pharmacological choice to manage his delirium?
    a. Dexmedetomidine
    b. Propofol
    c. Haloperidol
    d. Midazolam

6. A 55-year-old man is admitted to a trauma unit following a motor vehicle collision. On admission he is taken to operation theater for damage control surgery. Intraoperatively, he receives 10 units of packed red cells, 10 units of fresh frozen plasma and 10 pooled doses of platelets. The surgeon reports that the surgical field continues to ooze. A thromboelastogram report shows: R-time 10 minutes, K-time 3 minutes, angle 62°, maximum amplitude 71 mm, clot lysis at 60 minutes 11%. Given these results, what is the most appropriate blood product/medication to administer to improve hemostasis?
    a. Fresh frozen plasma
    b. Cryoprecipitate
    c. Platelets
    d. Recombinant factor VII

7. A 46-year-old 60-kg man meets with RTA and sustains a grade IV splenic laceration; he has hypotension so undergoes emergency damage control laparotomy. Postoperatively he is transferred to the trauma unit. His blood pressure is 80/40 mm Hg and heart rate is 125 beats/min. Urine output is 10 mL/hour. After resuscitation with crystalloid and blood products, blood pressure is 110/70 mm Hg, heart rate is 88 beats/min, and urine output is 100–120 mL/hour. Lactate level is mmol/L, and base deficit is -12 mmol/L. Which of the following is the most appropriate course of action at this time?
    a. Aggressive fluid resuscitation should be continued
    b. Base deficit should be corrected with the administration of sodium bicarbonate
    c. No further aggressive resuscitation should be done
    d. A Swan-Ganz catheter should be placed for better assessment of hemodynamics and thereby titrate his resuscitation

8. A 42-year-old man is transferred to the neurotrauma unit after emergent laparotomy for blunt trauma. In the operating room, he had been found to have liver, bowel, and

splenic injuries, requiring bowel resection and reanastamosis and splenectomy. He received 30 units of packed red blood cells, 14 units of fresh frozen plasma, 6 units of platelets, and 3 liters of crystalloid. In the trauma unit, he requires ongoing resuscitation for reversal of tissue hypoperfusion. Two hours later, his abdomen is distended and his bladder pressure is elevated. Which of the following signs would describe abdominal compartment syndrome?
a. Bladder pressure greater than 30 mm Hg
b. Central venous pressure (CVP) 25 mm Hg, elevated peak and plateau airway pressures, oliguria, bladder pressure 25 mm Hg
c. CVP 25 mm Hg, elevated peak and plateau airway pressures, oliguria, bladder pressure 6 mm Hg
d. CVP 8 mm Hg, elevated peak pressure, normal plateau airway pressure, normal urine output, bladder pressure 15 mm Hg

9. A 62-year-old man is admitted to the ICU following evaluation in the emergency department for a 3-hour history of pressure-like substernal chest pain with dyspnea. ECG reveals new T-wave inversions in the inferior leads. Coronary angiography reveals 80% occlusion of the proximal left anterior descending artery, proximal OM1, and mid-right coronary artery. He undergoes urgent coronary artery bypass graft without complication. Which of the following is the most appropriate decision about his antiplatelet therapy on arrival to the ICU?
a. Start aspirin and clopidogrel
b. There is no indication for antiplatelet therapy at this time
c. Start clopidogrel only
d. Start aspirin only

10. A 27-year-old man is admitted to ICU after an emergency craniotomy, splenectomy, and femoral fracture fixation. He also underwent left chest tube insertion for hemothorax. On hospital day 3, the chest radiograph still shows left chest opacification. Which of the following is the most effective management for this patient?
a. Insertion of a second chest tube
b. Video-assisted thoracoscopic surgery followed by evacuation of hemothorax
c. Intrapleural fibrinolysis with streptokinase
d. Increase the preexisting chest suction

11. A 58-year-old man with hepatitis C and hepatocellular carcinoma undergoes an orthotopic liver transplantation. He receives 14 units of packed red blood cells, 10 units of fresh frozen plasma, and 2 units of platelets intraoperatively. On arrival in the ICU, he is intubated, sedated, and hypotensive, requiring vasopressor support. Which one of the following signs is most associated with poor allograft function?
a. Elevated transaminases
b. Metabolic alkalosis
c. Ongoing coagulopathy
d. Hypercalcemia

CHAPTER 22 Postoperative Critical Care

12. A 60-year-old woman brought to ER with history of fall while climbing steps in garden. Her CT imaging of brain shows right temporoparietal SDH with mass effect. She underwent emergency craniotomy and transferred to trauma unit on volume control mode. On postoperative day 3, she develops acute respiratory distress syndrome, with a fever and worsening leukocytosis of 21,000/mm³. She has abdominal distention and does not tolerate Ryles tube feeding. Her FiO_2 requirement increases to 80%, positive end-expiratory pressure 12 cm H_2O, respiratory rate 18 breaths/min, and tidal volume is 420 mL (7 mL/kg). Arterial blood gas results: pH 7.32, partial pressure of carbon dioxide 50 mm Hg, partial pressure of oxygen 68 mm Hg, and oxygen saturation 90%. What is the next step in this patient's management?
    a. Change the mode of ventilation
    b. Prescribe start broad-spectrum antibiotics for probable diagnosis of ventilator-associated pneumonia (VAP)
    c. Wait for cultures of bronchoalveolar lavage specimen
    d. Abdominal and pelvic CT

13. Virtually all other conditions have the potential to benefit from a period of ICU management prior to definitive operation. Which are the two general surgery conditions which require surgery to control the underlying process and one cannot get ahead of the disease process with resuscitation prior to operation?
    a. Occlusive mesenteric ischemia and necrotizing soft tissue infection
    b. Duodenal and intestinal perforation
    c. Gallbladder stone
    d. Appendicitis and ileal perforation

14. Which is the following scoring system that predicts the cardiac risk in preoperative assessment?
    a. American Society of Anesthesiologists (ASA)
    b. Charlson Comorbidity Index
    c. Revised Cardiac Risk Index (RCRI)
    d. Physiological & operative severity score for enumeration of mortality (POSSUM)

15. A 54-year-old male undergoes pneumonectomy for emphysematous bullae that develops hypotension, which of the following is not sign of cardiac herniation?
    a. Acute obstructive shock
    b. Jugular venous distention
    c. Discoloration of the upper torso
    d. Discoloration of lower limbs

16. A 55-year-old man undergoes cardiac surgery. Which of the following is not a complication of cardiac bypass surgery?
    a. Cardiac tamponade
    b. Massive hemothorax
    c. Right heart failure
    d. Cardiac herniation

17. A 64-year-old female undergoes carotid artery endarterectomy. Postoperatively develops decrease in blood pressure. What is the most appropriate cause?
    a. Loss of cervical sympathetic tone
    b. Loss of chemoreceptor function
    c. Loss of baroreceptor function
    d. Hemorrhage or intracerebral bleed

18. A pregnant lady was in labor; she was receiving labor analgesia. Due to fetal distress, she underwent LSCS under epidural anesthesia. Postoperatively she had headache, photophobia and hyperesthesia of both lower limbs. What would be the most appropriate treatment of choice?
    a. Reassurance and review in 2 hours
    b. Neurosurgical consultation and emergency CT scan
    c. IV fluids
    d. Epidural saline

19. In a patient with a healthy heart transplant undergoing had to undergo major elective noncardiac surgery under general anesthesia. Which of the statement is appropriate?
    a. A resting heart rate of 50 beats/min is normal
    b. The cardiovascular response to laryngoscopy is absent
    c. Atropine will cause a tachycardia
    d. Iisoprenaline is the chronotrope of choice

ANSWERS

1. **Ans. (d)**

   Sessler DI. Temperature monitoring and perioperative thermoregulation. Anesthesiology. 2008;109(2):318-38.

   The gold-standard measure of core temperature is of blood by a pulmonary artery (PA) catheter. Other sites which correlation with the gold-standard measurement are esophagus, bladder, rectum, nasopharynx and infrared measures of forehead and tympanic membrane. Peripheral monitoring has poor correlation with core temperature. Thermistor-based temperature probes may be used to estimate core temperature. Common sites of use of infrared thermometers are the tympanic membrane and forehead. This sites are thought to be more indicative of brain temperature. Peripheral sites do not accurately correlate with core temperature and should not be used to guide therapeutic hypothermia.

2. **Ans. (b)**

   Webber S, Andrzejowski J, Francis G. Gas embolism in anesthesia. BJA CEPD Rev. 2002;2(2):53-7.

   PEEP reduces the risk of embolized air entering the heart. It increases right atrial pressure (RAP) but reduces left atrial pressure, so increasing the risk of pulmonary air embolism. Fluid loading increases pulmonary artery pressure, reducing the site to heart pressure gradient. In surgery, carrying a high risk of venous air embolism, a central venous line should be placed before the operation is commenced.

3. **Ans. (d)**

   Goodyear SJ, You H, saedon M, et al. Risk stratification by preoperative cardiopulmonary exercise testing improves outcomes following elective abdominal aortic aneurysm surgery: a cohort study. Med (Lond). 2013;2:10.

   Cardiopulmonary exercise testing (CPET) is a tool used to quantify the risk of perioperative complications and can be used to assess the need for postoperative critical care management. Patient does a static cycle ergometer and simultaneously gas analysis, 12-lead continuous ECG, noninvasive blood pressure and oxygen saturation measurements are performed. The oxygen consumption, carbon dioxide production, respiratory exchange ratio and the anaerobic threshold (AT) are calculated. As work increases, muscle uses more oxygen and this is provided by increasing the cardiac output and increasing the oxygen extraction ratio. VO_2 increases linearly with cardiac output until a peak oxygen extraction ratio of 75% is reached. At this point oxygen demand outstrips supply and the anaerobic threshold (AT) is reached. Patients who are taken up for major surgery should be able to perform >4 METs (metabolic equivalents), which is equivalent to climbing at least one flight of stairs. An AT of less than 11 mL/kg/min is predictive of an increased relative risk of cardiorespiratory morbidity and mortality following major surgery. These such patients will most likely to benefit from postoperative critical care admission. Contraindications to CPET are broadly the same as those to cardiac exercise ECG stress testing, and include severe aortic stenosis, acute myocardial infarction and acutely decompensated heart failure.

4. **Ans. (b)**

   The ARDS Definition Task Force, Ranieri VM, Rubenfeld GD, et al. Acute Respiratory Distress Syndrome: The Berlin Definition. JAMA. 2012;307(23):2526-33.

   The Berlin definition (2013) of ARDS no longer differentiates between ARDS and acute lung injury (ALI). Transfusion-related acute lung injury is defined as new-onset acute lung injury that occurs during or within 6 hours of transfusion, not explained by another acute lung injury risk factor. Ventilator-associated pneumonia is, by definition, only diagnosed after the patient has been ventilated for more than 48 hours. The good cardiac function as demonstrated by echocardiography suggests that cardiogenic pulmonary edema is unlikely and the stroke volume variation of 14% (assuming full mechanical ventilation) suggests that the patient is still fluid-responsive.

5. **Ans. (a)**

   Irwin SA, Pirrello RD, Hirst JM, et al. Clarifying delirium management: practical, evidenced-based, expert recommendations for clinical practice. J Palliat Med. 2013;16(4):423-35.

   Delirium is an independent predictor of increased mortality at 6 months and longer length of stay in ventilated intensive care patients. The Confusion Assessment Method for the ICU (CAM-ICU) and the Intensive Care Delirium Screening Checklist (ICDSC) are the most valid and reliable delirium monitoring tools in adult ICU patients. Three subtypes of delirium have been characterized: hyperactive, hypoactive, and mixed. Predisposing factors for the development of delirium, including severe infection and patient-ventilator dyssynchrony. Haloperidol is drug of choice for the management of hyperactive or mixed delirium; however, it carries a risk of QT prolongation and should not be used if the QTc is prolonged (>450 ms). Benzodiazepines should be used to manage specific delirium syndromes such as alcohol withdrawal and otherwise avoided as they can contribute to the delirium. Midazolam or propofol can be used as rescue therapy for achieving rapid tranquillization if other therapy is failing and the patient poses a danger to themselves or attending staff. Atypical antipsychotics, such as quetiapine, may reduce the duration of delirium in adult ICU patients, but parenteral formulations are not available. In mechanically ventilated adult ICU patients at risk of developing delirium, dexmedetomidine infusions administered for sedation may be associated with a lower prevalence of delirium compared with benzodiazepine infusions. As an α1-agonist, dexmedetomidine will have an antihypertensive effect which may also help in this case.

6. **Ans. (a)**

   Rippe I, Thakur M, Ahmed AB. A review of thromboelastography. Int J Periop Ultrasound Appl Technol. 2012;1(1):25-9.

   The R-time is prolonged in this patient which suggests a deficiency in clotting factors and FFP should be administered. Thromboelastography (TEG®) provides information on all phases of coagulation and due to the quick turnaround time can be used to reduce inappropriate transfusion. The principle of thromboelastography is that whole blood from the patient is added to activators and placed into a cup. A pin is immersed into the blood and the cup is rotated. As the blood clots the 100 rotational movement of the cup is transmitted to the pin. A transducer converts the torsion on the pin into a thromboelastograph. The R-time (reaction time) for whole blood is 4–8 minutes, and this is the time until initiation of fibrin formation (a 2-mm amplitude on the tracing). This reflects the concentration of soluble clotting factors in the plasma. The K-time for whole blood is 1–4 minutes; this is the time period for the amplitude of the tracing to increase from 2 mm to 20 mm. The angle (whole blood 47–74°) is the angle between a tangent to the tracing at 2 mm amplitude and the horizontal midline. The K-time and the angle measure clot kinetics and the rapidity of fibrin build-up and cross-linking. The maximum amplitude (MA, whole blood 55–73 mm) is the greatest vertical width achieved by the tracing and reflects the number and function of platelets and fibrinogen concentration. Clot lysis at 30 minutes (percentage in amplitude 30 minutes after MA) and at 60 minutes shows clot stability and fibrinolysis.

7. **Ans. (a)**
Hoste EA, Maitland K, Brudney CS, et al. Four phases of intravenous fluid therapy: a conceptual model. Br J Anaesth. 2014;113(5):740-7.

The optimal endpoints for trauma resuscitation are not known. But adequate resuscitation can be assessed by good urine output and vital signs. It is important to remember that if trauma patients are not resuscitated adequately their is risk of multiorgan failure and death. Thus, one should combine the clinical picture with multiple markers of hypoperfusion (vital signs, physical examination, urine output, lactate, base deficit, mixed venous oxygen saturation, etc.) while resuscitation of trauma patient. Base deficit has been studied in the trauma population, with a correlation to outcome. Furthermore, base deficit is a crude marker of hypoperfusion that can be highly influenced by treatment, such as chloride administration. A pulmonary artery catheter is not recommended in this patient.

8. **Ans. (b)**
Hunt L, Frost SA, Hillman K, et al. Management of intra-abdominal hypertension and abdominal compartment syndrome: a review. J Trauma Manag Outcomes. 2014;8(1):2.

This patient has classic signs of abdominal compartment syndrome. Blunt trauma to the abdomen requiring massive resuscitation. Normal intra-abdominal pressure is 5–7 mm Hg and should be measured at end-expiration, in the supine position, absent of abdominal muscle contraction, with a zeroed transducer at the level of the mid-axillary line. Without abdominal compartment syndrome, in such conditions as morbid in obesity and ascites can be associated with intra-abdominal hypertension. Abdominal compartment syndrome is the presence of intra-abdominal hypertension (>20 mm Hg) associated with new or worsening organ dysfunction. Abdominal compartment syndrome can affect most all organ systems. This patient may present with findings: elevated central venous pressure, increase in both peak and plateau airway pressures. Due to a reduction in perfusion pressure to the kidney, oliguria will occur. When bladder pressure is normal, other causes for deterioration should be sought, such as acute respiratory distress syndrome with concomitant acute cor pulmonale.

9. **Ans. (d)**

Berger JS, Frye CB, Harshaw Q, et al. Impact of clopidogrel in patients with acute coronary syndromes requiring coronary artery bypass surgery: a multicenter analysis. J Am Coll Cardiol. 2008;52(21):1693-701.

Antiplatelet therapy is needed to prevent graft occlusion.

The American Heart Association/American College of Cardiology guidelines recommend starting aspirin within 6 hours after surgery. If the patient is allergic to aspirin, clopidogrel may be used alone. Dual-antiplatelet therapy with aspirin and clopidogrel has not shown to have a greater benefit than aspirin alone.

10. **Ans. (b)**

DuBose J, Inaba K, Demetriades D, et al. Management of post-traumatic retained hemothorax: a prospective, observational, multicenter AAST study. J Trauma Acute Care Surg. 2012;72(1):11-22.

A CT is needed if there is persistent opacity in chest X-ray to rule out suspected hemothorax. The preferred method of evacuation of retained hemothorax is video-assisted thoracoscopic surgery (VATS) over a second chest tube.

11. **Ans. (c)**

Razonable RR, Findlay JY, O'Riordan A, et al. Critical care issues in patients after liver transplantation. Liver Transpl. 2011;17(5):511-27.

Indicators of satisfactory allograft after orthotopic liver transplant: good mental status, hemodynamic stability, good urine output, bile production (seen intraoperatively), correction of coagulopathy, improvement in electrolytes, and improvement of metabolic acidosis as the new liver is able to clear lactate and metabolize citrate. Factors pointing toward the new liver rejection: persistent metabolic acidosis, ongoing coagulopathy, hemodynamic instability, hypocalcemia due to citrate toxicity (especially in the setting of massive transfusion of blood products), hypoglycemia, hyperkalemia, increasing encephalopathy, and poor renal function.

In functioning new transplanted liver, transaminases immediately increase after surgery and often peak within 24 hours of transplant, then should begin to decrease.

12. **Ans. (d)**

Hudson LD, Milberg JA, Anardi D, et al. Clinical risks for development of the acute respiratory distress syndrome. Am J Respir Crit Care Med. 1995;151:293-301.

Sepsis is the most common cause of acute respiratory distress syndrome (ARDS). This patient probably had a preexisting community-acquired pneumonia, or now has an early ventilator-associated pneumonia. However, severe ARDS (P/F ratio is 68/0.8 = 85). But with gastrointestinal signs, there are high chances of concern of missed intra-abdominal catastrophe. Ventilation management is also important. Pulmonary embolism could be included in the differential diagnosis, but the feeding intolerance and leukocytosis excludes the diagnosis.

13. **Ans. (a)**

    Piper GL, Kaplan LJ. Critical Care of the Abdominal Surgery Patient; Intra-peritoneal Surgery; Emergency General Surgery; Elective General Surgery; 2016.

    These conditions have the potential to benefit from a period of ICU management prior to definitive operation as the vast majority of these are related to obstructive, inflammatory or infective processes.

14. **Ans. (c)**

    Yurtlu DA, Aksun M, Ayvat P, et al. Comparison of Risk Scoring Systems to Predict the Outcome in ASA-PS V Patients Undergoing Surgery: A Retrospective Cohort Study. Medicine (Boltimore). 2016;95(13):e3238.

    The American Society of Anesthesiologists' (ASA) physical status classification system is a widely used preoperative scoring system that describes the overall health of the patient and burden of comorbidities. The score is ideal in being simple to apply and requiring no laboratory data; however, it is also subject to substantial interobserver variation in score assignment. Despite this inherent subjectivity, the ASA classification has been recognized as a helpful predictor of potential postoperative morbidity and mortality. Another scoring system of preoperative comorbidities is the Charlson Comorbidity Index, which assigns weights to a variety of systemic diseases and predicts long-term survival. This score is usually considered more useful for research purposes than for risk stratification in real time. There are also organ system-specific scores, most notably the Revised Cardiac Risk Index (RCRI), a scoring system that incorporates six factors to predict the risk of major cardiac events after noncardiac surgery. The RCRI predicts only cardiac risk, while the ASA and Charlson Comorbidity Index do not incorporate variables specific to the surgical procedure.

15. **Ans. (d)**

    Iyer A, Yadav S. Postoperative Care and Complications after Thoracic Surgery. Principles and Practice of Cardiothoracic Surgery. 2013. [online] Available from https://www.intechopen.com/books/principles-and-practice-of-cardiothoracic-surgery/postoperative-care-and-complications-after-thoracic-surgery. [last accessed June, 2019].

    Cardiac herniation following pneumonectomy and pericardial patch breakdown is characterized by acute obstructive shock, jugular venous distention, and discoloration of the upper torso. The mortality rate is 50%; therefore, immediate recognition and surgical treatment are imperative.

16. **Ans. (d)**

    Simmons J, Adam LA. Chapter 112: Principles of Postoperative Critical Care. United States: McGraw-Hill Education; 2015.

    Cardiac tamponade, massive hemothorax, and right heart failure are significant causes of morbidity and mortality in cardiac surgery. Their presentations can be similar and distinguishing between the different causes is imperative to ensure that proper medical and/or surgical treatment is performed. Cardiac herniation is complication of neumonectomy of pericardial patch surgery.

17. **Ans. (c)**

Stoneham MD, Thompson JP. Arterial pressure management and carotid endarterectomy. Br J Anaesth. 2009;102(4):442-52.

Postoperative hypotension (a systolic blood pressure of less than 120 mm Hg) occurs in approximately 5% of patients. It responds well to fluids and low doses of phenylephrine infusions and usually resolves in 24–48 hours. Patients with significant postoperative hypotension should be investigated with serial ECGs and cardiac enzyme studies to rule out a myocardial infarction. Causes of hypotension include:
- Local anesthetic infiltration around the carotid sinus
- Carotid artery injury
- Excessive analgesia, e.g. morphine
- Bleeding.

18. **Ans. (c)**

Goswami D, Das J, Deuri A, et al. Epidural haematoma: Rare complication after spinal while intending epidural anaesthesia with long-term follow-up after conservative treatment. Indian J Anaesth. 2011;55(1):71-3.

Headache occurs in around 80% typically from 2 hours to 24 hours postpuncture. The headache is thought to be due to loss of CSF via the tear resulting in traction on the intracranial contents. A reduction in CSF pressure may lead to cerebral vasodilatation and headache. The presentation of the patient with headache, photophobia and hyperesthesia of both lower limbs may suggest spinal cord compression by an epidural hematoma or abscess. Epidural hematoma is very rare but classically presents with a sharp radiating back pain and a sensorimotor deficit.

Headache due to a CSF leak is not associated with neurological signs in the lower limbs, bladder or bowel function. Once symptoms have developed, urgent decompression is required within 8 hours to prevent permanent neurological damage.

19. **Ans. (d)**

Shaw IH, Kirk AJ, Conacher ID, et al. Anesthesia for patients with transplanted hearts and lungs undergoing non-cardiac surgery. Br J Anaesth. 1991 Dec;67(6):772-8.

The heart is denervated and will, therefore, only respond to circulating catecholamine. If there is no extra-adrenaline stimulus, the heart rate will be about 60 bpm. In the presence of adrenaline there will be a high-resting rate, typically 100–120 bpm. A slowing heartbeat is a sign of rejection. The cardiovascular responses to laryngoscopy are still evident via the adrenal axis but they are often delayed. There is no vagal tone in the transplanted heart therefore atropine is ineffective as a chronotope. Isoprenaline is the drug of choice in a bradycardia. Antirejection therapy should be monitored.

CHAPTER 23

Tropical Diseases

DHRUV CHAUDHARY

QUESTIONS

1. Which of the following conditions does not fulfill the criteria for dengue hemorrhagic fever?
   a. Fever + Thrombocytopenia + Positive Hess Test
   b. Fever + Thrombocytopenia + Hematemesis + Hypoproteinemia
   c. Fever + Thrombocytopenia + Positive Hess Test + Ascites
   d. Fever + Thrombocytopenia + Shock

2. Which of the following is not a sign of plasma leakage in dengue hemorrhagic fever?
   a. Presence of pleural effusion and ascites
   b. HCT rise ≥ 10% baseline or decrease after giving fluid therapy
   c. Signs of hypotension
   d. Decrease in serum albumin > 0.5 g/dL from baseline

3. Which of the following is not a characteristics laboratory finding of leptospirosis?
   a. Blood urea level—118 mg/dL
   b. S. Bilirubin (total)—4.8 mg/dL
   c. Total leukocyte count—13,000/mm3
   d. SGOT/SGPT—1102/701

4. Most widely used laboratory method for diagnosis of leptospirosis:
   a. Direct visualization by dark field microscopy of urine sample
   b. Isolation by blood or urine culture
   c. Polymerase chain reaction
   d. Microscopic agglutination test

5. Gold standard test for diagnosis of scrub typhus:
   a. Weil Felix
   b. IgM and IgG ELISA
   c. Polymerase chain reaction (PCR)
   d. Immunofluorescence assay (IFA)

6. A 10-week pregnant lady presented with high grade fever is found to be positive for *Plasmodium falciparum* infection. What treatment you will prescribe to her?
   a. Quinine + Clindamycin
   b. Clindamycin alone

    c. Artesunate oral therapy
    d. Quinine + Doxycycline

7. A 30-year-old veterinary physician is diagnosed to be suffering from leptospirosis. His wife is 8 months pregnant and is concerned that she may also encounter the disease. Which of the following drug can be used as a chemoprophylaxis of leptospirosis?
    a. Ceftriaxone
    b. Azithromycin
    c. Amoxicillin-clavulanic acid
    d. Cefotaxime

8. A 46-year-old male was admitted with history of fever for 15 days. For last 2 days his wife noted swelling of face initially followed by swelling of whole body. His urea was 46 mg/dL, creatinine 1.7 mg/dL. Which of the following electrolytes will help in predicting whether he was at risk of developing leptospiral nephropathy?
    a. Loss of sodium in urine
    b. Loss of calcium in urine
    c. Loss of magnesium in urine
    d. Loss of potassium in urine

9. A 64-year-old male died after suffering from multiorgan failure due to unknown cause. Which of the following pathological findings in his autopsy will go against the diagnosis of leptospirosis?
    a. Tubular necrosis in kidney
    b. Plugging of bile canaliculi in liver
    c. Disseminated intravascular coagulation
    d. Interface hepatitis

10. A registrar in ICU told the consultant in round that a patient of Weil's syndrome was admitted. Consultant was not satisfied with the answer and he told in reply that Weil's disease and syndrome are not synonymous. Which of the following is not a part of Weil's syndrome?
    a. Jaundice
    b. Altered sensorium
    c. Renal dysfunction
    d. Hemorrhagic diathesis

11. Leptospirosis is more prevalent in resource limited poor countries. Modified Faine's criteria in diagnosis of leptospirosis include all of the following *except*:
    a. Clinical criteria
    b. Serological criteria
    c. Laboratory criteria
    d. Epidemiological criteria

12. A 38-year-old lady was admitted with fever for 10 days, breathlessness for 2 days, and altered sensorium for 2 days. Neck rigidity was present. CSF was cloudy in nature with plenty of neutrophils. Patient was put on injection Ceftriaxone. A consultant is of the

view that doxycycline should be added as they encountered a number of patients with scrub typhus this season. Which of the following serum findings will help in justifying the physician's diagnosis of scrub typhus meningitis?
    a. Increased serum pyruvate transaminase
    b. Increased serum adenosine deaminase
    c. Increased serum glutamate oxaloacetate transaminase
    d. Increased serum pyruvate kinase

13. A pregnant lady (16 weeks) was suffering from fever for 10 days with loose motion for 3 days. On investigation, scrub typhus IgM was found to be positive. Which of the following is the drug of choice?
    a. Doxycycline
    b. Ceftriaxone
    c. Azithromycin
    d. Penicillin

14. CSF picture of scrub typhus meningitis closely mimics:
    a. Pyogenic meningitis
    b. Viral meningitis
    c. Tubercular meningitis
    d. Aseptic meningitis

15. A 42-year-old male was admitted with 10 days history of fever, pain in abdomen for 3 days, and vomiting for 2 days. His initial vital parameters were Pulse: 134/min, BP 80/46 mm Hg, RR: 34/min, Chest: Bilateral crepitation, Temperature: 102° F. His blood investigations were Hb: 16.3 g/dL, TLc: 10, 400 with polymorph 71%, Platelet: 1,20,000, Sodium: 126 mEq/L, Potassium: 2.8 mEq/L; pH: 7.27, PCO_2: 32 mm Hg, PO_2: 56 mm of H (FiO_2 0.5), urea: 62 mg/dL, creatinine: 2.3 mg/dL; Resident on duty asked his senior what could be the most probable differential diagnosis?
    a. Scrub typhus
    b. Leptospirosis
    c. Enteric fever
    d. Malaria

16. All of the following are true for dengue infection *except*:
    a. IgM after a slow rise will persist for life
    b. Antidengue IgG is detectable at the end of first week of illness
    c. IgM antibodies may remain elevated for 2–3 months after the illness
    d. Dengue NS1 antigen has been detected as early as 1 day post onset of symptoms

17. Dengue shock syndrome is characterized by all *except*:
    a. Hepatomegaly
    b. Pleural effusion
    c. Decreased hemoglobin
    d. Thrombocytopenia

18. Tourniquet test (Hess test) is positive in dengue, if it has:
    a. 10 or more petechiae/2.5 cm²
    b. 15 or more petechiae/2.5 cm²
    c. 20 or more petechiae/2.5 cm²
    d. Any number of petechiae

19. All of the following are true for dengue shock syndrome *except*:
    a. Susceptibility decreases considerably after 12 years of age
    b. Females are more often affected than males
    c. Dengue virus 1 infection followed by dengue virus 2 infection seems to be more dangerous than dengue virus 4 infection followed by dengue virus 2
    d. Southeast Asian dengue virus 2 variants have less potential to cause severe dengue than do others variants

20. Which of the following concerning the monitoring of dengue fever is not true?
    a. Leukopenia (< 5000/mm³) is rare
    b. An increase in the hematocrit with a rapid drop in the platelet count (≤ 100,000/mm³) is a warning sign
    c. An increased or persistently high hematocrit indicates severe plasma leakage
    d. A decrease in hematocrit may indicate a hemorrhage

21. Severe falciparum malaria is characterized by all of the following *except*:
    a. Arterial pH < 7.25
    b. Hematocrit < 15%
    c. Hyperglycemia
    d. Parasitemia > 10% in any patient

22. All of the following statements are correct regarding rapid diagnostic tests (RDTs) for malaria *except*:
    a. Sensitivity of RDTs is similar to or slightly lower than that of thick peripheral blood films
    b. PfHRP2 card test detects only *P. falciparum*
    c. PfHRP2 card test detects both *P. falciparum* and *P. vivax*
    d. PfHRP2 may remain positive for several weeks after acute infection

23. Which of the following statements regarding *P. falciparum* is false?
    a. Causes more severe disease in pregnancy
    b. Is the only malarial parasite causing >20% parasitemia
    c. Typically associated with thrombocytopenia
    d. Is the only cause of cerebral malaria

ANSWERS

1. **Ans. (a)**
   National guidelines for clinical management of Dengue fever. [online] Available from http://www. searo.who.int/india/publications/national_guidelines_clinical_management_dengue1.pdf. [Last accessed June, 2019].
   Anand AC and Garg HK. Approach to clinical syndrome of jaundice and encephalopathy in tropics. J Clin Exp Hepatol. 2015;5(Suppl 1):S116–S130.

   Signs of capillary leak must be present for diagnosis of dengue hemorrhagic fever. Evidence of hemorrhagic manifestation or a positive tourniquet test + thrombocytopenia ($\leq$ 100,000 cells/mm^3) + evidence of plasma leakage shown by hemoconcentration (> 20%) like ascites, pleural effusion, anasarca or hypoproteinemia.

2. **Ans. (b)**
   HCT rise $\geq$ 20% from baseline or decrease in 20% after giving fluid therapy is consistent with plasma leakage. New onset pleural effusion and ascites is considered as one of the most specific sign for the leaky capillaries.

3. **Ans. (d)**
   Bal AM. Unusual clinical manifestations of leptospirosis. J Postgrad Med. 2005;51(3):179-83.

   Classical Weil's disease is characterized by elevated level of blood urea level, conjugated and unconjugated hyperbilirubinemia with aminotransferase elevation but not more than 5 times of normal limit. Leukocytosis is more common finding than leukopenia. Mild to moderate rise in creatine kinase is because of myositis or muscle damage.

4. **Ans. (d)**
   Senaka R, Chaturaka R, Shiroma MH, Current immunological and molecular tools for leptospirosis: diagnostics, vaccine design, and biomarkers for predicting severity. Ann Clin Microbiol Antimicrob. 2015;14:351-5.

   Serological method is the most preferred technique for identification of leptospiral infection. Sample sent during acute phase may be negative because antibodies against leptospira appear during 2nd phase of illness so a paired sample must be sent for diagnosis. Seroconversion or four-fold increase in titer is highly suggestive of recent infection.

5. **Ans. (d)**
   Singhi S, Chaudhary Dhruva, Varghese GM, et al. Tropical fevers: Management guidelines. Indian J Crit Care Med. 2014;18(2):62-9.

   Sensitivity of PCR test is highest but sample for identification include eschar and blood, CSF where concentration decrease over 1 week. Currently indirect immunoperoxidase (IIP) is replacing IFA method because of low cost and similar specificity and sensitivity. Weil-Felix is the oldest method for diagnosing scrub which has a very poor sensitivity.

6. **Ans. (a)**
   Guidelines for treatment of malaria by WHO. 3rd Edition. [online] Available from: http://apps. who.int/iris/bitstream/10665/162441/1/9789241549127_eng.pdf. [Last accessed June, 2019].

Malaria infection in pregnant women is associated with high risks of both maternal and perinatal morbidity and mortality. Pregnant woman has 3–10 times higher risk of severe malaria than nonpregnant. In case of chloroquine-resistant *P. falciparum* infection, prompt treatment with either mefloquine or a combination of quinine sulfate and clindamycin is recommended. Mefloquine should be avoided in first trimester. Quinine therapy and clindamycin should be continued for 7 days.

7. **Ans. (b)**
   Kasper D, Fauci AS, Hauser SL, et al. Harrison's Principle of Internal Medicine, 19th edition. p. 1145.
   - Ceftriaxone, Amoxicillin or Cefotaxime all are used as treatment of leptospirosis.
   - Azithromycin or doxycycline can be used for chemoprophylaxis, however effectiveness in epidemic or endemic settings still remains unclear.

8. **Ans. (c)**
   Leptospiral nephropathy at earliest is associated with loss of magnesium in urine before other abnormalities develop.

9. **Ans. (d)**
   Interface hepatitis is usually a feature of autoimmune hepatitis and chronic hepatitis. It is usually not found in hepatitis due to acute causes or hepatic failure as a part of multiorgan failure.

10. **Ans. (b)**
    Palaniappan RU, Ramanujam S, Chang YF. Leptospirosis: pathogenesis, immunity, and diagnosis. Curr Opin Infect Dis. 2007 Jun;20(3):284-92.

    Altered sensorium does not classically constitute the triad of Weil's syndrome.

11. **Ans. (b)**
    Faine S. Guidelines for the control of leptospirosis. Geneva: World Health Organization; 1982. p. 67.

    World Health Organization (WHO) has introduced "Faine's criteria" for diagnosis of leptospirosis, based on clinical history (Part A) and epidemiological history (Part B) supported by laboratory parameters (Part C).

12. **Ans. (c)**
    Jamil MD, Hussain M, Lyngdoh M, Sharma S, Barman B, Bhattacharya PK. Scrub typhus meningoencephalitis, a diagnostic challenge for clinicians: A hospital based study from North-East India. J Neurosci Rural Pract. 2015;6(4):488-93.

    Increased serum glutamate oxaloacetate transaminase. Scrub typhus meningitis should be kept in differential diagnosis of meningoencephalitis in tropical countries. Elevated SGOT is a feature of scrub typhus.

13. **Ans. (c)**
    Rajan SJ, Sathyendra S, Mathuram AJ. Scrub typhus in pregnancy: Maternal and fetal outcomes. Obstet Med. 2016;Dec;9(4):164-166.

    Although doxycycline and azithromycin both are effective in treatment of scrub typhus, doxycycline is not used in treatment of scrub typhus in pregnancy. Doxycycline is avoided during pregnancy because other tetracyclines have been associated with transient suppression of bone growth and staining of developing teeth.

14. **Ans. (c)**

    Viswanathan S. Scrub Typhus Meningitis Versus Acute Bacterial Meningitis and Tuberculous Meningitis. Indian Pediatr. 2018;Jan15;35(1):25-26.

    Scrub typhus meningitis typically causes lymphocytic meningitis, CSF pleocytosis, CSF protein elevation resembling tubercular meningitis.

15. **Ans. (b)**

    Kasper D, Fauci AS, Hauser SL, et al. Harrison's principle of Internal Medicine 19th edition. p. 1140.

    Hypokalemia along with acute kidney injury is classically seen in leptospirosis.

16. **Ans. (a)**

    World Health Organization, Regional Office for South-East Asia. Comprehensive guidelines for prevention and control of dengue and dengue hemorrhagic fever by WHO. [online] Available from http://apps.searo.who.int/pds_docs/B4751.pdf. [Last accessed June, 2019].
    World Health Organization. National guidelines for clinical management of Dengue fever. [online] Available from http://www.searo.who.int/india/publications/national_guidelines_clinical_management_dengue1.pdf. [Last accessed June, 2019].

17. **Ans. (c)**

    World Health Organization, Regional Office for South-East Asia. Comprehensive guidelines for prevention and control of dengue and dengue hemorrhagic fever by WHO. [online] Available from http://apps.searo.who.int/pds_docs/B4751.pdf. [Last accessed June, 2019].

    World Health Organization. National guidelines for clinical management of Dengue fever. [online] Available from http://www.searo.who.int/ india/publications/national_guidelines_clinical_management_dengue1.pdf. [Last accessed June, 2019].

18. **Ans. (c)**

    World Health Organization, Regional Office for South-East Asia. Comprehensive guidelines for prevention and control of dengue and dengue hemorrhagic fever by WHO. [online] Available from http://apps.searo.who.int/pds_docs/B4751.pdf. [Last accessed June, 2019].
    World Health Organization. National guidelines for clinical management of Dengue fever. [online] Available from http://www.searo.who.int/ india/publications/national_guidelines_clinical_management_dengue1.pdf. [Last accessed June, 2019].

19. **Ans. (d)**

    World Health Organization, Regional Office for South-East Asia. Comprehensive guidelines for prevention and control of dengue and dengue hemorrhagic fever by WHO. [online] Available from http://apps.searo.who.int/pds_docs/B4751.pdf. [Last accessed June, 2019].

World Health Organization. National guidelines for clinical management of Dengue fever. [online] Available from http://www.searo.who.int/ india/publications/national_ guidelines_clinical_management_dengue1.pdf. [Last accessed June, 2019].

20. Ans. (a)
World Health Organization, Regional Office for South-East Asia. Comprehensive guidelines for prevention and control of dengue and dengue hemorrhagic fever by WHO. [online] Available from http://apps.searo.who.int/pds_docs/B4751.pdf. [Last accessed June, 2019].
World Health Organization. National guidelines for clinical management of Dengue fever. [online] Available from http://www.searo.who.int/ india/publications/national_ guidelines_clinical_management_dengue1.pdf. [Last accessed June, 2019].

21. Ans. (c)
Lewallen S, Bakker H, Taylor TE, et al. Retinal findings predictive of outcome in cerebral malaria. Trans R Soc Trop Med Hyg. 1996;90(2):144-6.
Kochar DK, Shubhakaran, Kumawat BL, et al. Ophthalmoscopic abnormalities in adults with falciparum malaria. QJM. 1998;91(12):845-52.
Jones RG, Sue-Ling HM, Kear C, et al. Severe symptomatic hypoglycemia due to quinine therapy. J R Soc Med. 1986;79(7):426-28.
Guidelines for treatment of malaria by WHO. 3rd Edition. [online] Available from http://apps.who.int/iris/bitstream/10665/162441/1/9789241549127_eng.pdf. [Last accessed June, 2019].

22. Ans. (c)
Lewallen S, Bakker H, Taylor TE, et al. Retinal findings predictive of outcome in cerebral malaria. Trans R Soc Trop Med Hyg. 1996;90(2):144-6.
Kochar DK, Shubhakaran, Kumawat BL, et al. Ophthalmoscopic abnormalities in adults with falciparum malaria. QJM. 1998;91(12):845-52.
Jones RG, Sue-Ling HM, Kear C, et al. Severe symptomatic hypoglycaemia due to quinine therapy. J R Soc Med. 1986;79(7):426-28.
Guidelines for treatment of malaria by WHO. 3rd Edition. [online] Available from http://apps.who.int/iris/bitstream/10665/162441/1/9789241549127_eng.pdf. [Last accessed June, 2019].

23. Ans. (d)
Lewallen S, Bakker H, Taylor TE, et al. Retinal findings predictive of outcome in cerebral malaria. Trans R Soc Trop Med Hyg. 1996;90(2):144-6.
Kochar DK, Shubhakaran, Kumawat BL, et al. Ophthalmoscopic abnormalities in adults with falciparum malaria. QJM. 1998;91(12):845-52.
Jones RG, Sue-Ling HM, Kear C, et al. Severe symptomatic hypoglycaemia due to quinine therapy. J R Soc Med. 1986;79(7):426-28.
Guidelines for treatment of malaria by WHO. 3rd Edition. [online] Available from http://apps.who.int/iris/bitstream/10665/162441/1/9789241549127_eng.pdf. [Last accessed June, 2019].

CHAPTER 24

Critical Care Pharmacology 2019

NATESH PRABHU R

BASIC PHARMACOLOGY AND CRITICALLY ILL PATIENTS

1. Choose the wrong statement.
   a. Steady state concentration of the drug is a function of the volume of distribution of drug
   b. The half-life of the drug depends on both volume of distribution and clearance of the drug
   c. Maintenance dose depends on the clearance of the drug
   d. Loading dose depends on the volume of distribution of drug

2. Choose the false statement regarding prescription of high protein bound antimicrobials in hypoalbuminemic critically ill patients.
   a. May need increase in the loading dose
   b. Increase in clearance of the drug should be anticipated
   c. The drug will be more effective
   d. May need reduction in dosing frequency

3. Choose the wrong statement regarding the pharmacokinetic property of antimicrobials in patients with septic shock.
   a. Volume of distribution (Vd) is affected when the drug is more lipid soluble
   b. Hydrophilic antimicrobials generally have less tissue penetration
   c. Renal function affects the elimination of hydrophilic drugs
   d. Hydrophilic drugs generally attain low plasma concentration with standard dose

4. Enhanced elimination of drugs during renal replacement therapy is influenced by many factors. All are factors that enhance elimination *except*:
   a. Low protein binding
   b. Low molecular weight
   c. High lipid solubility
   d. Duration and mode of renal replacement therapy

5. Choose the false statement regarding the efficacy of antimicrobials:
   a. Piperacillin-tazobactam concentration in plasma should be maintained at least 40% of the time above MIC
   b. Amikacin should attain around 10 times above MIC
   c. Meropenem concentration in plasma should be maintained at least 40% of the time above MIC
   d. Vancomycin follows AUC0-24/MIC and needs to maintain > 400

6. **True of augmented renal clearance:**
   a. Observed in patients with normal renal functions with a normal glomerular filtration rate
   b. May affect the efficacy of lipophilic drugs
   c. It is associated with low cardiac output state
   d. Low systemic vascular resistance and high renal blood flow contribute to ARC in patients with septic shock

7. **Choose the correct statement regarding mutant selection window and influence of antimicrobial choice and dosing in the development of drug resistance.**
   a. Antimicrobial concentration in plasma influences the development of resistant mutants
   b. Mutant selection window is a hypothetical window between MIC99 and MIC50
   c. The dose of a drug required to prevent the emergence of mutants is higher than required for its effect
   d. Synergistic effect of combination of antibiotics may prevent falling in MSW

8. **A 40-year-old male patient admitted after emergency surgery for perforation peritonitis with acute kidney injury and septic shock to the intensive care unit (ICU). On day 2 of ICU stay, his renal functions further worsened with a serum creatinine of 3.4 mg/dL, serum urea—102 mmol/dL, requiring renal replacement therapy (intermittent hemodialysis). His current antibiotics are piperacillin-tazobactam 4.5 g 6th hourly and amikacin 1 g 24 hourly. How will you optimize the antimicrobial dose?**
   a. Reduce the dose and frequency of piperacillin-tazobactam, and amikacin
   b. Reduce the dose and frequency of amikacin and continue the same dose of piperacillin-tazobactam
   c. Continue the same dose of amikacin and prescribe every 48–72 hours and reduced dose of piperacillin-tazobactam and maintain increased frequency
   d. Give the same dose of piperacillin-tazobactam, and amikacin

9. **A 35-year-old male patient admitted to ICU with community-acquired pneumonia with septic shock. He received empirical ceftriaxone 2 g and azithromycin in the emergency room and 2.5 L crystalloids over 4 hours time and on noradrenaline support of 0.1 mic/kg/min with urine output of 100 mL/hr for past 2 hours. His Hb: 10.2 g/dL, WBC count: 18,598 cells/mm³, platelets: 12,300 cells/mm³, creatinine: 1.2 mg/dL, serum albumin: 2.1 g/dL, pH: 7.10, and serum bicarbonate: 16 mmol/L. Choose the wrong statement.**
   a. Volume of distribution of antimicrobials may be increased in this patient warranting alteration in dosage
   b. Plasma concentration of antibiotics will be less due to altered protein binding
   c. Uremia and acidosis will decrease protein binding and increase Vd
   d. The patient may have increased clearance requiring a higher dose of ceftriaxone

10. **The 56-year-old male got admitted in the intensive care unit with pyelonephritis and septic shock with mild acute respiratory distress syndrome (ARDS). Blood culture and urine culture have grown *E. coli* sensitive to colistin (mic <1.0), resistant to piperacillin-tazobactam, meropenem, and amikacin.**

a. Colistin loading dose should be given in all patients irrespective of their renal impairment
b. An additional dose of colistin should be given to patients undergoing intermittent hemodialysis.
c. The more active form of colistin is formed in patients without renal impairment
d. Colistin is known to cause neurotoxicity

11. The 32-year-old male admitted with fever, headache for 3 days, and altered sensorium 1 day. The patient had one episode of generalized tonic-clonic convulsion. CSF—suggestive of bacterial meningitis. Further history and examination revealed right ear discharge for 1 week and ear pain for 5 days. Regarding antibiotic choice, which of the following antibiotic is not preferable?
    a. Meropenem
    b. Vancomycin
    c. Amikacin
    d. Ciprofloxacin

12. A 45-year-old female patient with uncontrolled diabetes and neutropenia postchemotherapy for acute leukemia is admitted with septic shock and acute kidney injury-II (AKIN). She had multiple uroscopies for renal calculi and had candiduria (*Candida albicans*) in the ward. All are appropriate antifungal therapy in this patient *except*:
    a. Fluconazole
    b. Caspofungin
    c. Amphotericin
    d. Voriconazole

13. A 40-year-old male came to emergency room (ER) with history of fever, jaundice and abdominal pain for 5 days and breathlessness and altered sensorium for 1 day. On examination, patient was febrile, HR: 120 bpm, RR: 32 breaths/min, and BP: 88/56 mm Hg. USG abdomen suggestive of distended biliary ducts and common bile duct. ERCP was done and a stent was placed in CBD after extracting CBD stone. Bile culture—*E. coli*, sensitive to piperacillin-tazobactam, meropenem, amikacin, ciprofloxacin, and cotrimoxazole. Which of the following is least preferred antibiotic for de-escalation in this patient?
    a. Piperacillin-tazobactam
    b. Amikacin
    c. Cotrimoxazole
    d. Ciprofloxacin

14. Which of the following is not a correct statement regarding amphotericin-B?
    a. Acute infusion-related events are less common with liposomal amphotericin compared to the conventional formulation
    b. Liposomal amphotericin does not cause increased liver enzymes
    c. Liposomal amphotericin-B dose modification is not needed with renal failure
    d. Good hydration reduces nephrotoxicity of standard amphotericin-B

15. A 30-year-old male patient admitted in ICU with perforation peritonitis and ARDS (postsurgery). The patient is currently on ECMO and receiving meropenem and morphine infusion. Choose the false statement regarding pharmacokinetic consideration in patients on ECMO.
    a. There will be increased Vd of meropenem
    b. There will be generally increased drug clearance when on ECMO
    c. The dose of sedatives for maintenance is increased during ECMO to maintain the same effect
    d. Highly lipophilic drugs have more circuit sequestration

16. Which is true regarding factors affecting the drug pharmacokinetics and pharmacodynamics in patients with advanced liver disease (cirrhosis)?
    a. For all orally administered drugs that have a high hepatic extraction ratio, the plasma concentration is increased in patients with liver cirrhosis
    b. Bioavailability is reduced for drugs with a low hepatic extraction ratio
    c. Renally excreted drugs are affected only when serum creatinine is elevated
    d. The initial loading dose is affected for all drugs with low hepatic extraction

17. Antimicrobial that requires dose modification in liver disease is:
    a. Ciprofloxacin
    b. Meropenem
    c. Tigecycline
    d. Liposomal amphotericin B

18. Nebulized antibiotic use in critically ill with pneumonia, pick up the correct statement.
    a. During nebulization, HME filters should be removed but can continue heated humidification
    b. Volume controlled mode with a lower respiratory rate is preferable during nebulization
    c. Continuous delivery nebulizer should be attached near Y piece for better effect
    d. Jet nebulizers are preferable to ultrasonic nebulizer

DRUG PHARMACOLOGY IN CRITICALLY ILL PATIENTS

19. Nebulized colistin methane sulfonate (CMS) use in critically ill with pneumonia, pick up the false statement.
    a. Achieves good alveolar concentration and less systemic absorption
    b. Colistin methane sulfonate can be used for nebulization purpose
    c. The dose of 2MU is suggested
    d. CMS is more stable with increased dilution

20. All are options for the treatment of pneumonia with methicillin-resistant *Staphylococcus aureus* (MRSA) except:
    a. Vancomycin
    b. Cotrimoxazole
    c. Linezolid
    d. Daptomycin

21. Arbekacin sulfate:
    a. Its broad-spectrum antibiotic with significant activity against pseudomonas, Acinetobacter and MRSA
    b. Its pharmacodynamic effects are based on concentration dependent killing
    c. Its active against MRSA is par with gentamicin but do not inhibit TSST-1, toxic shock syndrome toxin
    d. Nephrotoxicity is a known adverse effect

22. Best evidence for the use of angiotensin II in critically ill patients is:
    a. Restored glomerular perfusion pressure
    b. High cardiac output shock
    c. Shock and ARDS
    d. ACE inhibitor overdose

23. Choose false statement regarding meropenem vaborbactam.
    a. Vaborbactam is a non-beta-lactam nonsuicidal inhibitor of certain serine beta-lactamases
    b. Approved for complicated urinary tract infection with carbapenemase-producing *Enterobacteriaceae*
    c. It is active against all except KPC-producing *Enterobacteriaceae*
    d. The effluent flow rate appears to be the most important parameter affecting meropenem-vaborbactam filter clearance during CVVH

24. False about fosfomycin is:
    a. Oral fosfomycin is being in use for uncomplicated urinary tract infection (UTI)
    b. Fosfomycin causes more electrolyte imbalances
    c. Fosfomycin covers *Staphylococcus aureus* but not MRSA
    d. Parenteral fosfomycin has good tissue distribution and penetration

25. Incorrect statement regarding eravacycline is:
    a. Belongs to a group of tigecycline and is more potent
    b. Has broad spectrum activity covering MRSA, enterococcus, pseudomonas, and acinetobacter
    c. Switching over to oral formulation during recovery is a potential advantage
    d. Follows AUC/MIC for clinical efficacy

26. Pick false statement regarding noradrenaline.
    a. Noradrenaline increases only afterload and not preload to heart
    b. It increases vasomotor tone by acting on alpha-1 receptor
    c. Is vasopressor of choice for vasodilatory shock
    d. Affects inotropy of heart

27. What is the drug of choice for sedation in critically ill patients which has least delirium risk?
    a. Midazolam
    b. Lorazepam
    c. Dexmedetomidine
    d. Morphine

ANSWERS

1. Ans. (a)
Absorption, distribution, metabolism, and excretion are basic processes of pharmacokinetics of drugs. When a drug is infused, it distributes in the body—the volume of distribution (Vd), it indicates the extent of distribution of drug: volume of distribution (Vd). It is not actual volume rather apparent volume of distribution. Vd is influenced by the amount of drug infused and its concentration.[1]

Clearance: Elimination of drug corresponds to irreversible removal of drug from the volume containing it, i.e. amount of volume cleared of substance in unit time: clearance. How fast the drug is fully cleared depends on the half-life of the drug (The time required for the plasma drug concentration to fall by 50% is the elimination half-life). It takes approximately five half-lives to attain steady state or for full elimination and it depends on the Vd and clearance.

Steady state is a state where the amount of drug added is equal to the amount of drug removed and the concentration of drug remains constant. The steady state does not depend on Vd, i.e. changing Vd may not constantly affect the steady state except during the initial period. It is affected primarily by clearance.

Whenever Vd increases it will take more time to achieve steady state and requires a larger loading dose to achieve steady state quickly. When clearance of the drug is fast, frequent dosing of the drug will be required which influences the maintenance dose.

2. Ans. (d)
Hypoalbuminemia is common in critically ill patients, which affects all highly protein-bound drugs. Highly protein-bound drugs will have increased unbound fraction when serum albumin is very low which leads to enhanced Vd, drug effect and elimination.[2] This warrants higher loading and maintenance dose and increases the frequency of dosing as well.[3,4]

3. Ans. (a)
Pharmacokineties/Pharmacodynamies of antimicrobials are affected by pathophysiology and complications of the disease.[3] Patients with septic shock will have capillary leakage and low albumin concentration and they will receive fluid expansion, all of which will increase the volume of distribution of hydrophilic drugs, e.g. beta-lactams and aminoglycosides. This leads to low serum/plasma concentration thus needing higher loading and maintenance dose. Almost all hydrophilic drugs are eliminated by kidneys to a considerable extent which in turn affects its plasma concentration. Lipophilic drugs are not affected much by increased Vd as they have good tissue concentration and predominantly have hepatic clearance, e.g. fluoroquinolones and tetracyclines.[3]

4. Ans. (c)
The pharmacokinetics of drugs are altered by the presence of renal failure and renal replacement therapy.[5,6] For a drug to be cleared by dialysis, it should be available in free form (unbound—so more clearance for less protein-bound drugs), should have low

molecular weight, less volume of distribution and more water soluble. The magnitude of the elimination of drugs depends on the duration and mode of dialysis.[7] More elimination with continuous modality and a higher dose of dialysis.[6]

5. **Ans. (a)**
The clinical success of antimicrobials depends on the adequacy of plasma concentration, the drug achieves. Each antimicrobial follows a unique mechanism for bacterial killing. The antimicrobials that follow time-dependent killing should be maintained above required therapeutic concentration for a maximal period of time and antimicrobials that follow concentration-dependent killing should be maintained many fold higher levels than MIC values for great efficacy and drugs that follow AUC/MIC have properties mixture of both.[8,9]

Commonly used antimicrobials and its pharmacodynamic (PD) characteristics				
Drug class	Examples	Killing characteristics	PD parameter	Comments
Beta-lactams	Piperacillin-tazobactam Meropenem Ceftriaxone	Time-dependent	50% of time T > MIC 40% of T > MIC 50–70% of T > MIC	Bactericidal, G negative bacteria
Aminoglycosides	Amikacin	Concentration-dependent	8–10 times above MIC	Single high dose (G negative bacteria)
Glycopeptide	Vancomycin	Time + concentration	AUC/MIC = 400	

6. **Ans. (d)**
Augmented renal clearance (ARC) happens when there is increased glomerular filtration, commonly seen in high cardiac output and low systemic vascular resistance states both of which increase blood flow to kidneys. There is no standard definition for ARC, and it is referred to as augmented renal clearance when there is >10% increase in glomerular filtration or >130–150 mL/min of GFR. The commonly accepted definition is clearance of >130 mL/min. Commonly seen in sepsis, trauma and young adults. Urinary creatinine clearance 8th hourly is more feasible and accurate to diagnose ARC.[10] ARC leads to low plasma concentration and increased elimination of hydrophilic drugs necessitating higher dosage. Though the concept of ARC is increasingly recognized, it has not been translated yet into clinical practice to change the dose of renally eliminated drugs. Practical point is to dose the drug higher and more frequent when ARC is diagnosed. As studies are sparse better to go for therapeutic monitoring of drugs and dose accordingly.[10]

7. **Ans. (b)**
The mutant selection window (MSW) is a hypothetical concept that postulates that for any antimicrobial-pathogen interaction there exists an antimicrobial concentration range in which selective amplification of drug-resistant mutants develop. It lies between MIC99 and mutant prevention concentration (MPC).[11] MPC-MIC of the least drug-susceptible mutant subpopulation. MIC99: minimal concentration of an antimicrobial

that inhibits 99% colony formation. So MSW—has a lower boundary with minimal concentration and the upper boundary of maximal concentration, within which the chance of developing resistant mutants is high. Higher plasma concentration above MPC, no/lesser development of resistant strains, more could be adverse effects of antibiotics. Combining antimicrobials which are synergic, may close each other selection window[12] and help to prevent the emergence of resistant strain with less dose of either and may also prevent adverse effects.

8. Ans. (c)
Dosing antimicrobials depend on its pharmacodynamic mechanism of efficacy,[8] i.e. the effect of antimicrobials either depend on:
 a. Time above minimum inhibitory concentration MIC (T > MIC): Time-dependent antibiotics
 b. Concentration achieved above MIC (C_{max} > MIC): Concentration-dependent antibiotics
 c. The area under curve of 24 hours combination of above two (AUC 0-24/MIC).

For good efficacy the drug that follows T >MIC, it should be given as an infusion or more frequently so that the concentration of drug in plasma is always >MIC and for concentration-dependent antibiotics, the large dose should be given.

The drugs eliminated predominantly by kidney accumulate during renal failure, which warrants dose reduction. All dialysis modalities are effective in removing hydrophilic drugs which have low protein binding and high renal clearance.[6] Amikacin is a concentration-dependent antibiotic and water soluble so ideal dose adjustment in renal failure is to maintain the same dose and reduce the frequency, monitoring the trough levels before the next dose, e.g. 1 g every 48–72 hourly. Piperacillin-tazobactam is time-dependent and water soluble. Ideal dose adjustment is to maintain frequent dosing and reduced dose, e.g. piperacillin-tazobactam 2.25 g 6–8 hourly as an infusion. (Same dose and reduced frequency 4.5 g 12 hourly by prolong infusion). Also, do consider giving dose post dialysis or an additional dose after dialysis. The amount/percentage of the drug to be given post dialysis depends on the PK/PD properties of the individual drug.

9. Ans. (b)
The pharmacokinetics of antimicrobials are altered in critically ill patients especially in patients with sepsis.[13] Patients with sepsis will have increased capillary permeability and will receive fluid expansion and both will lead to increased Vd as in this patient. Also, the patient may have hypoalbuminemia leading to an increased free fraction of drugs which add to increased Vd of highly protein-bound drugs. Moreover, acidosis and uremia cause reduced protein binding and further adding to an increased free fraction of protein-bound drugs. Clearance of renally eliminated drugs may be either increased (ARC) or decreased (if renal impairment) in patients with sepsis. Hydrophilic and highly protein bound antibiotic (ceftriaxone) will have increased Vd and increased clearance (if ARC) warranting increased initial and maintenance dose.

10. **Ans. (c)**
Colistin (polymyxin E) is the active form of colistin methane sulfonate (CMS) also called colistimethate. CMS converts into an active form by hydrolysis. When CMS is infused, most of CMS is eliminated by kidney and rest is converted into active form, so in patients with renal failure, more CMS will be retained and available for conversion into active form and hence more effect rather in patients with normal renal functions.[14]

Mechanism of action: Colistin has a positive charge, it electrostatically gets attached to negatively charged lipopolysaccharides in the outer membrane of gram-negative bacteria and destroys leading to the death of bacteria. It follows concentration dependent, C_{max} > MIC for great efficacy.

Colistin accumulates in renal tubules causing renal tubular damage and causes nephrotoxicity. Colistin is known to cause neuropathy, neuromuscular weakness, and even neuromuscular paralysis.

Dosing: A loading dose of 9MU achieves the target concentration quickly compared to conventional dosages and to start maintenance dose after 12–24 hours.[15,16] It is more commonly accepted to give colistin maintenance dose as two or three divided doses. Few suggest different loading dose for the varied degree of renal impairment based on creatinine clearance. Colistin is eliminated in urine and dose modification is required in renal failure patients. Creatinine clearance >50 mL/min—(-12 MU, 30–50 mL/min—5.5–7.5 MU and 10–30 mL/min—5 MU per day dose is suggested.[17] It gets adsorbed to dialysis filter and eliminated during dialysis. It is recommended giving an additional dose (30–50% of total dose) after dialysis to maintain target concentration (1 MU = 30 mg, CBA = 80 mg, CMS, CBA: colistin base activity).[18]

11. **Ans. (c)**
Acute bacterial meningitis is an emergency and may lead to neurologic complication and increased morbidity. An early empirical and effective antibiotic is crucial for successful treatment. The antibiotic of choice should have activity against anticipated bacteria and should achieve good tissue concentration, i.e. good CNS/CSF penetration. Majority of antibiotics have less blood-brain barrier penetration. The penetration increases with inflamed meninges and with a higher dosage. Certain antimicrobials have good CSF penetration, e.g. ciprofloxacin, fluconazole. Certain antimicrobials have less penetration in intact meninges and slightly better when inflamed (30–40%), e.g. meropenem and vancomycin. Certain antimicrobials have poor penetration even in strong meningeal irritation, e.g. aminoglycosides.[19]

12. **Ans. (b)**
All immunocompromised patients with persistent candida in urine warrant further investigation and treatment.[20] The choice of antifungal in patients with septic shock is echinocandin as recommended by IDSA. Choice of therapy should also be based on the adequacy of tissue penetration in interest. Echinocandins attain good concentration at renal parenchyma but very low concentration in human urine.[21] Echinocandins do

not have good penetration in the urinary tract or CSF and not a choice if lower UTI or meningitis is suspected. Rest other drugs attain good urinary concentration and are effective against Candida.

13. **Ans. (b)**
De-escalation is commonly done when the clinical improvement of patient happens, the organism is sensitive to narrow-spectrum antibiotics. Antibiotic of choice should have good tissue penetration, less adverse effects and more effective. Aminoglycosides attain fewer bile levels compared to serum and hence less biliary concentration and are not preferred.[22]

14. **Ans. (b)**
Conventional or standard amphotericin-B is known to cause more febrile reactions, renal toxicity.[23] Febrile reactions reduce with subsequent infusions and may be reduced with a slower rate of infusion. Acute infusion-related events are common with liposomal preparations due to compliment activation. Nephrotoxicity of standard amphotericin can be reduced with good pre- and posthydration.[24] Liposomal preparations are not superior if the patient is not tolerant or refractory to standard preparations. Renal toxicity is more common with standard preparations and can be prevented with pre- and posthydration. Dose modification is not required for liposomal amphotericin-B in patients with renal impairment[23] and the dose depends on characteristics of fungus, requiring higher dose in case of mucormycosis compared to Candida.

Liposomal amphotericin caused elevated liver enzymes and increased bilirubin levels, and the mechanism is not fully clear.

Drug	Mechanism of action	Monitoring	Antidote	Comments
Dabigatran	Direct thrombin	aPTT, ECT, dTT	Idarucizumab	Renally eliminated, dialysis may help
Rivaroxaban	Factor Xa inhibition	PT, Anti-Xa		PCC, aVII
Apixaban	Factor Xa inhibition	Anti-Xa		PCC, aVII
Edoxaban	Factor Xa inhibition	Anti-Xa		PCC, aVII

(ECT: Ecarin clotting time; dTT: Dilution thrombin time; PCC: Prothrombin concentrate; aVII: Activated factor VII)

15. **Ans. (b)**
Pharmacokineties/Pharmacodynamies of drugs are altered by ECMO due to various factors.[26] Volume of distribution is generally increased in patients on ECMO, by increasing dilution of drug in priming solution, increased circuit sequestration and by other physiological changes. Highly lipophilic drugs have more circuit sequestration and almost all sedatives like midazolam, morphine, propofol, dexmedetomidine require increased loading and daily dose. The clearance of the drug is generally reduced on ECMO, commonly due to reduced perfusion to the liver and kidney. At present, the meropenem is dosed as in other critically ill patients not on ECMO and preferable to monitor drug concentration.

16. **Ans. (a)**
Many factors affect PK/PD of drugs in patients with cirrhosis/advanced chronic liver disease like hepatic extraction ratio, blood flow to the liver, protein binding of the drug, the severity of liver disease/Child-Pugh score, renal function.[27] Drugs with a high extraction ratio achieve high plasma concentration and its oral bioavailability increases many folds needing reduced loading and maintenance dose of such drugs, e.g. morphine. Drugs with low hepatic extraction ratio, the oral bioavailability is not affected compared to patients with normal liver. Such drugs with high protein binding (>90%) have high free fraction and reduced total concentration and same free concentration.

Many patients with liver cirrhosis have altered renal plasma flow and glomerular filtration. Serum creatinine could be low due to less production and low muscle mass[28] in such patients and there is a potential chance of overestimation of renal functions. The drugs with predominant renal excretion should be given with reduced dose even when the serum creatinine is normal to avoid high plasma concentration and intern adverse effects. Loading dose should be reduced only for drugs with high extraction ratio and maintenance dose should be reduced to drugs that have either high/intermediate/low extraction ratio or which have major metabolism in the liver.

17. **Ans. (c)**
For majority of antimicrobials the data is sparse regarding dose modification in patients with liver disease. Drugs that have a high hepatic extraction ratio or high protein binding needs dose modification. Certain drugs can have hepatotoxicity at higher plasma concentration. Tigecycline maintenance dose should be reduced especially in patients with Child Pugh C, 100 mg followed by 25 mg 12th hourly. Drugs like chloramphenicol achieve very high plasma concentration and lead to more bone marrow suppression.[29]

18. **Ans. (b)**
Humidification affects nebulization efficiency; it increases the size of the particle due to water absorption and it has been shown that dry circuit is better than a humidified circuit for better nebulization.[30] So, HME filters should be removed and heated humidifiers should be switched off during nebulization. Theoretically, laminar flow increases drug deposition at lungs and the delivery is better when the flow is low, lower respiratory rate, and long enough inspiratory time. Volume controlled mode, with low respiratory rate and long inspiratory time, is preferred and it is shown that it performs better than pressure controlled mode.[31]

19. **Ans. (d)**
Nebulized colistin is commonly used for patients with pneumonia multidrug-resistant bacteria. It is given in vibrating mesh/ultrasonic nebulizers. CMS is commonly used for nebulization and once diluted with water or saline; it can spontaneously convert to active form colistin A by hydrolysis. The hydrolysis is time and concentration dependent, more dilution and more time more is the conversion.[32] Currently, the dose of 2 MU is practiced and recent studies have shown good lung concentration with 0.5 MU.[33,34]

20. **Ans. (d)**

Vancomycin and teicoplanin are preferred first line for treatment of MRSA. Linezolid is an alternative, which can be given orally and achieve good lung penetration. Various groups of antimicrobials have varied potency and efficacy against MRSA, doxycycline, cotrimoxazole, ciprofloxacin, quinupristin, daptomycin, etc.[35] Daptomycin though is active against MRSA, it gets degraded by alveolar surfactant in lungs so not effective for pneumonia.[36]

21. **Ans. (c)**

Arbekacin sulfate belongs to the aminoglycoside group (kanamycin family) derived from dibekacin. It is in use in Japan since 1990 and Korea since 2000. It is a broad spectrum antibiotic covering both gram-positive and gram-negative bacteria. It is active against Pseudomonas, *Acinetobacter baumanii*, MRSA including TSST-1 producing strains. It has efficacy against aminoglycoside modifying enzymes and thus cover multidrug-resistant bacteria that are resistant to amikacin and gentamicin. It has very good coverage against MRSA much better than gentamicin and other aminoglycoside antibiotics. It follows C_{max}/MIC and AUC/MIC and currently being dosed with 5-6 mg/kg. Nephrotoxicity is well-known complication and seen more with higher doses.[37]

22. **Ans. (b)**

Angiotensin II is emerging noncatecholamine vasopressor for refractory vasodilatory shock. The action mimics physiologic angiotensin II. It has shown to restore perfusion pressure in high output shock states like distributive shock and shown to increase glomerular perfusion pressure. ATHOS-3 trial showed increased mean arterial pressure compared to placebo and a trend toward mortality reduction.[38] Post hoc analysis showed improved glomerular perfusion[39] and better vasoconstrictor effect in a patient with ARDS[40] possible could be due to deficient ACE or deficiency. Other clinical scenarios where angiotensin II has shown benefits are in patients with ACE inhibitor overdose, patients with ARDS with shock.[41]

23. **Ans. (c)**

Meropenem-vaborbactam[42] is a fixed-dose combination antimicrobial effective against KPC *Enterobacteriaceae*. Vaborbactam is non-beta-lactam, nonsuicidal serine beta-lactamase active against all beta-lactamases, especially against KPC. It prevents degradation of meropenem and extends its spectrum. Both are eliminated by kidney requiring dose modification with impaired renal function. More drug will be eliminated with increasing effluent flow and gets cleared with dialysis.[43] It is mainly approved for complicated UTI, pyelonephritis, etc.

24. **Ans. (c)**

Fosfomycin is bactericidal to most gram positive (including MRSA) and gram-negative bacteria (including pseudomonas but not Acinetobacter) by inhibiting phosphoenolpyruvate synthase.[47] Oral formulation is in use for uncomplicated UTIs and it has excellent urinary tract penetration and eliminated predominantly in urine. Parenteral fosfomycin has attracted great interest due to emerging resistant bacteria. It has shown good efficacy in treating MDR gram-negative bacteria with urinary, CNS and respiratory infections. Dose of 12–16 g/day is given by IV infusion and dose reduction is done when creatinine clearance <50 mL/min. Fosfomycin causes more sodium load and more incidence of hypokalemia.[47]

25. **Ans. (b)**
Eravacycline is a novel drug, a synthetic fluorocycline antibacterial agent that is structurally similar to tigecycline. It has more potent coverage against both gram-positive (including MRSA) and gram-negative bacteria (not Pseudomonas) than tigecycline.[48] It is a potential option for multidrug-resistant bacteria. AUC/MIC best describes the mechanism for its efficacy and phase I and II trials have proven efficacy with both oral and parenteral formulations. The most common adverse effects are nausea, vomiting, and GI upset. A recent randomized controlled trial showed noninferiority of eravacycline (dose 1 mg/kg 12th hourly IV) with ertapenem in patients with complicated intra-abdominal infections.[49] Clinical studies are emerging and there is sparse literature on its efficacy especially in critically ill patients.

26. **Ans. (a)**
Noradrenaline/Norepinephrine is catecholamine potent peripheral vasoconstrictor acting on alpha-1 receptor. It also has some action on beta-1 receptors thus affects contractility of heart. Noradrenaline increases venous tone and increased venous returns to heart and thus preloads.[50,51] Because of potent vasoconstriction it is preferred in vasodilatory states like sepsis.[52]

27. **Ans. (c)**
The risk factors for delirium in the intensive care unit are multifactorial. Almost all sedatives increase the risk of developing delirium and more prevalent with benzodiazepines. Trials that compared various sedatives and analgesics showed less risk with propofol and dexmedetomidine. In MENDS[55] and DEXCOM[56] study dexmedetomidine reduced the duration of delirium when compared with lorazepam and morphine respectively. In a study that compared dexmedetomidine with propofol for sedation in postcardiac surgical patients showed reduced, a delayed onset and lesser duration of delirium in the dexmedetomidine group.[57]

REFERENCES

1. Fan J. Pharmacokinetics. 2014;87:93-120.
2. Roberts JA, Pea F, Lipman J. The clinical relevance of plasma protein binding changes. Clin Pharmacokinet. 2013;52(1):1-8.
3. Blot SI, Pea F, Lipman J. The effect of pathophysiology on pharmacokinetics in the critically ill patient—Concepts appraised by the example of antimicrobial agents. Adv Drug Deliv Rev. 2014;77:3-11.
4. Udy AA, Roberts JA, Lipman J. Clinical implications of antibiotic pharmacokinetic principles in the critically ill. Intensive Care Med. 2013;39(12):2070-82.
5. Choi G, Gomersall CD, Tian Q, et al. Principles of antibacterial dosing in continuous renal replacement therapy. Blood Purif. 2010;30(3):195-212.

6. Pea F, Viale P, Pavan F, et al. Pharmacokinetic considerations for antimicrobial therapy in patients receiving renal replacement therapy. Clin Pharmacokinet. 2007;46(12):997-1038.
7. Atkinson AJ Jr. Pharmacokinetics in Patients requiring renal replacement therapy. In: Atkinson AJ Jr., Abernethy D, Daniels C, Dedrick R, Markey S (Eds). Principles of Clinical Pharmacology, Second Edition. USA: Academic Press Elsevier Inc.; 2007. pp. 21-59.
8. Kuti JL. Optimizing antimicrobial pharmacodynamics: A guide for your stewardship program. Rev Médica Clínica Las Condes. 2016;27(5):615-24.
9. Moore RD, Lietman PS, Smith CR. Clinical response to aminoglycoside therapy: Importance of the ratio of peak concentration to minimal inhibitory concentration. J Infect Dis. 1987;155(1):93-9.
10. Udy AA, Roberts JA, Boots RJ, et al. Augmented renal clearance: implications for antibacterial dosing in the critically ill. Clin Pharmacokinet. 2010;49(1):1-16.
11. Drlica K, Zhao X. Mutant selection window hypothesis updated. Clin Infect Dis. 2007;44(5):681-8.
12. Xu X, Xu L, Yuan G, et al. Synergistic combination of two antimicrobial agents closing each other's mutant selection windows to prevent antimicrobial resistance. Sci Rep. 2018;8(1):1-7.
13. Roberts JA, Abdul-Aziz MH, Lipman J, et al. Individualised antibiotic dosing for patients who are critically ill: Challenges and potential solutions. Lancet Infect Dis. 2014;14(6):498-509.
14. Nation RL, Velkov T, Li J. Colistin and polymyxin B: Peas in a pod, or chalk and cheese? Clin Infect Dis. 2014;59(1):88-94.
15. Karaiskos I, Friberg LE, Pontikis K, et al. Colistin population pharmacokinetics after application of a loading. Antimicrob Agents Chemother. 2015;59(12):7240-8.
16. Nation RL, Garonzik SM, Thamlikitkul V, et al. Dosing guidance for intravenous colistin in critically-ill patients. Clin Infect Dis. 2016;64(5):565-71.
17. Nation RL, Garonzik SM, Li J, et al. Updated US and European dose recommendations for intravenous colistin: How do they perform? Clin Infect Dis. 2016;62(5):552-8.
18. Nation RL, Li J, Cars O, et al. Framework for optimisation of the clinical use of colistin and polymyxin B: The Prato polymyxin consensus. Lancet Infect Dis. 2015;15(2):225-34.
19. Nau R, Sörgel F, Eiffert H. Penetration of drugs through the blood-cerebrospinal fluid/blood-brain barrier for treatment of central nervous system infections. Clin Microbiol Rev. 2010;23(4):858-83.
20. Pappas PG, Kauffman CA, Andes DR, et al. Clinical Practice Guideline for the Management of Candidiasis : 2016 Update by the Infectious Diseases Society of America. Clin Infect Dis. 2016;62(4):1-50.
21. Felton T, Troke PF, Hope W. Tissue penetration of antifungal agents. Clin Microbiol Rev. 2014;27(1):68-88.
22. Dooley JS, Hamilton-Miller JM, Brumfitt W, et al. Antibiotics in the treatment of biliary infection. Gut. 1984;25(9):988-98.
23. Stone NR, Bicanic T, Salim R, et al. Liposomal amphotericin B (AmBisome(®)): A review of the pharmacokinetics, pharmacodynamics, clinical experience and future directions. Drugs. 2016;76(4):485-500.

24. Patel GP, Crank CW, Leikin JB. An evaluation of hepatotoxicity and nephrotoxicity of liposomal amphotericin B (L-AMB). J Med Toxicol. 2011;7(1):12-5.
25. Lefevre ER, Wondergem MJ, Ten Tusscher BL. Direct oral anticoagulants and critical care: a review of literature and current opinion. Neth J Crit Care. 2018;26(5):174-9.
26. Cheng V, Abdul-Aziz MH, Roberts JA, et al. Optimising drug dosing in patients receiving extracorporeal membrane oxygenation. J Thorac Dis. 2018;10(Suppl 5):S629-41.
27. Delcò F, Tchambaz L, Schlienger R, et al. Dose adjustment in patients with liver disease. Drug Saf. 2005;28(6):529-45.
28. Takabatake T, Ohta H, Ishida Y, et al. Low serum creatinine levels in severe hepatic disease. Arch Intern Med. 1988;148:1313-5.
29. Periáñez-párraga L, Martínez-lópez I, Ventayol-bosch P, et al. Drug dosage recommendations in patients with chronic livwr disease. Rev Esp Enferm Dig. 2012;104(4):165-84.
30. Ari A, Areabi H, Fink JB. Evaluation of aerosol generator devices at 3 locations in humidified and non-humidified circuits during adult mechanical ventilation. Respir Care. 2010;55(7):837-44.
31. Dugernier J, Reychler G, Wittebole X, et al. Aerosol delivery with two ventilation modes during mechanical ventilation: a randomized study. Ann Intensive Care. 2016;6(1):73.
32. Wallace SJ, Li J, Rayner CR, et al. Stability of colistin methanesulfonate in pharmaceutical products and solutions for administration to patients. Antimicrob Agents Chemother. 2008;52(9):3047-51.
33. Matthieu B, Matthieu J, Nicolas G, et al. Comparison of intrapulmonary and systemic pharmacokinetics of colistin methanesulfonate (CMS) and colistin after aerosol delivery and intravenous administration of CMS in critically ill patients. Antimicrob Agents Chemother. 2014;58(12):7331-9.
34. Boisson M, Grégoire N, Cormier M, et al. Pharmacokinetics of nebulized colistin methanesulfonate in critically ill patients. J Antimicrob Chemother. 2017;72(9):2607-12.
35. Chukwunonso E, Veronica B, Chiagozie E, et al. Methicillin-resistant Staphylococcus Aureus: A mini review. Int J Med Res Heal Sci. 2018;7(1):122-7.
36. Silverman JA, Mortin LI, VanPraagh ADG, et al. Inhibition of daptomycin by pulmonary surfactant: In vitro modeling and clinical impact. J Infect Dis. 2005;191(12):2149-52.
37. Matsumoto T. Arbekacin: Another novel agent for treating infections due to methicillin-resistant Staphylococcus aureus and multidrug-resistant Gram-negative pathogens. Clin Pharmacol Adv Appl. 2014;6:139-48.
38. Khanna A, English SW, Wang XS, et al. Angiotensin II for the treatment of vasodilatory shock. N Engl J Med Overseas Ed. 2017;377(5):419-30.
39. Tumlin JA, Murugan R, Deane AM, et al. Outcomes in patients with vasodilatory shock and renal replacement therapy treated with intravenous angiotensin II. Crit Care Med. 2018;46(6):949-57.
40. Busse LA, Gong T, Thompson M. Outcomes in patients with acute respiratory distress syndrome receiving angiotensin II for vasodilatory shock. Crit Care. 2018;22(Suppl 1):82.
41. Bussard RL, Busse LW. Angiotensin II: A new therapeutic option for vasodilatory shock. Ther Clin Risk Manag. 2018;14:1287-98.

42. Petty LA, Henig O, Patel TS, et al. Overview of meropenem-vaborbactam and newer antimicrobial agents for the treatment of carbapenem-resistant enterobacteriaceae. Infect Drug Resist. 2018;11:1461-72.
43. Sime FB, Pandey S, Karamujic N, et al. Ex vivo characterization of effects of renal replacement therapy modalities and settings on pharmacokinetics of meropenem and vaborbactam. Antimicrob Agents Chemother. 2018;62(10):1-10.
44. Välitalo PA, Ahtola-Sätilä T, Wighton A, et al. Population pharmacokinetics of dexmedetomidine in critically ill patients. Clin Drug Investig. 2013;33(8):579-87.
45. Miller JL, Allen C, Johnson PN. Neurologic withdrawal symptoms following abrupt discontinuation of a prolonged dexmedetomidine infusion in a child. J Pediatr Pharmacol Ther. 2019;15(1):38-42.
46. Haenecour AS, Seto W, Urbain CM, et al. Prolonged dexmedetomidine infusion and drug withdrawal in critically ill children. J Pediatr Pharmacol Ther. 2017;22(6):453-60.
47. Michalopoulos AS, Livaditis IG, Gougoutas V. The revival of fosfomycin. Int J Infect Dis. 2011;15(11):e732-9.
48. Zhanel GG, Cheung D, Adam H, et al. Review of eravacycline, a novel fluorocycline antibacterial agent. Drugs. 2016;76(5):567-88.
49. Solomkin J, Evans D, Slepavicius A, et al. Assessing the efficacy and safety of eravacycline vs ertapenem in complicated intra-abdominal infections in the investigating Gram-Negative Infections Treated with Eravacycline (IGNITE 1) trial a randomized clinical trial. JAMA Surg. 2017;152(3):224-32.
50. Hamzaoui O, Georger JF, Monnet X, et al. Early administration of norepinephrine increases cardiac preload and cardiac output in septic patients with life-threatening hypotension. Crit Care. 2010;14(4):R142.
51. Monnet X, Jabot J, Maizel J, et al. Norepinephrine increases cardiac preload and reduces preload dependency assessed by passive leg raising in septic shock patients. Crit Care Med. 2011;39(4):689-94.
52. Rhodes A, Evans LE, Alhazzani W, et al. Surviving Sepsis Campaign: International Guidelines for Management of Sepsis and Septic Shock: 2016. Intensive Care Med. 2017;43(3):304-77.
53. Myburgh JA, Higgins A, Jovanovska A, et al. A comparison of epinephrine and norepinephrine in critically ill patients. Intensive Care Med. 2008;34(12):2226-34.
54. Annane D, Vignon P, Renault A, et al. Norepinephrine plus dobutamine versus epinephrine alone for management of septic shock: A randomised trial. Lancet. 2007;370(9588):676-84.
55. Pandharipande PP, Pun BT, Herr DL, et al. Effect of sedation with dexmedetomidine vs lorazepam on acute brain dysfunction in mechanically ventilated patients the MENDS randomized controlled trial. JAMA. 2007;298(22):2644-53.
56. Shehabi Y, Grant P, Wolfenden H, et al. Prevalence of delirium with dexmedetomidine compared with morphine based therapy after cardiac surgery a randomized controlled trial (DEXmedetomidine COmpared to Morphine-DEXCOM Study). Anesthesiology. 2009;111:1075-84.
57. Djaiani GN, Rao V. Dexmedetomidine versus propofol sedation reduces delirium after cardiac surgery: A randomized controlled trial. Anesthesiology. 2016;124:362-8.

CHAPTER 25

HRCT Thorax

BALASAHEB PAWAR

QUESTIONS

1. A 48-year-old male, case of acute myeloid leukemia, admitted with fever. He has received induction chemotherapy. Laboratory investigation showed ANC of 126/mm³. Started on IV meropenem. Persisted to have fever after 7 days and also has cough, and pleuritic chest pain with mild hemoptysis. HRCT thorax was advised. HRCT image is shown below. Which of the following statements is not correct?

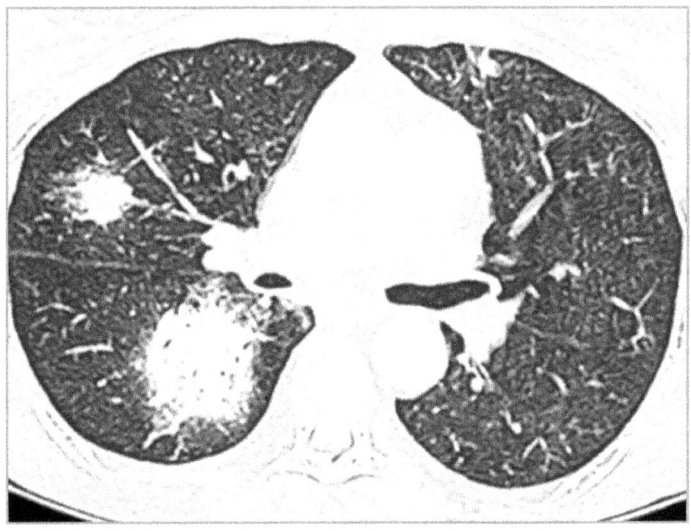

   a. The halo sign has been pathophysiologically characterized as a discrete nodule of angioinvasive aspergillosis with infarction and coagulative necrosis surrounded by alveolar hemorrhage
   b. Halo sign is seen in 100% of patient after 2 week of illness
   c. This sign is seen only in initial 10 days of angioinvasion after which it disappears
   d. Macronodules are the most common finding in invasive pulmonary aspergillosis

2. A 62-year-old female brought to emergency room (ER) with history of vehicular accident. On arrival to ER, she was tachypneic and had subcutaneous air over chest wall. After initial stabilization, computed tomography (CT) scan of chest was done. The CT scan image is shown. Which of the following statements is not true?

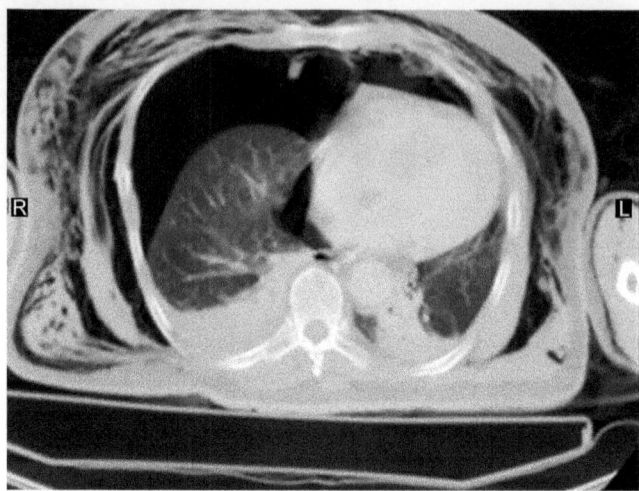

a. Trauma-related pneumothorax is most commonly caused by a disruption of closed airway spaces, such as the alveoli, due to a sudden increase in intrathoracic pressure or to a direct impact or deceleration force to the chest wall
b. Tracheobronchial injuries are always associated with pneumothorax
c. CT is more sensitive in detecting pneumothoraces as 78% of them are believed to be missed on chest radiograph (occult pneumothoraces)
d. Trauma-related pneumothorax occurs in 30–40% of cases of polytrauma

3. Mosaic attenuation is the presence of regions of differing attenuation appearing as black and white areas on HRCT. Following all are the causes of mosaic attenuation, *except*:

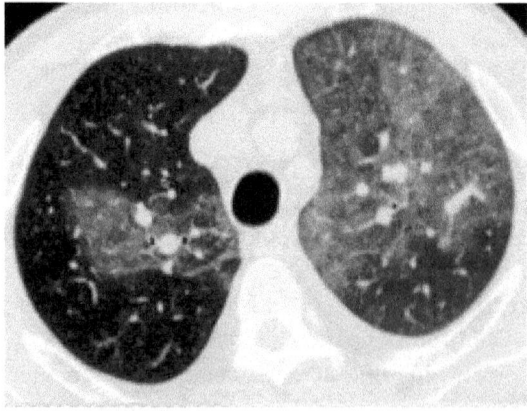

a. Bronchiolitis obliterans
b. Miliary tuberculosis
c. Chronic pulmonary embolism
d. Idiopathic pulmonary arterial hypertension

4. A 39-year-old female known case of SLE, on Wysolone 30 mg OD, is admitted with cough, fever, and breathlessness. She is tachypneic and SpO_2 on room air is 82%. After initial stabilization, high-resolution computed tomography (HRCT) chest was done. What is the most likely diagnosis?

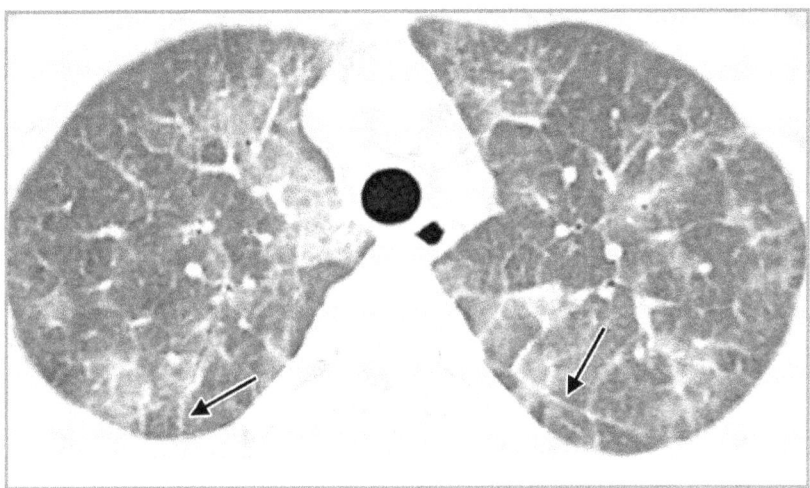

   a. Pulmonary edema
   b. *Pneumocystis jirovecii* pneumonia
   c. Pulmonary embolism
   d. Idiopathic pulmoanry fibrosis

5. A 62-year-old female shifted to intensive care unit (ICU) with acute onset of breathlessness. She was in wards, postoperative day 4. She underwent fracture fixation surgery for fracture neck femur. CTPA was advised to rule out pulmonary embolism. Which of the following statements is not true about CTPA?

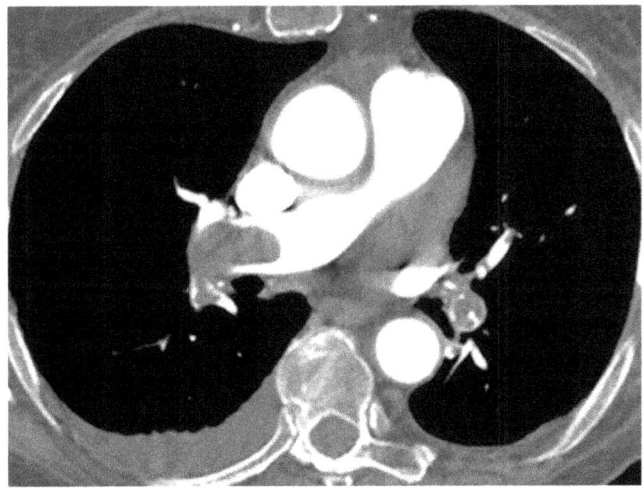

a. CT provides several parameters for estimating the severity of PE and risk-stratification, such as right heart strain, clot burden, and lung perfusion
b. Respiratory motion artifacts are the most common cause of an indeterminate CTPA and can be a cause of misdiagnosis of pulmonary embolism
c. CTPA has high sensitivity and specificity, with PIOPED II trial demonstrating sensitivity of 98% and specificity of 72%
d. Direct findings of acute PE in CT include a central filling defect within a vessel surrounded by contrast material yielding a "polo mint" appearance when orthogonal to the long axis of the vessel or a "railway sign" when observed parallel to the vessel long axis

6. A 63-year-old woman presented to ER with a nonproductive cough and shortness of breath, which she had experienced intermittently for 1 month. She had no fever, chills or night sweats. She had type 2 diabetes mellitus and hypertension. She is treated for carcinoma breast with surgery and chemotherapy 1 year back. Her routine workup and 2D echo is normal. HRCT thorax was done. HRCT image is shown below. Which statement of the following is not true?

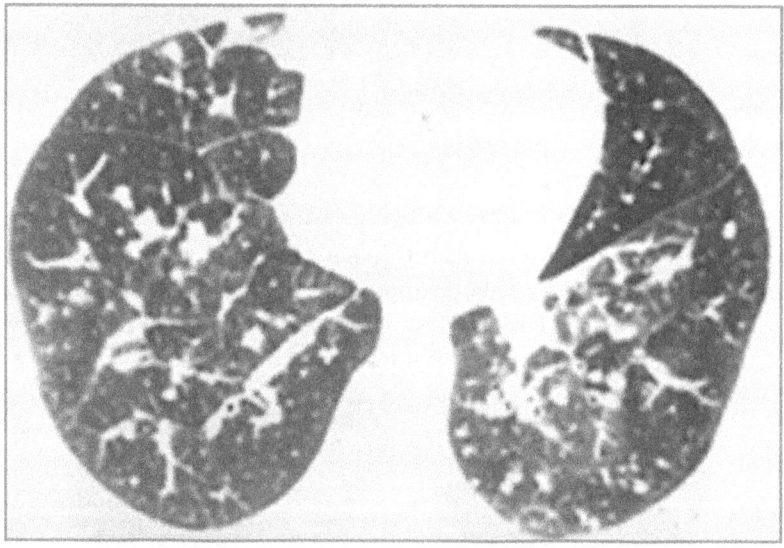

a. Computed tomographic (CT) findings of smooth or irregularly thickened interlobular septum ("nodular" appearance) are more characteristic of lymphangitic carcinomatosis than tumor embolism
b. Progressive unexplained dyspnea and hypoxemia in a patient with malignancy should raise the clinical suspicion for pulmonary tumor embolism or lymphangitic carcinomatosis
c. Follicular carcinoma of thyroid is the most common cause of lymphangitic carcinomatosis
d. Lung biopsy is the diagnostic test of choice for pulmonary tumor emboli and lymphangitic carcinomatosis

7. A 37-year-old male, known case of mesangial proliferative glomerulonephritis on Wysolone, admitted with on and off fever and cough for last 3 weeks and breathlessness. His HRCT was done, what is the diagnosis?

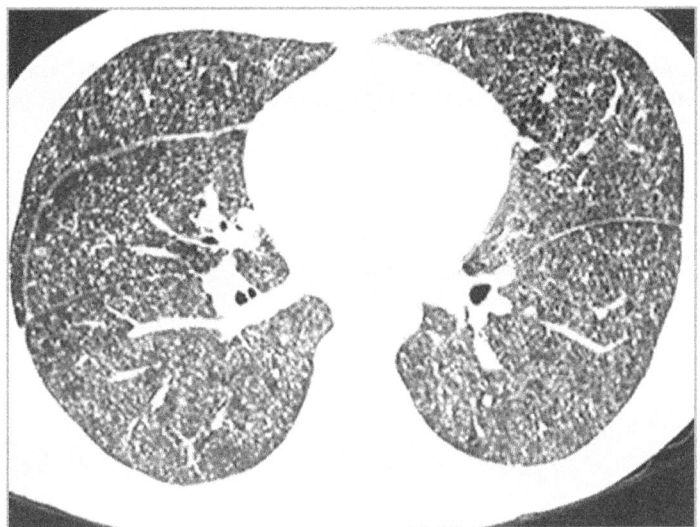

   a. Sarcoidosis
   b. Miliary tuberculosis
   c. Respiratory bronchiolitis
   d. Hypersensitivity pneumonitis

8. A patient, 62 years of age and known case of rheumatoid arthritis, on methotrexate, HCQ, admitted with cough and progressive worsening of breathlessness. HRCT image is shown below. Which of the following statements is not true about the management of this patient?

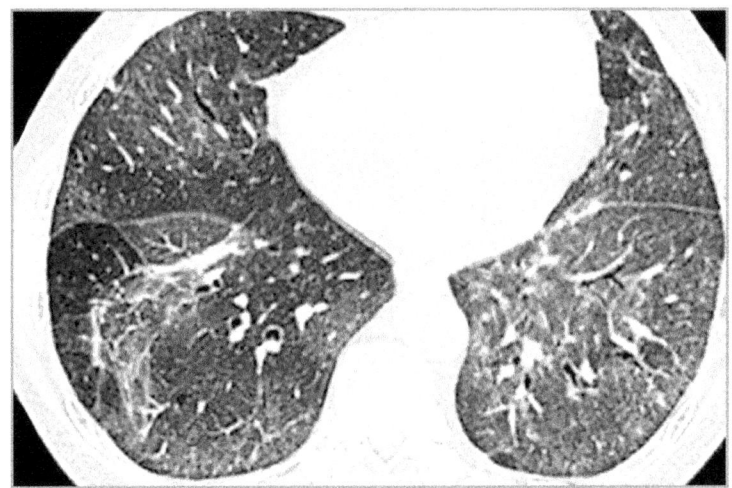

a. The predominant finding is ground-glass opacities
b. Bronchoalveolar lavage (BAL) is indicated to rule out infectious causes
c. Nonspecific interstitial pneumonia (NSIP) is very likely diagnosis by looking at HRCT
d. HRCT is classical usual interstitial pneumonia (UIP) and pulse methylprednisolone is treatment of choice

9. A 36-year-old man is admitted with cytomegalovirus pneumonia following renal transplantation. High-resolution CT image is shown below. What is the predominant HRCT pattern in this image?

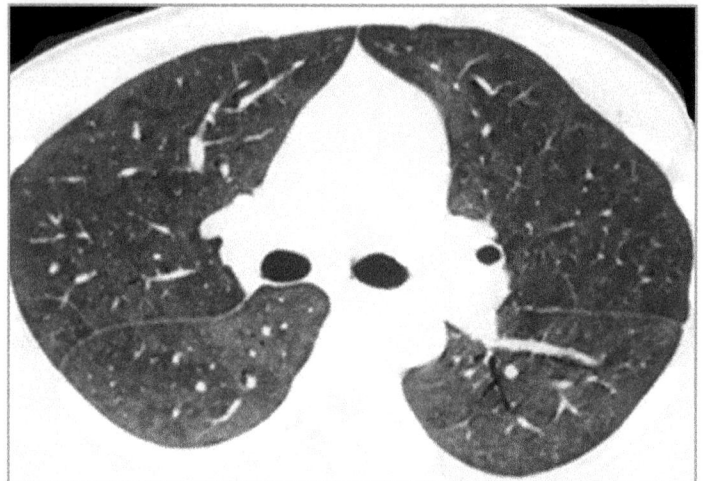

a. Tree in bud appearance
b. Consolidations
c. Honeycombing
d. Ground-glass opacities

ANSWERS

1. **Ans. (b)**

   Greene RE, Schlamm HT, Oestmann JW, et al. Imaging findings in acute invasive pulmonary aspergillosis: clinical significance of the halo sign. Clin Infect Dis. 2007;44(3):373-9.

   The halo sign represents pulmonary hemorrhage, coagulative necrosis surrounding the central necrotic nodule containing aspergillus hyphae.

   This sign is seen only in initial 10 days of angioinvasion after which it disappears.

   Other causes of halo sign: The halo sign has been reported in infections due to *Coccidioides immitis* and *Candida* species, *Nocardia* species, *Mycobacterium tuberculosis*, cytomegalovirus, and herpes simplex virus, and angioinvasive bacterial infections, such as those caused by *Pseudomonas aeruginosa*.

   Noninfectious causes of the halo sign include bronchioloalveolar cell carcinoma, lymphoproliferative disorders, metastatic angiosarcoma, Kaposi sarcoma, Wegener granulomatosis, eosinophilic lung disease, and organizing pneumonia (17–19).

   In one study, the sign was seen only in 61% of patients.

2. **Ans. (a)**

   Oikonomou A, Prassopoulos P. CT imaging of blunt chest trauma. Insights Imaging. 2011;2(3):281-95.

   Trauma-related pneumothorax occurs in 30–40% of cases, and it is most commonly associated with rib fractures that lacerate the lung. Less commonly, pneumothorax may be caused by a disruption of closed airway spaces, such as the alveoli, due to a sudden increase in intrathoracic pressure or to a direct impact or deceleration force to the chest wall. Tracheobronchial injuries are also always associated with pneumothorax. CT is more sensitive in detecting pneumothoraces, as 78% of them are nowadays believed to be missed on chest radiograph (occult pneumothoraces). Pneumothorax in supine polytrauma patients tends to accumulate at the anterior and medial aspect of the lung, rendering it difficult to recognize on a supine chest radiograph, although it might be visible on an upright chest radiograph.

3. **Ans. (b)**

   The term mosaic attenuation is used to describe density differences between affected and nonaffected lung areas.

   There are patchy areas of black and white lung.

   Mosaic attenuation can be produced due to one of the following reasons:
   1. Infiltrative process adjacent to normal lung
   2. Normal lung appearing relatively dense adjacent to lung with air trapping
   3. Hyperperfused lung adjacent to hypoperfused lung due to chronic thromboembolic disease

4. **Ans. (b)**

   Ground-glass opacity (GGO) is either due to filling of the alveolar spaces with pus, edema, hemorrhage, inflammation or tumor cells or thickening of the interstitium or alveolar walls below the spatial resolution of the HRCT as seen in fibrosis. So, ground-glass opacification may either be the result of air space disease (filling of the alveoli) or interstitial lung disease (i.e. fibrosis). Acutely GGOs can appear in acute pulmonary edema, acute respiratory distress syndrome (ARDS), alveolar hemorrhage, acute hypersensitivity pneumonitis, *pneumocystis jirovecii* pneumonia and other bacterial pneumonia.

Immunocompromised host-like HIV, patients on steroids presenting with hypoxic respiratory failure and having bilateral GGOs on HRCT, *p. jirovecii* pneumonia is most likely diagnosis.

5. **Ans. (b)**
The diagnostic criteria for acute pulmonary embolism include the following:
1. Arterial occlusion with failure to enhance the entire lumen due to a large filling defect; the artery may be enlarged compared with adjacent patent vessels.
2. A partial filling defect surrounded by contrast material, producing the "polo mint" sign on images acquired perpendicular to the long axis of a vessel and the "railway track" sign on longitudinal images of the vessel.
3. A peripheral intraluminal filling defect that forms acute angles with the arterial wall.

Patient should be able to tolerate a short breathhold in inspiration and follow breathing directions adequately to minimize motion artifact.

CT provides several parameters for estimating the severity of PE and risk stratification, such as right heart strain, clot burden, and lung perfusion. Features of right heart strain include—increased right ventricle (RV)/left ventricular (LV) ratio (>1 in axial plane, >0.9 in 4-chamber reconstruction), flattening of interventricular septum and reflux of contrast material into the IVC and hepatic veins. RV/LV ratio >1.1 has been associated with increased risk of death within 30 days.

The PIOPED II study, which used a composite gold standard, showed that CTPA has a sensitivity of 83% and specificity of 96% for the detection of pulmonary embolism and that combined CTPA and CT venography have a sensitivity of 90% and specificity of 95% for the detection of venous thromboembolic disease.

6. **Ans. (c)**
Lymphangitic carcinomatosis results from hematogenous spread to the lung, with subsequent invasion of interstitium and lymphatics.

The presenting symptoms are dyspnea and cough and can predate the radiographic abnormalities.

In many cases, however, the patients are asymptomatic.

Lymphangitic carcinomatosis is seen in carcinoma of the lung, breast, stomach, pancreas, prostate, cervix, thyroid, and metastatic adenocarcinoma from an unknown primary.

7. **Ans. (b)**
HRCT image shows predominant nodular pattern. The distribution of nodules shown on HRCT is the most important factor in making an accurate diagnosis in the nodular pattern. In most cases, small nodules can be placed into one of three categories: perilymphatic, centrilobular, or random distribution.

Perilymphatic distribution: In patients with a perilymphatic distribution, nodules are seen in relation to pleural surfaces, interlobular septa, and the peribronchovascular interstitium. Nodules are almost always visible in a subpleural location, particularly in relation to the fissures.

Perilymphatic nodules are most commonly seen in sarcoidosis. They also occur in silicosis, coal-worker's pneumoconiosis, and lymphangitic spread of carcinoma.

Centrilobular distribution: In certain diseases, nodules are limited to the centrilobular region.

Unlike perilymphatic and random nodules, centrilobular nodules spare the pleural surfaces. The most peripheral nodules are centered 5–10 mm from fissures or the pleural surface. Centrilobular nodules are seen in hypersensitivity pneumonitis, respiratory bronchiolitis in smokers, and infectious airways diseases (endobronchial spread of tuberculosis or nontuberculous mycobacteria, bronchopneumonia).

Random distribution: Nodules are randomly distributed relative to structures of the lung and secondary lobule. Nodules can usually be seen to involve the pleural surfaces and fissures, but lack of the subpleural predominance is often seen in patients with a perilymphatic distribution. These types of nodules are seen in hematogenous metastases, miliary tuberculosis, miliary fungal infections, and Langerhans cell histiocytosis (early nodular stage).

The HRCT image shows randomly distributed nodules, diagnostic of miliary tuberculosis.

8. **Ans. (d)**
Histopathological patterns of interstitial lung disease (ILD) associated with RA include the following:
- Nonspecific interstitial pneumonia
- Usual interstitial pneumonia, which is the pattern associated with idiopathic pulmonary fibrosis
- Organizing pneumonia
- Lymphocytic interstitial pneumonia
- Desquamative interstitial pneumonia
- Diffuse alveolar damage, the pathological correlation of acute interstitial pneumonia
- Drug-induced lung disease.

It is important to determine whether the patient is experiencing a first presentation of new interstitial disease, an exacerbation of previously unknown interstitial disease (usually UIP pattern), or one of these possibilities combined with a superimposed comorbid disease not directly due to RA. Investigations evaluating the various pulmonary manifestations of RA are designed to exclude the possibility that another lung disease or extra-pulmonary process is etiologic or coexistent, such as:
- Infection (especially in immunosuppressed host)
- Hypersensitivity pneumonitis due to inhalational agent
- A new or intercurrent ILD, such as acute interstitial pneumonitis or vasculitis, if symptoms are rapidly progressive
- Heart failure, pulmonary embolism, cancer, or recurrent gastroesophageal aspiration.

9. **Ans. (d)**
Miller WT, Shah RM. Isolated Diffuse Ground-Glass Opacity in Thoracic CT: Causes and Clinical Presentations. Am J Roentgenol. 2005;184:613-22.

Ground-glass opacity (GGO) is defined as increased attenuation of the lung parenchyma without obscuration of the pulmonary vascular markings on CT images. GGO may be the result of a wide variety of interstitial and alveolar diseases and frequently represents a nonspecific finding. GGOs often will be present in the company of other interstitial or alveolar findings on CT. As an alveolar finding, GGO represents partially filled alveoli and often is found at the margins of the consolidated lung. With interstitial diseases, it has been associated with active inflammation in some cases. In other situations, GGO adjacent to interstitial abnormalities represents fine fibrosis, below the resolution of CT images.

Many patients with *Cytomegalovirus* (CMV) viremia will have normal imaging studies. However, in those with imaging findings, CMV pneumonia usually will appear as diffused GGO on CT scans. In some cases, small (<5 mm) nodules may be detected and in more severe cases, diffuse consolidation may be present.

CHAPTER 26

Chest X-Ray

SUBHAL DIXIT, KHALID ISMAIL KHATIB

QUESTIONS

1. A 65-year-old, male patient, with past history of transanterior myocardial infarction, presents with severe dyspnea, SpO$_2$ of 80%, and bilateral extensive crepitations over lungs. 2D Echo reveals LVEF of 30%. His CXR will not reveal:
   a. Kerley B lines
   b. Increased vascularity of upper lobes (inverted moustache sign)
   c. Oligemia of the lung fields
   d. None of the above

2. In a normal CXR, the left border of the heart is made up of the following structures, from top to bottom:
   a. Arch of aorta/aortic knuckle, pulmonary trunk, left atrium, left ventricle
   b. Left atrium, left ventricle, arch of aorta/aortic knuckle, pulmonary trunk
   c. Left ventricle, arch of aorta/aortic knuckle, pulmonary trunk, left atrium
   d. Pulmonary trunk, left atrium, superior vena cava

3. In a normal CXR, the right border of the heart is made up of the following structures, from top to bottom
   a. Superior vena cava, right atrium, inferior vena cava
   b. Right atrium, superior vena cava, inferior vena cava
   c. Superior vena cava, inferior vena cava, right atrium
   d. Arch of aorta, superior vena cava, inferior vena cava, right atrium

4. The heart shadow is magnified in the:
   a. PA view as compared to the AP view
   b. AP view as compared to the PA view
   c. PA view as compared to the lateral view
   d. AP view as compared to the lateral view

5. A 35-year-old male patient, presented with shortness of breath increasing over the last 15 days and mild fever on and off for these 15 days. Respiratory system examination revealed stony dull note on right side with absent breath sounds. CXR revealed right-sided pleural effusion. Thoracic paracentesis was done. 15 minutes after the paracentesis, patient started complaining of chest pain (on right side of the chest) and increased breathlessness. CXR taken is shown in Figure 1.

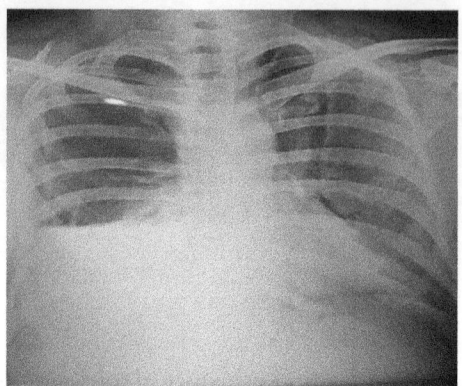

Figure 1: Chest X-ray of the patient described in Question 5.

What is the next step?
a. High flow O_2 and observe
b. Repeat thoracic paracentesis
c. Decortication of the lung
d. Intercostal drain insertion on the right side

6. A 60-year-male, presented with shortness of breath and palpitations since 3–4 days. He gives history of similar complaints on and off for the last several years. On examination, he has irregularly irregular pulse and a diastolic murmur at the apex. His CXR AP view is shown in Figure 2. What is the diagnosis?

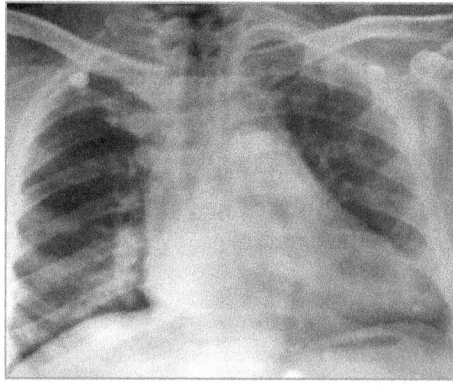

Figure 2: Chest X-ray of the patient described in Question 6.

a. Aortic regurgitation
b. Aortic stenosis
c. Tricuspid stenosis
d. Mitral stenosis

7. A 48-year-old male presented with history of low-grade fever and cough for 3 weeks and dyspnea on exertion since 5 days. His CXR is shown in Figure 3. Describe the relation of the pulmonary shadow to the heart:

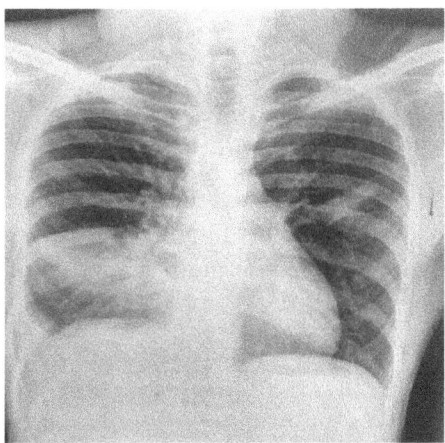

Figure 3: Chest X-ray of the patient described in Question 7.

   a. Pulmonary shadow is anterior to the heart
   b. Pulmonary shadow is posterior to the heart
   c. Pulmonary shadow is adjacent to the heart
   d. None of the above

8. A 58-year-old male presented with acute onset (2–3 days) of high-grade fever, cough, dyspnea, and chest pain. Cough was productive and sputum was "currant jelly" in color. He had leukocytosis and his CXR showed "Bulging Fissure" sign. Name the organism most likely to be isolated on sputum culture?
   a. *Mycobacterium tuberculosis*
   b. Non-tuberculous mycobacteria
   c. *Haemophilus influenzae*
   d. *Klebsiella pneumoniae*

9. A 32-year-old male patient, presents with history of fever, cough and breathlessness for the past 10 days. His CXR is as shown in Figure 4. The differential diagnosis includes

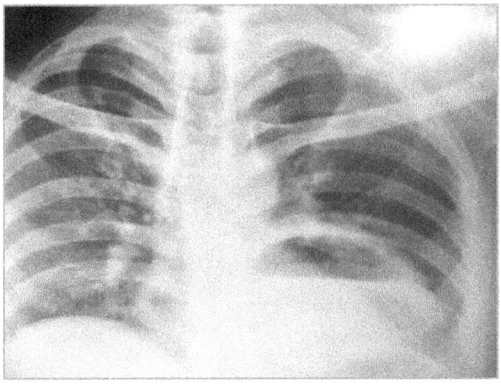

Figure 4: Chest X-ray of the patient described in Question 9.

a. Aspergillosis/Aspergilloma
b. Lung abscess
c. Pulmonary tuberculosis
d. Bronchogenic carcinoma
e. All of the above

10. A 70-year-old male, presented to the emergency department with complaints of cough and increasing dyspnea for last 1 month. The CXR shows a right-sided opaque hemithorax (OH) (Figure 5). The differential diagnoses of OH with mediastinal shift on the affected side are:

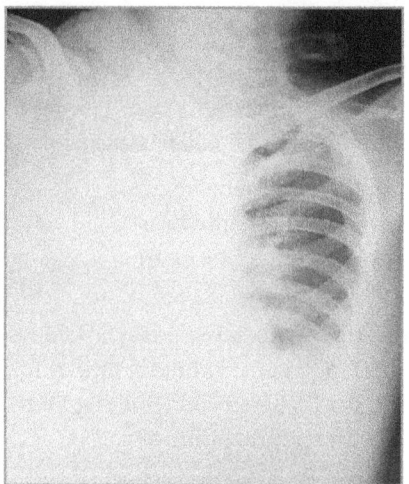

Figure 5: CXR shows a right-sided opaque hemithorax

a. Pulmonary agenesis
b. Pneumonectomy
c. Atelectasis due to foreign body/endobronchial tumor
d. Pneumonia

Answers

1. **Ans. (d)**

   Sethi S. Review of Radiology, 5th edition. New Delhi: Peepee Publishers and Distributors; 2014. pp. 32-3.

   Thomason JW, Ely EW, Chiles C, et al. Appraising pulmonary edema using supine chest roentgenograms in ventilated patients. Am J Respirat Crit Care Med. 1998;157 (5 Pt 1):1600-8.

   Milne EN, Pistolesi M, Miniati M, et al. The radiologic distinction of cardiogenic and noncardiogenic edema. Am J Roentgenol 1985;144(5):879-94.

   In patients with left ventricular failure/pulmonary edema, the radiology findings will depend on the level of elevation of pulmonary capillary wedge pressure (PCWP). With a marginal elevation of the PCWP (9-12 mm Hg), the chest X-ray (CXR) picture will be normal. In the early stage of LVF/Pulmonary edema (PCWP= 12-19 mm Hg), dilated upper lobe pulmonary veins will be evident on the CXR (cephalization of pulmonary vasculature or inverted moustache sign or stag antler's sign). When the PCWP rises further (20-24 mm Hg), interstitial edema manifests as Kerley B lines in the CXR. In florid pulmonary edema (PCWP >25 mm Hg), the CXR will reveal the typical "Batwing appearance" due to alveolar edema manifesting as perihilar fluffy opacities (*see* Figure 6).

   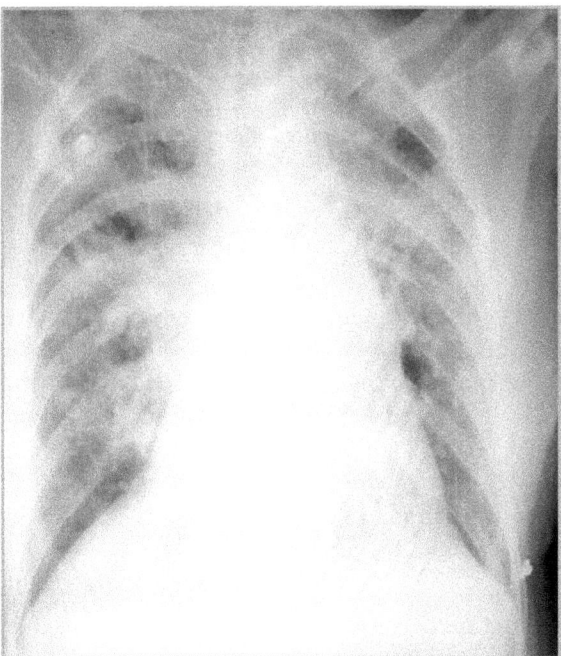

   Figure 6: CXR showing Batwing appearance.

2. **Ans. (a)**

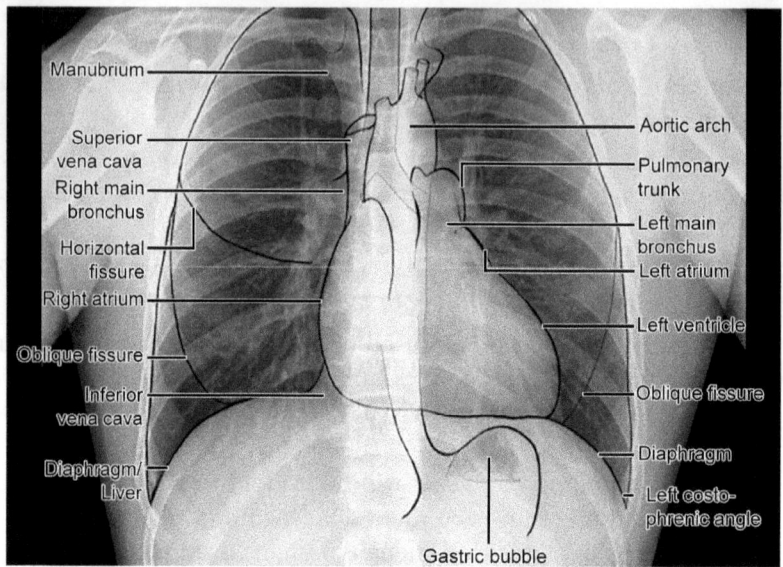

Figure 7: Normal CXR showing left and right borders of the heart with different structures.

The top of the left border of the heart is made up by the aortic arch, below which is the pulmonary trunk. The pulmonary trunk arches over the left atrium. The lower part of the left border of the heart is made up entirely of the left ventricle (*see* Figure 7).

3. **Ans. (a)**

The top of the right border of the heart is made up by the superior vena cava (SVC). Below the SVC is the right atrium which is followed by the Inferior vena cava making up the rest of the right border of the heart (*see* Figure 7).

4. **Ans. (b)**

https://www.med-ed.virginia.edu/courses/rad/cxr/technique3chest.html. [Last Accessed March 2019].

When taking the PA view, the patient stands facing the X-ray film cassette, while the X-ray tube is at a distance of 72 inches (6 feet). Due to the distance there is less divergence of the X-ray beam and hence there is lesser magnification of the structures closer to the X-ray tube. In an AP view (usually taken with the patient in supine position), the patient faces the X-ray tube, which is about 4 feet away. This leads to magnification of the anterior structures (heart). Therefore, one must not comment on cardiomegaly on AP view. The appearance of the pulmonary vasculature is also different as the effect of gravity is eliminated, as the patient is in supine position.

5. **Ans. (d)**

Awad N, Kasargod V. Clinical profile, etiology, and management of hydropneumothorax: an Indian experience. Lung India. 2016;33:278.

The CXR reveals a hydropneumothorax with collapse of the underlying lung. Treatment of hydropneumothorax is placement of intercostals drain (ICD) and connecting it to underwater seal. The ICD may be required for longer duration.

6. **Ans. (d)**
   Chadha S, Shetty V, Sadiq A, et al. Left heart border straightening in severe mitral stenosis. QJM. 2013;106(8):775-6.

   Thibault GE. Studying the classics. N Engl J Med. 1995;333(10):648-52.

   The structural changes due to long-standing mitral stenosis are due to pulmonary hypertension. There is increase in the size of the left atrium and also the left atrial appendage, and this affects the structures surrounding it (tracheal bifurcation).

   The CXR shows straightening of the left cardiac border (due to enlargement of left atrial appendage) with double density shadow of the left atrium with obtuse angle of the carina (due to elevation of left main bronchus). These are all indicative of long standing mitral stenosis. The acute worsening of the patient seems to be due to the onset of atrial fibrillation.

7. **Ans (b)**
   Longuet R, Phelan J, Tanous H, et al. Criteria of the silhouette sign. Radiology. 1977;122:581-5.

   ScienceDirect. Silhouette Sign. [online] Available from https://www.sciencedirect.com/topics/medicine-and-dentistry/silhouette-sign. [Last Accessed May, 2019].

   The pulmonary lesion is posterior to the heart as the right border of the heart is seen separated from the lesion by a thin rim of air in the lungs (denoted by two arrows in the Figure 8). This is confirmed by taking a lateral view which shows a loculated pleural effusion posterior to the mediastinum, including the heart (black arrow in Figure 9). This CXR demonstrates the principle behind the "Silhouette sign". If there is a radiopaque mass in the thorax which is in contact with the cardiac border, there will be a loss of the cardiac silhouette, i.e. the cardiac border will not be seen separate from the opacity. Whenever this mass is posterior to the heart, the cardiac border will be seen distinctly. The silhouette sign was popularized by the Felson brothers.

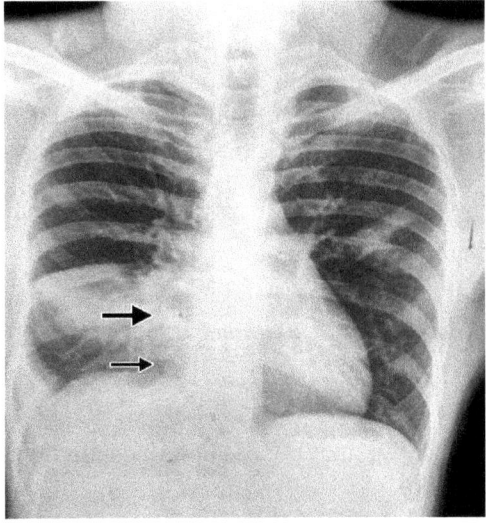

Figure 8: Chest X-ray showing the pulmonary lesion and heart is separated from the lesion by a thin rim of air in the lungs (denoted by two arrows).

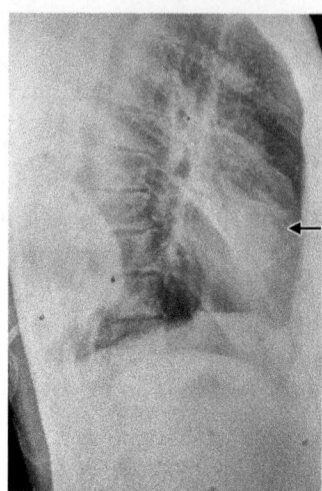

Figure 9: Chest X-ray showing silhouette sign.

8. **Ans. (d)**

   Ko WC, Paterson DL, Sagnimeni AJ, et al. Community-acquired Klebsiella pneumoniae bacteremia: global differences in clinical patterns. Emerg Infect Dis. 2002;8(2):160.

   Mandell LA, Wunderink RG, Anzueto A, et al. Infectious Diseases Society of America/American Thoracic Society consensus guidelines on the management of community-acquired pneumonia in adults. Clin Infect Dis. 2007;44(Suppl 2):S27.

   The genus Klebsiella consists of *K. pneumoniae*, *K. oxytoca* and *K. granulomatis*. These organisms belong to the family of *Enterobacteriaceae*. *K. pneumoniae* can cause many infections in humans (community- or hospital-acquired) including pneumonias, urinary tract infections, and bacteremia. Community-acquired pneumonia caused by *K. pneumoniae* is the typical lobar pneumonia with a predilection for the upper lobe and production of the typical currant-jelly sputum (thick, mucoid and hemorrhagic) due to inflammation, hemorrhage, and necrosis of the lung parenchyma. It is usually seen in patients with associated comorbid conditions (alcoholism, diabetes mellitus, and chronic lung diseases). The CXR in a patient may demonstrate the bulging fissure sign due to the large amount of inflammation and necrosis. There may be presence of complications such as pleural effusions and empyema.

9. **Ans. (e)**

   Abramson S. "The air crescent sign," Radiology. 2001;218(1):230-2.

   Fred HL, Gardiner CL. The air crescent sign: causes and characteristics. Tex Heart Inst J. 2009;36(3):264-5.

   A cavity filled with fluid and air may be seen in various conditions including aspergilloma, angioinvasive aspergillosis, a cavity caused by pulmonary tuberculosis, bronchial carcinoma which has necrosis in the center, etc. The CXR appearance is sometimes called the "air crescent sign".

10. **Ans. (d)**

Marchiori E, Hochhegger B, Zanetti G. Opaque hemithorax. J Bras Pneumol. 2017;43(3):161.

Vaidya VN, Vohra PA, Ghugare BW. Opaque hemithorax: Clinical, histological and radiological assessment of 30 cases at a tertiary care hospital: a preliminary study. West Afr J Radiol. 2017;24:34-7.

The causes of opaque hemithorax (OH) are classified according to volume of the affected hemithorax which determines the position of the mediastinum. This is best indicated by the position of the trachea. The various causes of OH are given in Table 1.

S. No.	Volume of the affected hemithorax	Position of the mediastinum	Tracheal position	Causes
1.	Increased	Toward unaffected side	Pushed toward unaffected side	a. Large pleural effusions, b. Large thoracic masses
2.	Unchanged or Normal	Normal	Central	a. Pneumonia affecting the entire lung parenchyma (usually seen in children) b. Carcinoma of the bronchus, accompanied by pleural effusion and atelectasis (usually seen in adults)
3.	Decreased/Reduced	Toward affected side	Pulled toward affected side	a. Pulmonary agenesis b. Pneumonectomy c. Atelectasis due to bronchial obstruction by a foreign body or an endobronchial tumor

Table 1: Causes of opaque hemithorax.

CHAPTER 27

Arterial Blood Gases

SUSHMA K GURAV

QUESTIONS

1. Carbonic anhydrase is present at all places *except:*
   a. Plasma
   b. Renal tubular cells
   c. Red blood cells
   d. Lung parenchyma

2. Choose the incorrect statement about anion gap out of the followings:
   a. In lactic acidosis, anion gap is increased
   b. Anion gap is decreased in hypercalcemia
   c. Anion gap is increased in lithium toxicity
   d. Anion gap is decreased in ketoacidosis

3. A 54-year-old female presents to emergency department with history of nausea and recurrent vomiting since 3 days. She gives history of consumption of several aspirin tablets for joint pain, ABG: pH: –7.56, pCO_2: 32, HCO_3: 33 mEq/L. Interpret the findings.
   a. Valid ABG, metabolic alkalosis with respiratory alkalosis
   b. Invalid ABG, respiratory alkalosis, metabolic acidosis
   c. Valid ABG, metabolic acidosis, metabolic acidosis

4. A person was admitted in a coma. Analysis of the arterial blood gave the following values: PCO_2 16 mm Hg, HCO_3^- 5 mmol/L and pH 7.1. What is the underlying acid-base disorder?
   a. Metabolic acidosis
   b. Metabolic alkalosis
   c. Respiratory acidosis
   d. Respiratory alkalosis

5. A young woman brought to emergency room. She was found comatose, sleeping pill bottle was found near her. Relatives do not have information of number pills consumed and timing of consumption of pills. An arterial blood sample yields the following values: pH –6.90, HCO_3^- 13 mEq/L, $PaCO_2$ 68 mm Hg. This patient's acid-base status is most accurately described as:
   a. Uncompensated metabolic acidosis
   b. Uncompensated respiratory acidosis
   c. Simultaneous respiratory and metabolic acidosis
   d. Respiratory acidosis with partial renal compensation

6. A 42-year-old man was brought to ER after he was found lying in an alley with an empty liquor bottle nearby O/E blood pressure: 120/80, pulse: 110, RR: 28, temperature: 37° F. He was unresponsive, pupils reacting to light, Labs
   pH: 7.1; pCO_2: 36 mm Hg; pO_2 90 mm Hg;
   Na–145 mEq/L/K–4.5 mEq/L/CL –97/BUN-23/Creatinine 1.3 mg/dL
   BSL 110 mg, Lactates: 1 mmol; ketones negative; salicylates; negative;
   a. Primary disorder : Metabolic acidosis
   b. Primary disorder : Respiratory acidosis
   c. Mixed respiratory alkalosis and metabolic acidosis
   d. Primary disorder : Metabolic alkalosis

7. In same case, respiratory acidosis has occurred as a result of compensation. What is the anion gap and what is Δgap and final acid-base diagnosis?
   a. Anion gap: 30 Δgap: 10 (Metabolic acidosis, respiratory alkalosis, metabolic alkalosis)
   b. Anion gap: 39 Δgap: 9 (Metabolic acidosis, respiratory acidosis, metabolic alkalosis)
   c. Anion gap: 38 Δgap: 12 (High anion gap, metabolic acidosis, respiratory acidosis, metabolic alkalosis)
   d. Anion gap: 12 Δgap: 0 (Metabolic acidosis, respiratory alkalosis)

8. A 26-year-old, engineering student, was rushed to the hospital due to vomiting and a decreased level of consciousness. On examination, the patient had slow, and he is lethargic and irritable in response to stimulation. He appears to be dehydrated—his eyes are sunken and mucous membranes are dry. He has a two weeks history of polydipsia, polyuria, and weight loss. Measurement of arterial blood gas shows pH 7.0, PaO_2 90 mm Hg, $PaCO_2$ 23 mm Hg, and HCO_3 12 mmol/L; other results are Na^+ 126 mmol/L, K^+ 5 mmol/L, and Cl^- 95 mmol/L. What is your assessment?
   a. Respiratory acidosis uncompensated
   b. Respiratory acidosis partially compensated
   c. Metabolic alkalosis uncompensated
   d. Metabolic alkalosis partially compensated

9. A cigarette vendor was brought to the emergency department of a hospital after she fell into the ground and hurt her left leg. O/E: She is tachycardic and tachypneic. Pain killers were carried out to lessen her pain. Suddenly, she started complaining that she is still in pain and now experiencing muscle cramps, tingling, and paraesthesia. Measurement of arterial blood gas reveals pH 7.6, PaO_2 120 mm Hg, $PaCO_2$ 31 mm Hg, and HCO_3 25 mmol/L. What does this mean?
   a. Respiratory alkalosis uncompensated
   b. Respiratory acidosis partially compensated
   c. Metabolic alkalosis uncompensated
   d. Metabolic alkalosis partially compensated

10. A 72-year-old male with COPD presents with breathlessness and fever
    pH: 7.25; pCO_2: 80; HCO_3: 34; pO_2: 39; SaO_2: 54%
    Pulse 130/min; blood pressure 130/110 mm Hg; temperature 38.6°C; respiratory rate 32/min, TLC 18000' sodium 140 mEq/L; HCO_3^- 36; Cl^- 89; K 4.1 mEq/L

a. Acute respiratory acidosis
b. Acute respiratory acidosis and metabolic alkalosis
c. Chronic respiratory acidosis and metabolic acidosis
d. Chronic respiratory acidosis and metabolic alkalosis

11. A 32-year-old male was admitted with history diarrhea since two days investigations. Sodium 134 mEq/L, potassium 2.9 mEq/L, Cl^- 108, pH 7.31; pCO_2 33; HCO_3 16; pO_2 93 mm Hg. What is the acid-base disorder?
    a. High anion gap metabolic acidosis
    b. Metabolic alkalosis and respiratory acidosis
    c. Metabolic alkalosis and respiratory alkalosis
    d. Normal anion gap acidosis

ANSWERS

1. **Ans. (a)**
   Erythrocytes, skeletal muscles, renal tubules, gastric mucosa, pancreatic cells.
   Carbonic anhydrase accelerates the hydration/dehydration reaction between CO_2, HCO_3^- and H^+.

2. **Ans. (d)**
   Raised anion gap can result from either a decrease in unmeasured cations or an increase in unmeasured anions. In practice, it is almost exclusively the result of increased unmeasured anions derived from metabolic acids. Metabolic acidosis is thus the most common cause of raised anion gap.

   In metabolic acidosis, there is reduction in serum bicarbonate (HCO_3^-) concentration. To maintain electrochemical neutrality this reduction in measured anion (bicarbonate) is accompanied by either an increase in serum chloride (Cl^-), the only other measured anion, or much more commonly, an increase in unmeasured anions.

   In the first case, because the reduction in measured bicarbonate is matched by the increase in measured chloride, the anion gap remains unchanged and normal; this type of metabolic acidosis is called normal anion gap (hyperchloremic) metabolic acidosis. In the second case, because there is an increase in unmeasured anions, the metabolic acidosis is termed increased anion gap metabolic acidosis.

   Lactic acidosis is associated with increase in the anion gap. Accumulation of lactic acid reduction in the concentration of bicarbonate resulting from buffering protons of lactic acid is matched by an increase in the concentration of the "unmeasured" anion lactate.

   Lithium is a cation, it can lower the serum anion gap when present in sufficient concentration.

   Marked increments in the level of cations that normally are present in serum but not used to calculate the serum anion gap, such as calcium and magnesium, theoretically can lower the serum anion gap. In patients with hypercalcemia as a result of primary hyperparathyroidism, the serum anion gap was reduced by approximately 2.4 mEq/L.

   In diabetic ketoacidosis (DKA), the increased anion gap is due to increased serum concentration of the "unmeasured" anions, β-hydroxy butyrate and acetoacetate.

3. **Ans. (a)**
   Step 1: Validity: $24 \times 32/33 = 24$,
   Step 2: pH is 7.5, so alkalosis
   Step 3: pH and HCO_3 in same direction-metabolic alkalosis
   Step 4: Expected $CO_2 = 7 \times 33 + 21 \pm 2 = 44 \pm 2$, but CO_2 is 32. Thus, associated respiratory alkalosis.

4. **Ans. (a)**
   To follow the steps of solving ABG.

5. **Ans. (c)**

6. **Ans. (a)**
   Step 1: $H^+ = 2 \times 3/12 = 70$ ABG valid

Step 2: pH is 7.1, so it is academia
Step 3: pH and HCO_3 both are in same direction, so the primary disorder is metabolic acidosis.

7. **Ans. (c)**
   Respiratory compensation: $pCO_2 = 1.5 \times 12 = 8 \pm 2 = 26 \pm 2$
   Actual pCO_2 is 36, so is associated respiratory acidosis.
   $AG = 145 - (12 + 97) = 36$
   High anion gap metabolic acidosis,
   Δgap = Ag excess-HCO_3 deficit (24–12 = 12), so associated metabolic alkalosis

8. **Ans. (d)**
   The student was diagnosed having diabetes mellitus. The results show that he has metabolic acidosis (low HCO_3^-) with respiratory compensation (low CO_2).

9. **Ans. (a)**
   The primary disorder is acute respiratory alkalosis (low CO_2) due to the pain and anxiety causing her to hyperventilate. There has not been time for metabolic compensation.

10. **Ans. (c)**
    Step 1: $H^+ = 2 \times 80/34 = 56.5$ (valid)
    Step 2: Acidosis
    Step 3: Respiratory acidosis, as pH and pCO_2 in opposite direction
    Step 4: Acute or chronic (remember 1, 3, 2, starting with respiratory acidosis)
    Chronic respiratory acidosis with metabolic acidosis.

11. **Ans. (d)**
    Step 1: Valid ($H^+ = 2 \times 33/16 = 49$)
    Step 2: Acidosis
    Step 3: pH and pCO_2 in same direction—metabolic
    Step 4: $AG = 134 - (108 + 16) = 10$ nonanion gap
    Table 1 for validity of ABG (reference: **Interpretation of Arterial Blood Gases (ABGs) David A Kaufman**)

pH	Approximate [H⁺] mmol/L
7.00	100
7.05	89
7.10	79
7.15	71
7.20	63
7.25	56
7.30	50
7.35	45
7.40	40
7.45	35
7.50	32
7.55	28
7.60	25
7.65	22

CHAPTER 28

USG and ECHO

SHRIKANT SRINIVASAN

QUESTIONS

1. The following electrocardiogram (ECG) was recorded in a 25-year-old patient in intensive care unit (ICU) who was alert and conscious with a blood pressure of 100/50 mm Hg.

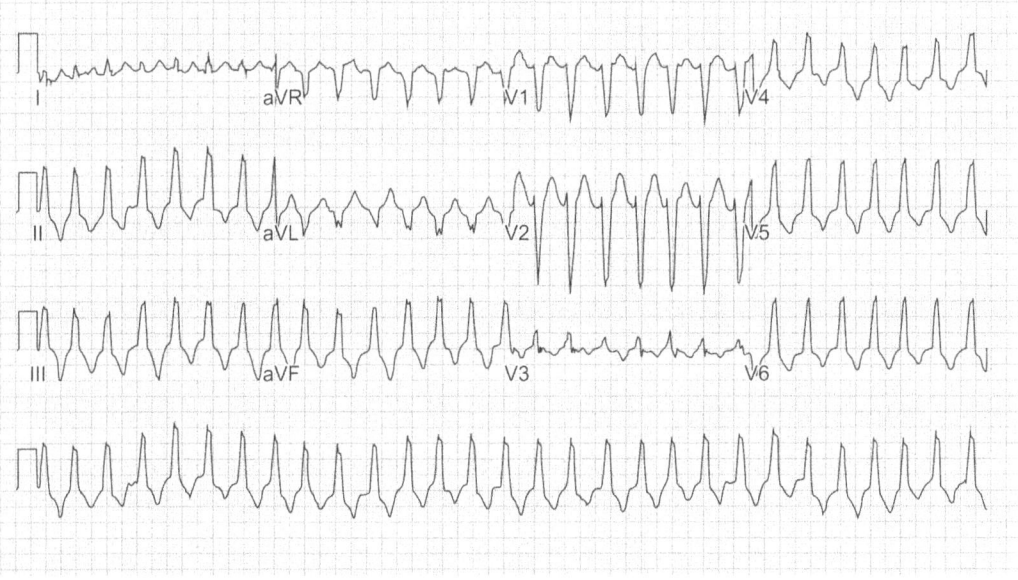

All of the following are features of ventricular tachycardia (VT), *except*:
a. Presence of capture or fusion beats
b. Positive or negative concordance throughout precordial leads
c. R-S interval distance <100 ms
d. Broad QRS complexes

2. A 47-year-old female patient was admitted to the intensive care unit with presumed urosepsis on noradrenaline support (15 µg/min). The lady had received resuscitation with 1 liter of fluid on arrival in the emergency department. The junior resident wanted to decide, if the patient would require further fluids, and proceeded to perform a passive leg raise (PLR) maneuver. Pre-PLR VTI was 21.6 cm, which increased to 26.5 cm after PLR. As the senior registrar in charge of the ICU, you would interpret the results as the need for treating the patient with:

a. Give more crystalloids
b. Restrict fluids, increase noradrenaline dose
c. Add dobutamine
d. Give starch-based fluids

3. The ECG shown below is of a 76-year-old male presenting with acute appendicitis requiring surgery. He is hemodynamically stable. Kindly comment on the ECG diagnosis.

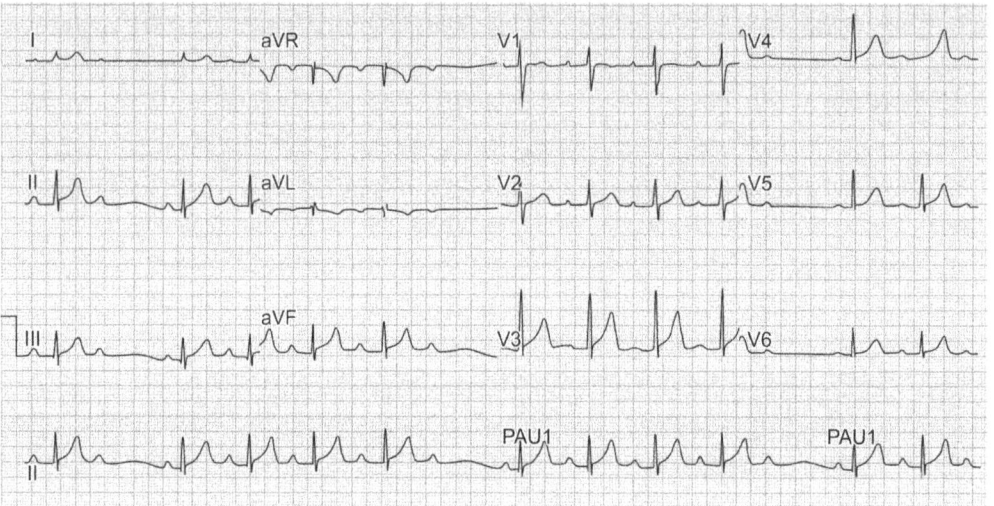

a. 1st degree heart block
b. Mobitz type 1
c. Mobitz type 2
d. 3rd degree heart block

4. The following ECG was recorded in a 40-year-old female admitted with severe trauma.

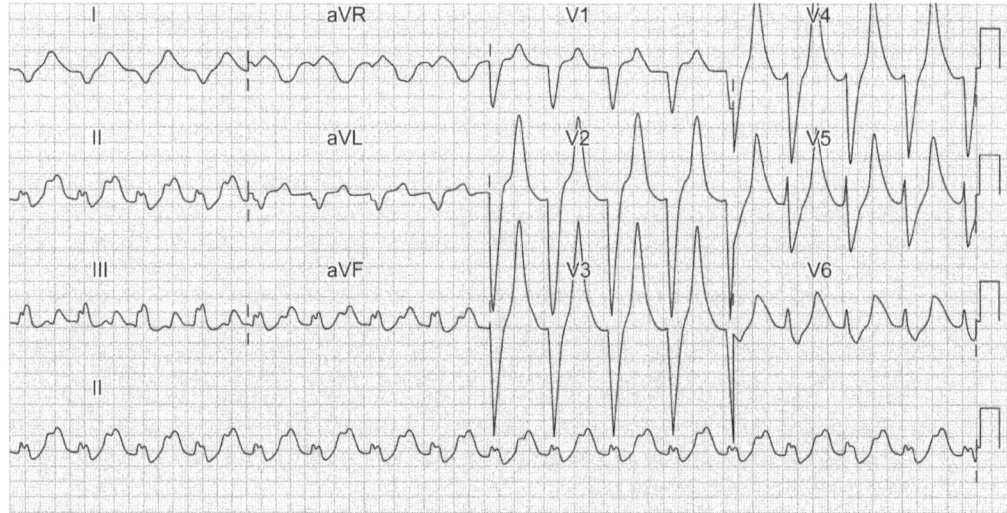

What is the possible underlying metabolic abnormality in this patient?
a. Hyperkalemia
b. Hypercalcemia
c. Hypomagnesemia
d. Hypermagnesemia

5. The following ECG was obtained from a 58-year-old patient who presented with chest pain of 3-hour duration in the emergency department.

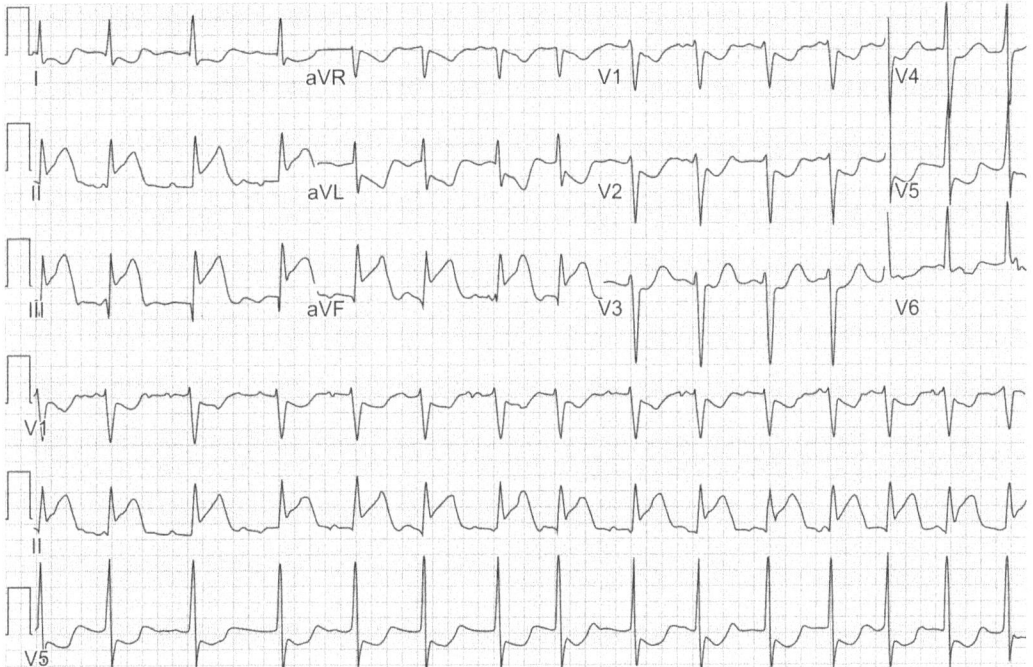

The ECG suggests possibility of:
a. Anterior wall of LV
b. Inferior wall infarction
c. Lateral wall infarction
d. Pericardial effusion

6. McConnell's sign in echocardiography is a characteristic feature classically described in patients with:
a. Cardiac tamponade
b. Severe hypovolemia
c. Pulmonary embolism
d. Infective endocarditis

7. The characteristic 2D ECHO finding of McConnell's sign is:
a. Global hypokinesia of LV
b. Hypokinesia and dilatation of right ventricle

c. Hypokinesia of LV apex and good contraction of LV base
d. Hypokinesia of RV-free wall with good contraction at RV apex

8. Diastolic collapse of the right ventricle is classically seen in patients with:
   a. Cardiac tamponade
   b. Right ventricular infarction
   c. Left ventricle free wall rupture
   d. Hypovolemic shock

9. A 51-year-old male patient is admitted to the ICU with a presumptive diagnosis of H1N1 infection leading to ARDS and is being ventilated following low tidal volume protocol (PaO_2: 60 mm Hg, $PaCO_2$: 62 mm Hg on PRVC mode, FiO_2: 70%, tidal volume: 280 mL, and respiratory rate: 28 breaths/min).
   The consultant in charge asks you to assess the function of the right heart.
   Which of the following parameters is used to assess the function of the right heart in echocardiography?
   a. E/A ratio
   b. TAPSE
   c. e/e' ratio
   d. S/D ratio

10. An 80-year-old male, known case of chronic obstructive pulmonary disease, is admitted to the ICU with community-acquired pneumonia and suddenly develops a tachycardia. Her 12-lead ECG is shown below:

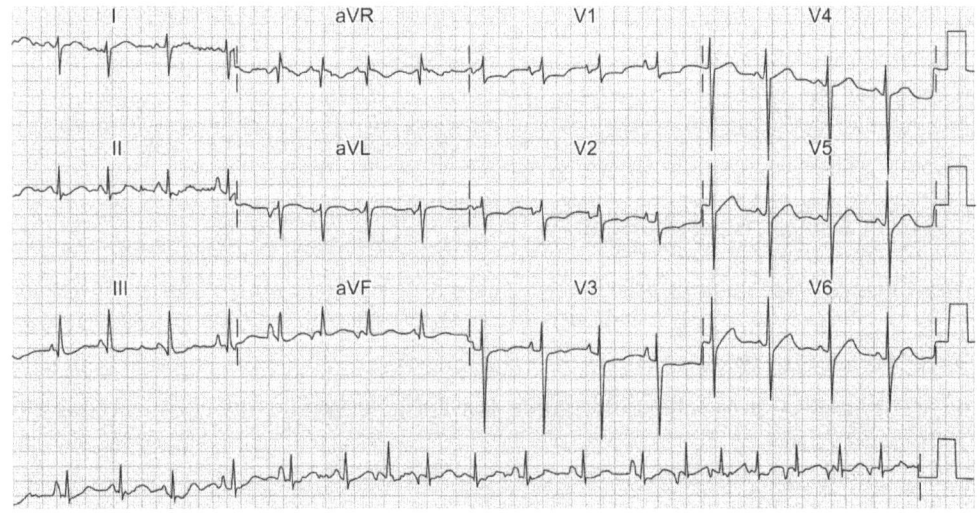

What is the likeliest diagnosis based on the ECG:
a. Atrial fibrillation
b. Atrial flutter
c. Junctional tachycardia
d. Multifocal atrial tachycardia

11. All of the following features support a diagnosis of pericarditis in ECG, *except*:
    a. PR segment depression
    b. Reciprocal ST changes
    c. Concave ST segment elevation
    d. Notching of J point

12. A 37-year-old female patient presents to the hospital with suicidal ingestion of paracetamol leading to acute liver failure. Initial CT done on D1 shows normal gray–white differentiation. On day 3 of illness, the lady develops a drop in sensorium following a seizure. A CT scan is repeated, which shows evidence of cerebral edema.

    The ONSD cutoff measured at bedside in such a patient corresponding to an intracranial pressure greater than 20 mm Hg is:
    a. 4 mm
    b. 5.2 mm
    c. 3 mm
    d. 7 mm

13. This is an ECG of a 70-year-old woman who presented to the ER with complaints of anorexia and multiple episodes of vomiting. She has a deranged renal function on arrival (serum creatinine—1.7 mg/dL) with metabolic acidosis (pH—7.25). Which of the following conditions can be associated with the following ECG?

    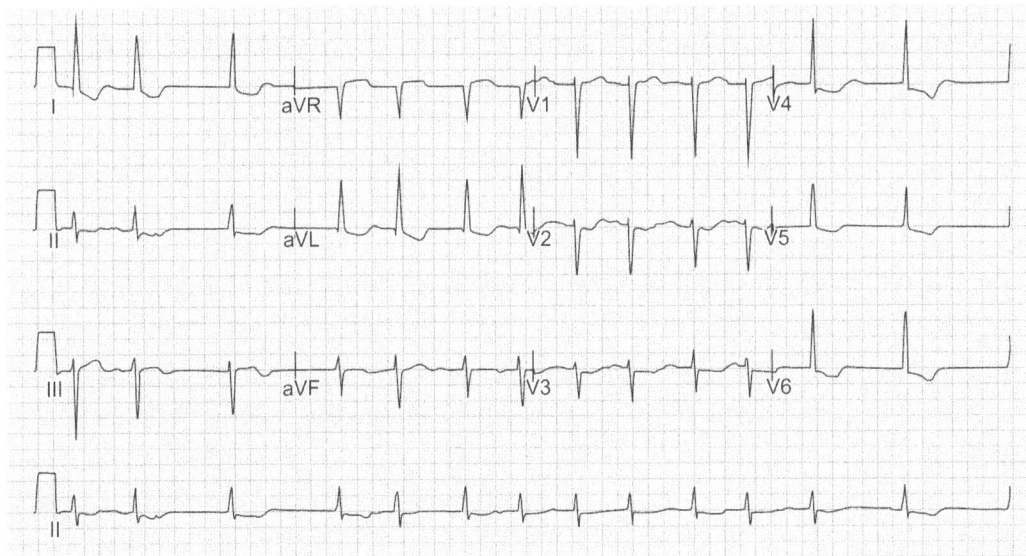

    a. Hyperkalemia
    b. Metabolic acidosis
    c. Digoxin toxicity
    d. Tricyclic antidepressant toxicity

14. The following ECG is of 72-year-old man who has been posted for an emergency fixation of a lower extremity fracture following a fall at home. Which among this is the most probable diagnosis?

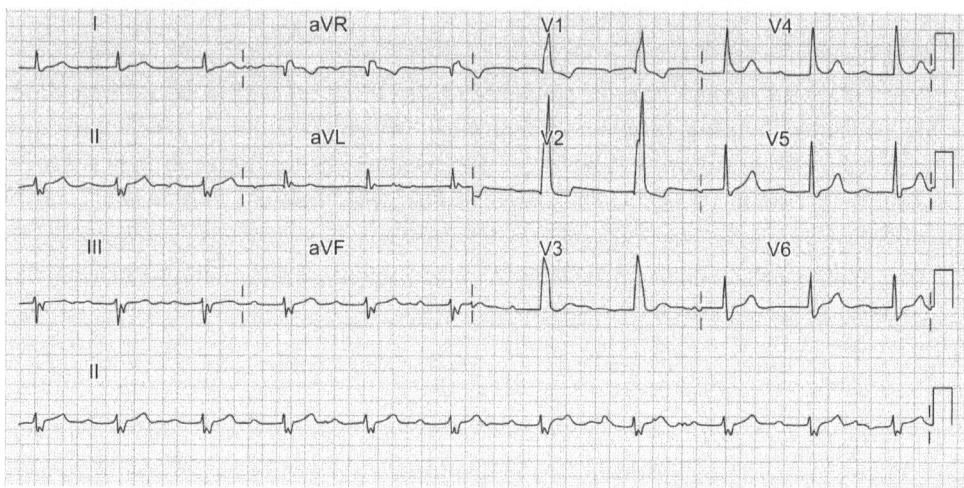

   a. RBBB
   b. LBBB
   c. Bifascicular block
   d. Trifascicular block

15. A 47-year-old male patient presents with central chest pain radiating to the left arm. An ECG is performed, shown below. The likely site of infarction is:

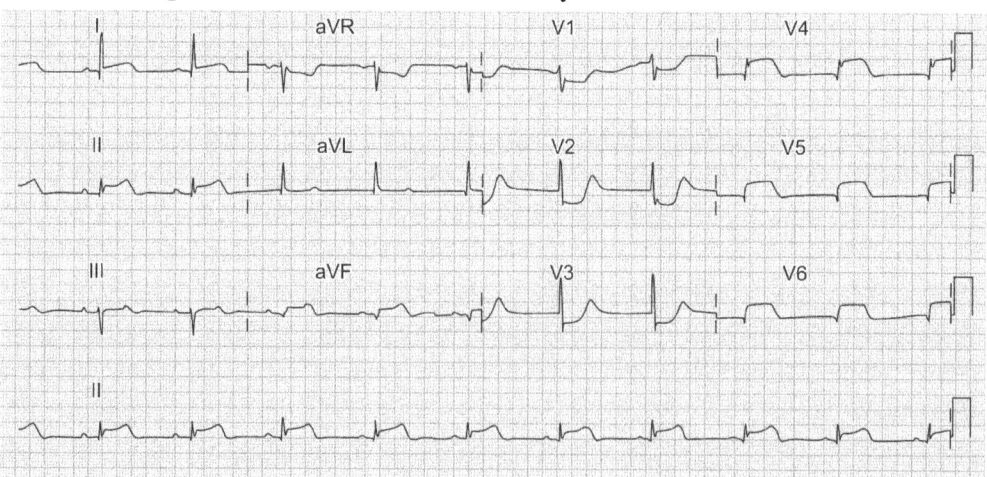

   a. Anterior
   b. Anteroseptal
   c. Septal
   d. Posterior

16. A 28-year-old young female presents with sudden onset of palpitations in the emergency department. ECG done at the bedside shows narrow complex tachycardia (HR—152 beats/min and BP 110/60 mm Hg). Intravenous adenosine is ordered by the emergency medicine registrar. Following adenosine flush the rhythm changes to the following as shown in the underlying figure:

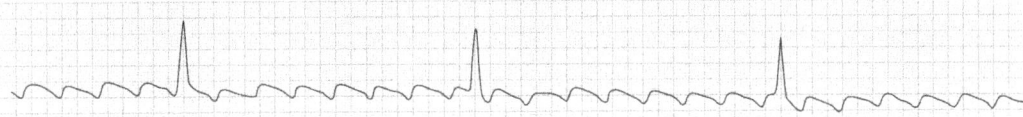

What is the underlying anomaly in this ECG?
a. Atrial flutter
b. Atrial fibrillation
c. Multifocal atrial tachycardia
d. Junctional tachycardia

17. A 64-year-old lady presents with intermittent palpitations and a transient loss of consciousness. The ECG is shown below:

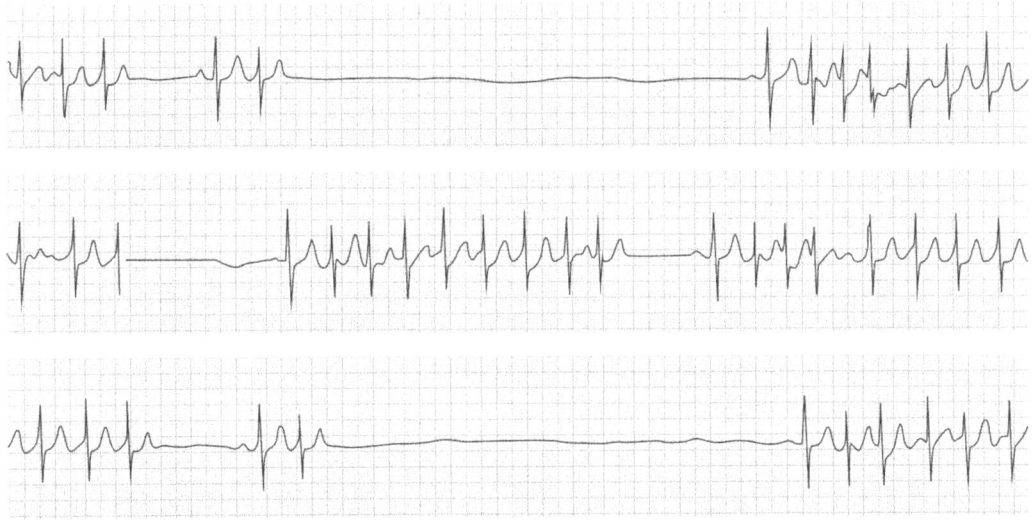

The most likely diagnosis is:
a. Pulseless electrical activity
b. Sick sinus syndrome
c. Polymorphic ventricular tachycardia
d. Sinus arrhythmia

18. The following ECG was obtained from a 55-year-old lady admitted in the cardiothoracic ICU. She had previously undergone aortic valve replacement for infective endocarditis. Suggest the abnormality seen in the ECG:

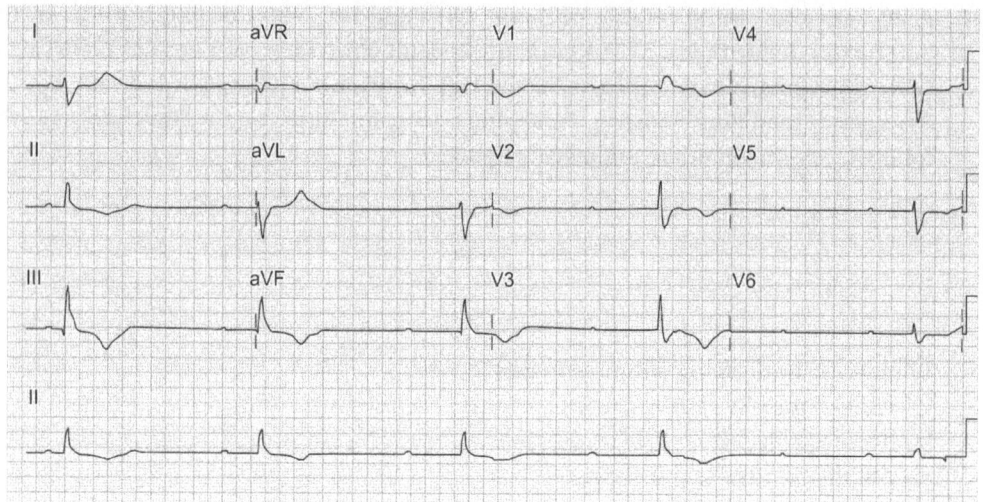

a. Mobitz 2nd degree, type 1 heart block
b. Mobitz 2nd degree, type 2 heart block
c. 3rd degree heart block
d. Sick sinus syndrome

19. Osborn wave (positive deflection of the J point) is seen in all of the following conditions, *except*:
    a. Hypokalemia
    b. Hypothermia
    c. Hypercalcemia
    d. Intracranial hypertension

20. A 50-year-old male patient presents to the emergency department with complaints of chest pain associated with worsening shortness of breath. The ECG ordered by the emergency medicine resident is shown below.
    What is the most likely abnormality?

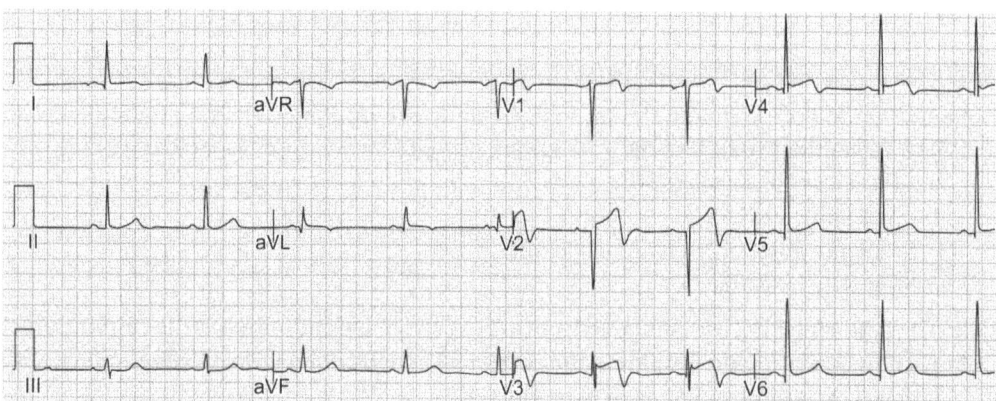

a. RCA stenosis
b. LCX stenosis
c. LAD stenosis
d. Triple vessel disease

21. Which of the following criteria is classically used to diagnose acute myocardial infarction in the presence of preexisting left bundle branch block?
    a. Sgarbossa criteria
    b. Wellens criteria
    c. Smith's criteria
    d. Wenckebach's criteria

22. All of the following views are included in the E-FAST in trauma patients, *except*:
    a. Subxiphoid view
    b. Anterior thoracic view
    c. Pelvic view
    d. Parasternal view

23. A 15-year-old male patient presents to the emergency department following sudden onset of chest pain. The ultrasound image is shown below.

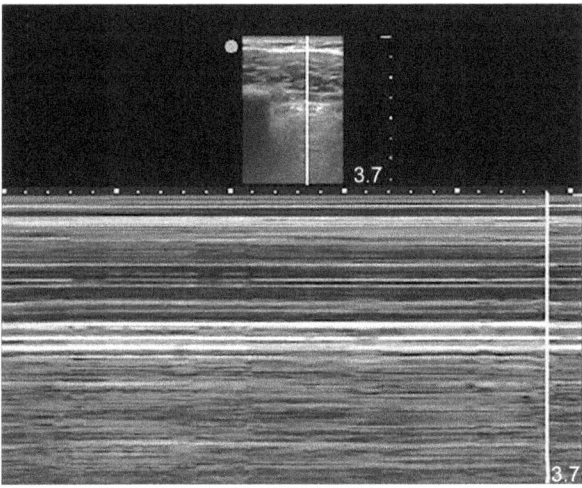

What is the most likely diagnosis?
a. Pleural effusion
b. Normal lung
c. Pulmonary embolism
d. Pneumothorax

24. A 55-year-old bed-bound male patient with advanced pancreatic cancer on palliative chemotherapy presents with worsening shortness of breath of 3-hour duration. ECG shows sinus tachycardia (HR—108 beats/min, BP—90/65 mm Hg). The parasternal short-axis echocardiographic view of the patient is shown below.

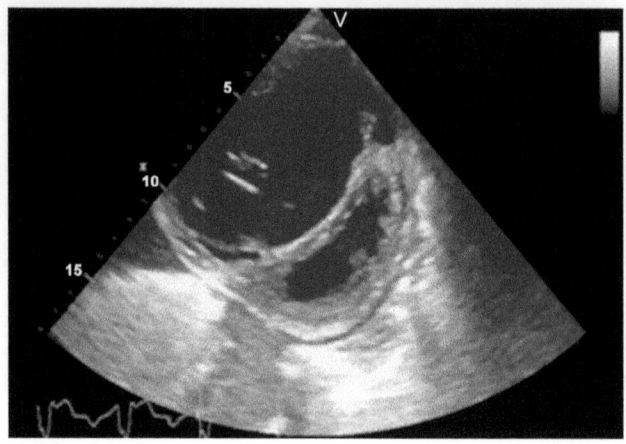

What could be a possible diagnosis in this patient?
a. Hypovolemia
b. Pulmonary embolism
c. Pericardial effusion
d. Pleural effusion

25. Which of the following on lung sonography is a sign of alveolar flooding?
a. A line
b. B line
c. Z line
d. E line

26. Lindegaard ratio measured using transcranial Doppler (TCD) is used to detect vasospasm. It measures the blood flow velocity ratio of which of the following arteries?
a. MCA:ICA
b. ICA:MCA
c. ECA:ICA
d. ICA:MCA

27. Which of the following modes of echocardiography is used to assess high-velocity blood flows such as those of stenosis and regurgitation?
a. M mode
b. Continuous wave Doppler
c. Pulse wave Doppler
d. TDI

28. The relationship between stroke volume (SV) and velocity across the left ventricular outflow tract (LVOT) is given by which of the following formula?
a. SV= LVOT VTI × LVOT CSA
b. SV= LVOT VTI × HR
c. SV= LVOT VTI × LVOT CSA/HR
d. SV = LVOT VTI / LVOT CSA

29. All of the following are ultrasonographic measures, which are used to predict liberation from mechanical ventilation, *except*:
    a. Lung ultrasound score (LUS)
    b. Diaphragmatic thickness fraction (DTF)
    c. P0.1
    d. Diaphragmatic excursion

30. All are dynamic measures of fluid responsiveness, *except*:
    a. Velocity time integral (VTI)
    b. Pulse pressure variation (PPV)
    c. Global end-diastolic volume (GEDV)
    d. Stroke volume variation (SVV)

31. The seagull sign classically described while scanning the abdominal aorta is formed by which of the following two arteries?
    a. Hepatic artery, splenic artery
    b. Splenic artery, superior mesenteric artery
    c. Right and left renal artery
    d. Bifurcation of aorta into common iliac arteries

ANSWERS

1. **Ans. (c)**
   ECG features of VT:
   - Absence of typical RBBB or LBBB morphology
   - Extreme axis deviation ("northwest axis")—QRS is positive in aVR and negative in I + aVF.
   - Very broad complexes (>160 ms)
   - **AV dissociation** (P and QRS complexes at different rates)
   - **Capture beats**—occur when the sinoatrial node transiently "captures" the ventricles, in the midst of AV dissociation, to produce a QRS complex of normal duration.
   - **Fusion beats**—occur when a sinus and ventricular beat coincides to produce a hybrid complex.
   - **Positive or negative concordance** throughout the precordial (chest) leads, i.e. leads V1-6 show entirely positive (R) or entirely negative (QS) complexes, with no RS complexes seen.
   - **Brugada sign**—the distance from the onset of the QRS complex to the nadir of the S-wave is >100 ms
   - **Josephson sign**—notching near the nadir of the S-wave
   - **RSR' complexes with a taller left rabbit ear.**

2. **Ans. (a)**
   An increase in VTI more than 12.5% in response to a PLR test is a sensitive and specific marker of fluid responsiveness.

3. **Ans. (b)**
   Progressive prolongation of PR interval followed by dropping of a beat is suggestive of Mobitz type 1, 2nd degree heart block.

4. **Ans. (a)**
   ECG changes in hyperkalemia are:
   - Peaked T waves
   - Prolonged PR segment
   - Loss of P waves
   - Bizarre QRS complexes
   - Sine wave pattern

5. **Ans. (b)**
   ECG changes in inferior wall MI are:
   - ST elevation in leads II, III, and aVF
   - Progressive development of Q waves in II, III, and aVF
   - Reciprocal ST depression in aVL (± lead I)

6. **Ans. (c)**
   McConnell's sign, where only the RV apex wall contracts with hypokinesia of lateral wall. It is specific for right heart strain and typically indicates a large PE.

7. **Ans. (d)**
   McConnell's sign, the characteristic ECHO finding is hypokinesia of lateral wall of right ventricular with preserved contraction of right ventricular apex.

CHAPTER 28 USG and ECHO

8. **Ans. (a)**
   Echocardiography features of cardiac tamponade are:
   Late RA diastolic collapse
   Early RV diastolic collapse
   Swinging heart
   Dilated IVC with reduced variability

9. **Ans. (b)**
   Tricuspid annular plane systolic excursion (TAPSE) is commonly recommended for estimating the right ventricular systolic function using M mode with the cursor placed over the lateral tricuspid annulus. A value greater than 16 mm is considered normal.

10. **Ans. (d)**
    ECG features of multifocal atrial tachycardia (MAT) are:
    - Heart rate >100 bpm (usually 100–150 bpm; may be as high as 250 bpm).
    - Irregularly irregular rhythm with varying PP, PR, and RR intervals.
    - At least, **three distinct P-wave morphologies** in the same lead.
    - Isoelectric baseline between P-waves (i.e. no flutter waves).

11. **Ans. (d)**
    ECG features of pericarditis are:
    - Widespread concave ST elevation and PR depression throughout most of the limb leads (I, II, III, aVL, and aVF) and precordial leads (V2-6).
    - Reciprocal ST depression and PR elevation in lead aVR (±V1).
    - Sinus tachycardia is also common

12. **Ans. (b)**
    ONSD cutoff of 5.2 mm was found to be 93% sensitive and 74% specific for elevated intracranial pressure.

13. **Ans. (c)**
    Digoxin effect refers to the presence on the ECG of:
    - Downsloping ST depression with a characteristic "Salvador Dali sagging" appearance
    - Flattened, inverted, or biphasic T waves
    - Shortened QT interval.

14. **Ans. (d)**
    He has trifascicular block as the ECG shows a combination of bifascicular block plus a 1st degree heart block.

15. **Ans. (d)**
    As the posterior myocardium is not directly visualized by the standard 12-lead ECG, reciprocal changes of STEMI are sought in the anteroseptal leads V1-3.
    Posterior MI is suggested by the following changes in V1-3:
    - Horizontal ST depression
    - Tall, broad R waves (>30 ms)
    - Upright T waves
    - Dominant R wave (R/S ratio >1) in V2

16. **Ans. (a)**
    ECG features of atrial flutter are:
    Narrow complex tachycardia
    - Regular atrial activity at ~300 bpm
    - Flutter waves ("sawtooth" pattern)—best seen in leads II, III, aVF—may be more easily spotted by turning the ECG upside down
    - Flutter waves in V1 may resemble P waves
    - Loss of the isoelectric baseline.

17. **Ans. (b)**
    Multiple ECG abnormalities can be seen in sinus node dysfunction including:
    - Sinus bradycardia
    - Sinus arrhythmia—associated with sinus node dysfunction in the elderly in the absence of respiratory pattern association
    - Sinoatrial exit block
    - **Sinus arrest—pause >3 seconds.**
    - Atrial fibrillation with slow ventricular response
    - Bradycardia-tachycardia syndrome.

18. **Ans. (c)**
    - Regular P-P interval
    - Regular R-R interval
    - No definite relation between P waves and R waves.

19. **Ans. (a)**
    Osborn waves are seen in the following conditions:
    These are characteristically seen in hypothermia (typically T<30°C), but they are not pathognomonic. J waves may be seen in a number of other conditions:
    - Normal variant
    - Hypercalcemia
    - Medications
    - Neurological insults such as intracranial hypertension, severe head injury, and subarachnoid hemorrhage
    - Le Syndrome d'Haïssaguerre (idiopathic VF).

20. **Ans. (c) (Wellens sign)**
    Wellens syndrome is a pattern of deeply inverted or biphasic T waves in V2-3, which is highly specific for a critical stenosis of the left anterior descending artery (LAD).

21. **Ans. (a)**
    Modified Sgarbossa criteria:
    - ≥1 lead with ≥1 mm of concordant ST elevation
    - ≥1 lead of V1-V3 with ≥1 mm of concordant ST depression
    - ≥1 lead anywhere with ≥1 mm STE and proportionally excessive discordant STE, as defined by ≥25% of the depth of the preceding S-wave.

22. **Ans. (d)**
    The E-FAST views include scanning the following areas:
    - The hepatorenal interface (Morison's pouch) and the right diaphragm
    - The splenorenal interface and left diaphragm
    - Pelvis in both planes—(1) longitudinal and (2) transverse
    - Pericardial: Subxiphoid or intercostal views of the pericardium
    - Pleura bilaterally.

23. **Ans. (d)**
    Sonographic features of pneumothorax:
    Findings consistent with a normal lung-pleural interface are absent, including:
    - Absence of lung sliding
    - Absence of B-lines (a type of "comet-tail" artefact consisting of vertical lines due to visceral pleural interlobular septa)
    - Presence of A lines instead (horizontal lines)
    - Loss of "waves on a beach" sign in M-mode.
    Positive findings seen in pneumothorax are:
    - "Lung point" sign—where normal pleural interface contacts the boundary of the pneumothorax
    - "Stratosphere" aka "bar code" sign on M-mode.

24. **Ans. (b)**
    The given image is a parasternal short-axis view showing an enlarged right ventricle pushing the septum inferiorly toward the left ventricle resulting in a "D"-shaped septum, which is characteristically seen in pulmonary embolism and other right ventricle overload states.

25. **Ans. (b)**
    The B lines are the ultrasound equivalent of the Kerley B lines found on chest X-ray. Bilateral B lines are commonly present in lungs with interstitial edema. They originate at the pleural line and traverse the entire ultrasound screen vertically to the bottom of the screen.

26. **Ans. (a)**
    Lindegaard Ratio = mean velocity in the MCA/mean velocity in ipsilateral extracranial internal carotid artery. High velocities in the MCA (>120 cm/s) may be due to hyperemia or vasospasm. the Lindegaard Ratio helps distinguish these conditions.

27. **Ans. (b)**
    Continuous wave Doppler:
    - Transducer is continuously transmitting and receiving Doppler signal
    - Good resolution of high velocities
    - No information about location of the signal
    - Measures:
        - Velocities of regurgitation
        - Systolic flow through the aortic valve.

28. Ans. (a)
Cardiac output (CO) is the volume of blood pumped out of the heart per minute. It is measured in liters/min, CO can be calculated using heart rate (HR) and stroke volume (SV).

$CO = SV \times HR$

Echocardiography can be used to measure SV using a method called pulsed waveform Doppler. This method allows approximation of the stroke volume by taking two measurements:
1. The left ventricular outflow tract (LVOT) area.
2. The range of velocities of blood flow across the LVOT, also known as velocity time integral (VTI).

$SV = LVOT\ area \times VTI$

29. Ans. (c)
Airway occlusion pressure (P 0.1) is the pressure generated at the airways during the first 100 ms of an inspiratory effort against an occluded airway. It is used to assess neural respiratory drive and is an index to facilitate liberation from mechanical ventilation.

30. Ans. (c)
Global end-diastolic volume (GEDV) is the combined end-diastolic volumes of all the four cardiac chambers. GEDV has been demonstrated to be a reliable preload marker and a static marker of fluid responsiveness.

31. Ans. (a)
The "seagull sign" in abdominal ultrasound identifies the celiac trunk and its division into hepatic and splenic arteries creating the wings of the seagull.

Exam Paper

KHALID ISMAIL KHATIB

QUESTIONS

1. Which of the following is the best test to confirm the correct placement of a nasogastric (NG) tube?
   a. Injection of 50 mL of air with auscultation over the stomach (Whoosh test)
   b. Chest X-ray
   c. Aspiration of at least 10 mL through the NG tube
   d. Checking the pH of the aspirate
   e. Abdominal X-ray

2. A 45-year-old male shifted to ICU postoperatively following surgery on cervical spine for prolapsed intervertebral disc. He was given general anesthesia. After 2 hours, he develops severe tachycardia (150 beats per minute) and develops fever (40°C). The first step in the immediate treatment should be:
   a. Dantrolene sodium 2–3 mg/kg as an initial bolus
   b. Dantrolene sodium 1 mg/kg as an initial bolus
   c. Send urine sample for myoglobin
   d. Measurement of arterial blood pH
   e. Insertion of central venous line

3. A 20-year-old female develops polyuria (urine output 6 L/24 h) following pituitary adenoma surgery. Her urine examination reveals osmolarity of 320 and specific gravity of 1.001. The most appropriate treatment is:
   a. 0.9% sodium chloride infusion up to 7 L/24 h
   b. Intravenous glucose
   c. Intravenous DDAVP
   d. Intravenous glucose and potassium

4. A 30-year-old male was brought to casualty with complaints of severe abdominal pain since 3 hours duration. Pain started after a party, where alcohol was served. On examination, patient was conscious, anxious and in pain. Heart rate was 118/min, BP 140/100 mm Hg, RR 28/min and oxygen saturation 100% on room air. ABG was normal and lab reports showed elevated serum amylase and lipase (> 5 times baseline). Which one of the following is the recommended investigation for an initial assessment?
   a. Ultrasound of abdomen
   b. X-ray of abdomen
   c. CT scan of abdomen
   d. MRI scan of abdomen

5. A 45-year-old male, K/C/o hypertension was admitted with sudden onset vomiting, giddiness and loss of balance. His CNS examination reveals GCS of 15/15 with bilateral cerebellar signs. CT brain shows cerebellar vermis bleeding of 4.5 cm in diameter and no evidence of coning. His vital signs are normal. What will you do in the next 24 hours?
   a. Close neuromonitoring and repeat neuroimaging, if GCS declines
   b. Urgent craniotomy and clot evacuation
   c. Elective hyperventilation for 24 hours and CT scan at 24 hours
   d. Stereotactic surgery and aspiration of the blood clot

6. A 60-year-old male, admitted to ICU postoperatively following laparotomy for blunt trauma abdomen. The perioperative course was uncomplicated. He is a chronic heavy smoker and has COPD, which is treated with a salbutamol inhaler and oral deriphyllin 300 mg bd. On the second postoperative day, the patient suddenly develops atrial fibrillation with fast ventricular rate (150 to 175 beats/min). He develops hypotension (blood pressure 80/30 mm Hg). Which of the following is the most appropriate immediate management is?
   a. Check the serum K^+ and Mg^+ levels
   b. Synchronized DC shock
   c. Commence oxygen 6 L/min using a non-rebreathing mask
   d. Give amiodarone 300 mg bolus over 60 minutes
   e. Intravenous digoxin

7. A 50-year-old female, K/C/o bipolar disorder on lithium is admitted for LRTI with respiratory failure. On the next day, she develops broad QRS tachycardia on monitor and ECG shows Torsades de pointes. Which of the following antiarrhythmic treatment should be administered to this patient?
   a. Isoprenaline infusion
   b. Intravenous lidocaine 2 mg/kg
   c. Intravenous phenytoin 15 mg/kg
   d. Intravenous magnesium 2 g
   e. Intravenous potassium chloride

8. The laboratory test used to differentiate between DIC versus dilutional coagulopathy is:
   a. Hemoglobin
   b. D-dimer
   c. Platelet count
   d. Bleeding time
   e. INR

9. A 15-year-old male patient presents to the emergency department with H/o ascending paralysis of all 4 limbs since last 30 hours. History of flue like symptoms. Which of the following treatment should be offered to him?
   a. Noninvasive ventilation
   b. Intravenous steroids
   c. Physiotherapy
   d. Intravenous immunoglobulin

10. A 35-year-old male admitted with H/o high-grade fever with rigors followed by altered sensorium. His peripheral smear shows *Plasmodium falciparum*. Lab investigation reveals elevated S creatinine (3.5 mg/dL), $PaO_2/FiO_2 < 100$, abnormal LFTs (elevated S bilirubin and SGOT/SGPT). He is diagnosed to have severe falciparum cerebral malaria with multiorgan dysfunction syndrome (MODS). He should be treated with the following:
    a. Intravenous artesunate
    b. Artemether plus doxycycline through Ryles tube
    c. Intravenous chloroquine
    d. Mefloquine through Ryles tube

11. Which of the following is the best test to confirm the correct placement of a central venous catheter?
    a. Aspiration of dark colored blood
    b. Measure the pH and CO_2 levels of the aspirated blood
    c. Chest X-ray
    d. Absence of pulsation of blood after syringe is disconnected from needle

12. A 28-year-old male is admitted to SICU following resuscitation in emergency department with H/o fall from height resulting in polytrauma (multiple long bone fractures with pelvic fracture with hemoperitoneum). The following day, he deteriorates and requires intubation and ventilation for evolving ARDS. Later he requires hemodialysis for acute renal failure and also requires inotropic support. Which of the following scoring systems will most accurately reflect the severity of his current clinical state and probability of mortality?
    a. Sequential organ failure assessment (SOFA) score
    b. Acute physiology and chronic health evaluation (APACHE) II score
    c. Acute physiology and chronic health evaluation (APACHE) III score
    d. Simplified acute physiology score (SAPS)
    e. Injury severity score (ISS)

13. Which of the following serious complication can occur in the first 3 days in a patient admitted with subarachnoid hemorrhage secondary to a ruptured intracranial aneurysm?
    a. Rebleeding
    b. Cerebral vasospasm
    c. Hypertension
    d. Hydrocephalus
    e. Pulmonary edema

14. A 60-year-old female, K/C/o mixed connective tissue disorder (MCTD) on steroids and azathioprine presents to the emergency department with H/o left sided chest pain, dyspnea and low grade fever. Her systemic examination reveals a pericardial rub. 12-lead ECG shows diffuse ST elevation with tachycardia (HR—110/min). The most likely diagnosis is:
    a. Congestive cardiac failure
    b. Pericardial effusion
    c. Cardiac tamponade
    d. Myocardial infarction
    e. Pericarditis

15. Therapeutic hypothermia has been shown to be of benefit in all of the following clinical situations, *except*:
    a. Out of hospital cardiac arrest
    b. Traumatic brain injury
    c. Heat stroke
    d. Coagulopathy of trauma shock

16. Which of the following laboratory results makes a diagnosis of type 2 heparin-induced thrombocytopenia (HIT) more likely?
    a. Platelet count of 102×10^9/L, 6 days after starting heparin
    b. Lowest platelet count of 12×10^9/L during the treatment period
    c. Detection of PF4-heparin IgA antibodies
    d. Platelet count of 297×10^9/L, 2 days after stopping heparin administration

17. A 22-year-old female, primigravida, is admitted to ICU with history of headache and giddiness. Her BP is found to be 190/110 mm Hg. She is treated with magnesium sulfate and subsequently she undergoes a cesarean section performed under epidural anesthesia. 24 hours later she becomes lethargic and confused. She has reduced muscle tone and reflexes. Her ECG shows a prolonged P-R interval and widened QRS. What is the most likely diagnosis?
    a. Pulmonary embolism
    b. Amniotic fluid embolism
    c. Hypermagnesemia
    d. Hyponatremia
    e. Hyperkalemia

18. Which one of the following is an absolute contraindication to fibrinolysis in patients with ST elevation myocardial infarction?
    a. Previous fibrinolysis 2 months ago
    b. Resuscitation from cardiac arrest within the last hour
    c. Diabetic retinopathy
    d. Ischemic stroke 2 months ago
    e. Pregnancy of 30 weeks gestation

19. Initial therapy in status epilepticus includes all the following, *except*:
    a. Phenytoin
    b. Lorazepam
    c. Phenobarbitone
    d. Carbamazepine

20. In patients with dengue fever, platelet transfusion may be considered in clinically stable patients when platelet counts are:
    a. 50,000/µL
    b. 25,000/µL
    c. 75,000/µL
    d. 5,000-10,000/µL

21. Which anticoagulant drug should be used in a pregnant woman in her first trimester for the treatment of deep vein thrombosis (DVT)?
    a. 5000 units of unfractionated heparin subcutaneously twice a day
    b. Enoxaparin 1 mg/kg subcutaneously every 12 hours
    c. Intravenous heparin infusion
    d. Oral warfarin therapy

22. Which of the following is not a *criterion* for the diagnosis of brain death?
    a. Absent pupillary reflexes
    b. Absent spinal reflexes
    c. Absent brainstem reflexes
    d. Absent oculovestibular reflex

23. Which of the following is not an effective method to decrease an elevated $PaCO_2$?
    a. Increase tidal volume
    b. Increase frequency
    c. Decrease circuit dead space
    d. Increase PEEP
    e. Increase inspiratory pressure

24. Abdominal compartment syndrome (ACS) is less likely in patients with the following:
    a. 20% burns
    b. Liver transplantation
    c. Pancreatitis
    d. Sepsis with extensive fluid resuscitation

25. In acute pancreatitis Ranson's score is calculated at:
    a. Admission and 24 hours
    b. Admission and 72 hours
    c. Admission and 48 hours
    d. At 24 and 48 hours

26. In which of the following conditions is sodium bicarbonate not indicated?
    a. Tricyclic antidepressant overdose
    b. Severe hyperchloremic acidemia
    c. Diabetic ketoacidosis
    d. Hyperkalemia with cardiac toxicity

27. Static compliance depends on all of the following, *except*:
    a. Tidal volume
    b. PEEP
    c. Peak inspiratory pressure
    d. Plateau pressure

28. Which is the most appropriate action to reduce intrinsic peep?
    a. Increase PEEP
    b. Reduce RR
    c. Decrease tidal volume
    d. Increase inspiratory time

29. In the Richmond agitation scale +3 denotes:
    a. Combative
    b. Very agitated
    c. Agitated
    d. Restless

30. All of the following are signs of pneumothorax on a supine X-ray in a patient on mechanical ventilation, *except*:
    a. Deep sulcus sign at costophrenic angle
    b. A sharp outline of the pericardial fat (pericardial fat pad sign)
    c. Oligemic lung field
    d. Lucency over liver and upper abdomen not explained by an abdominal structure

31. All are major criteria for the diagnosis of fat embolism, *except*:
    a. Axillary or subconjunctival petechiae
    b. Hypoxemia ($PaO_2 < 60$ mm Hg)
    c. Fat globules present in the sputum
    d. Central nervous system depression disproportionate to the hypoxemia

32. Which of the following medication should be avoided in patients with myasthenia gravis to prevent exacerbation of muscle weakness?
    a. Aminoglycosides
    b. Paracetamol
    c. Quinolones
    d. Aspirin

33. Metabolic alkalosis is caused by all of the following, *except*:
    a. Diuretic use
    b. Nasogastric drainage
    c. Diarrhea
    d. Vomiting
    e. Hyperaldosteronism

34. Which of the following treatments would be the most effective in reducing absorption of paracetamol in patients with ingestion of 50 tablets of paracetamol?
    a. Activated charcoal
    b. N-acetyl cysteine
    c. Induced emesis
    d. Gastric lavage
    e. Methionine

35. The following are criteria for the diagnosis of hepatorenal syndrome, *except*:
    a. Cirrhosis without ascites
    b. Creatinine >1.5 mg/dL
    c. Absence of shock
    d. Absence of hypovolemia (no response to diuretic withdrawal and albumin volume expansion)
    e. No nephrotoxic drugs

36. Bedside index of severity in acute pancreatitis (BISAP) score comprises all of the following, *except*:
    a. BUN > 25 mg/dL
    b. Impaired renal status
    c. SIRS
    d. Age > 60 years
    e. Presence of pleural effusion

37. All are measures to treat abdominal compartment syndrome, *except*:
    a. Adequate sedation and analgesia
    b. Diuretics
    c. Nasogastric/colonic decompression
    d. Decompressive laparotomy with temporary abdominal closure (TAC) techniques in patients requiring open abdomen
    e. Positive cumulative fluid balance

38. In Class III hemorrhagic shock, the approximate loss of blood is:
    a. 10–15% of circulating blood volume
    b. 20–25% of circulating blood volume
    c. 30–40% of circulating blood volume
    d. 50-60% of circulating blood volume

39. Which of the following drug is not useful for pharmacological treatment of hypertensive crises in the ICU?
    a. Amlodipine
    b. Nitroglycerine
    c. Sodium nitroprusside
    d. Hydralazine

40. A 40-year-old male, admitted with H/o reduced appetite, nausea, swelling over feet for 1 week. His investigations reveal S creatinine of 8 md/dL and S potassium of 7.5 mEq/L. All the following drugs are useful for the treatment of hyperkalemia in patients with renal failure, *except*:
    a. NaHCO$_3$
    b. Inhaled β-receptor agonists
    c. Cation exchange resins
    d. Intravenous insulin
    e. β-receptor antagonists

41. A 25-year-old male, admitted with H/o road traffic accident suffering from traumatic brain injury and fracture femur. His HR is 138/min and BP is 70/30 mm Hg. Which of the following fluid should not be used for resuscitation?
    a. 0.9% normal saline
    b. Ringers lactate
    c. 20% albumin

42. A 38-year-old male is admitted with acute severe pancreatitis. Which one of the following intervention/treatment will you administer at the earliest?
    a. Antibiotics in first 30 minutes
    b. Aggressive fluid resuscitation
    c. Maintaining glycemia
    d. Early nutrition

43. A 60-year-old female, admitted with ischemic stroke due to right middle cerebral artery infarct. Which of the following vital signs needs immediate correction?
    a. HR 58/min
    b. BP 160/80 mm Hg
    c. CVP 12 cm of water
    d. Temperature of 102°C

44. One unit of single donor platelets is equivalent to:
    a. 5–10 units of random donor platelets
    b. 10–15 units of random donor platelets
    c. 16–20 units of random donor platelets
    d. 20–25 units of random donor platelets

45. Which of the following electrolyte abnormality is not found in rhabdomyolysis?
    a. Hyperkalemia
    b. Hyperphosphatemia
    c. Hypercalcemia
    d. Hyperuricemia

46. A 21-year-old female, 28 weeks pregnant admitted with acute liver failure and hepatic encephalopathy. All of the following tests will be abnormal, *except*:
    a. Transaminases (SGOT/SGPT)
    b. Prothrombin time
    c. INR
    d. Troponin T
    e. Alkaline phosphatase

47. Choose the drug used for the immediate treatment of anaphylactic shock following intravenous contrast injection:
    a. Dopamine
    b. Antihistamines
    c. Dobutamine
    d. Isoprenaline
    e. Epinephrine

48. The most common cause of death in patients with dengue hemorrhagic fever is:
    a. Gastrointestinal bleeding
    b. Intracranial bleeding
    c. Shock
    d. Multiorgan dysfunction syndrome

49. The patient is diagnosed with acute fulminant hepatic failure when onset of encephalopathy is:
    a. Within 10 days of symptom onset
    b. Within 12 days of symptom onset
    c. Within 15 days of symptom onset
    d. Within 20 days of symptom onset

50. An 18-year-old male, was found submerged under water for approximately 15 minutes. He was rescued by emergency responders. On examination, his temperature was 30°C with dilated and fixed pupils. Describe the next appropriate step in his treatment:
    a. Phenobarbitone
    b. Hyperventilation
    c. Intravenous high dose steroids
    d. Cardiopulmonary resuscitation
    e. Immediate rewarming

ANSWERS

1. (b)
2. (a)
3. (c)
4. (a)
5. (b)
6. (b)
7. (d)
8. (b)
9. (d)
10. (a)
11. (c)
12. (a)
13. (a)
14. (e)
15. (d)
16. (a)
17. (c)
18. (d)
19. (d)
20. (d)
21. (b)
22. (b)
23. (d)
24. (a)
25. (c)
26. (c)
27. (c)
28. (b)
29. (b)
30. (c)
31. (c)
32. (a)
33. (c)
34. (a)
35. (a)
36. (b)
37. (e)
38. (c)
39. (a)
40. (e)
41. (c)
42. (b)
43. (d)
44. (a)
45. (c)
46. (d)
47. (e)
48. (d)
49. (a)
50. (d)

EU GSPR Authorised Reprsentative
Logos Europe, 9 rue Nicolas Poussin
1700, La Rochelle, France
Phone: +33 (0) 6 67 93 73 78
E-mail: contact@logoseurope.eu

www.ingramcontent.com/pod-product-compliance
Ingram Content Group UK Ltd.
Pitfield, Milton Keynes, MK11 3LW, UK
UKHW050456150426
5217IPUK00025B/1710